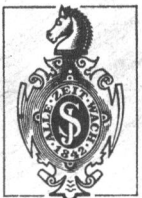

Urs Heim · Karl M. Pfeiffer

Small Fragment Set Manual

Technique Recommended by the ASIF-Group

ASIF: Swiss Association for the Study of Internal Fixation

In Collaboration with H. Ch. Meuli

Translated by R. Kirschbaum · R. L. Batten

With 157 Figures (414 Separate Illustrations)

Springer-Verlag
Berlin Heidelberg New York 1974

Priv.-Doz. Dr. U. Heim
Chirurgische Abteilung, Kreuzspital, Loestr. 99, CH-7000 Chur

Priv.-Doz. Dr. K. M. Pfeiffer
Leiter der Chirurgischen Universitäts-Poliklinik, Kantonsspital,
CH-4004 Basel

Dr. H. Ch. Meuli
Lindenhofspital, CH-3000 Bern

Library of Congress Cataloging in Publication Data
Heim, U.
Small fragment set manual.
Translation of Periphere Osteosynthesen.
Bibliography: p.
1. Bone-grafting. I. Pfeiffer, Karl Martin, joint author. II. Meuli, H. Ch., joint author.
III. Arbeitsgemeinschaft für Osteosynthesefragen. IV. Title.
RD123.H4513   617'.3   74-13966   ISBN 0-387-06904-6

ISBN-13: 978-3-540-06904-1   e-ISBN-13: 978-3-642-96227-1
DOI: 10.1007/978-3-642-96227-1

Foreword

Operation on fractures of shafts and joints is chiefly indicated in the upper arm, forearm, femur and tibia. Injuries in these areas can almost always be successfully treated by the techniques described in the "ASIF Manual of Internal Fixation," followed by early exercises. The fixation of small fragments which are of such biomechanical importance, has hitherto given indifferent results, especially when the distal parts of the hand and foot are involved.

The implants and instruments developed by Dr. Heim and tried out by ASIF members during recent years have now been assembled into a "small fragment set," which is now available. These implants have significantly expanded the scope of ASIF instrumentation for internal fixation. Pannike first compared the application of the small fragment set with the conventional methods used in hand surgery. Heim and Pfeiffer in cooperation with Meuli, illustrate in this Volume the small fragment set, elucidating in a didactic manner the composition of the set, the indications for its use, and its method of application to all suitable fractures. Enough good results have been secured to establish the usefulness of this development.

The following volume may therefore be regarded as an important supplement to the ASIF Manual. It makes it clear again that every internal fixation requires a high level of technical skill, a sense of responsibility, and very gentle handling of the soft tissues.

Basel/Switzerland   M. Allgöwer
Autumn 1974   M. E. Müller
                                                     H. Willenegger

Preface

ASIF techniques continue to develop. The same excellent results can be obtained in small bones as in fractures of larger ones, providing that the indications are correct and the operations carefully carried out.

Even when familiar with the methods of internal fixation, many surgeons have reservations about operating on small bones. Professor Allgöwer therefore encouraged us to publish the results we had obtained after several years experience. The intention was to arouse interest in the small fragment set and to deal systematically with its proper use. This work has led to the following volume. We have used the previously published "Manual of Internal Fixation" as our model. The "Small Fragment Manual" may be considered as a sequel to the "Manual of Internal Fixation," extending its field of application.

Many friends and colleagues have kindly helped us with their experience and criticism. We are especially indebted to Professors M. Allgöwer, M. E. Müller and H. Willenegger for their support and suggestions. For allowing us access to the case records and X-rays of their patients, we are grateful to the members of ASIF, the Doctors W. Bandi, H. Bloch, R. Hochuli and Professor H. Willenegger.

Special credit is due to our illustrator, Mr. Oberli for the high educational value of the figures.

We also record our appreciation of the cooperation of the publisher, whose advice and skill in lay-out has resulted in a book of such excellent quality.

Chur and Basel/Switzerland Autumn 1974   U. Heim
                                              K. M. Pfeiffer

Contents

I. Introduction and Objectives

Practical experience has shown the need for adding smaller implants to the standard instrument set of ASIF (AO)*.

In certain situations there were clear deficiencies in the technical equipment developed between 1958 and 1960. This applied first of all to the fixation of thin, loose fragments detached from large cylindrical bones; the wide drill holes in these small fragments endangered their vitality and the conical screw head threatened to split them (Spycher). The prominent screw head also proved occasionally to be a disadvantage, particularly over diaphysial crests.

The almost inflexible and rather thick plates were too large for application to the metaphysial areas of the upper limb and the lower tibia, leading to disproportion between skeleton and implant; this was detrimental to soft parts, especially the skin.

Comminuted fractures of smaller joints, such as the elbow and ankle, the long term prognosis of which depends very much upon exact reduction and fixation, were unsuitable for fixation with the bulky cancellous screws. Here treatment was limited to the use of Kirschner wires, which cannot give enough stability.

Both clinical experience and experimental work (Schenk, Perren) have repeatedly shown that entirely displaced and loose fragments of cortical bone are rapidly revitalized, provided that an exact and stable reduction has been performed in living tissue. This knowledge led to the introduction of separate small implants in complex internal fixations. Thus the painstakingly precise reassembly of comminuted fragments, for a time derided as "radiological cosmetics", received a fresh impetus.

* ASIF = Association for the study of internal fixation.
AO = Arbeitsgemeinschaft für Osteosyntheseverfahren.

Standard methods of internal fixation have little application to the skeleton of the hand and foot with their narrow, short cylindrical bones. In 1946, Kilbourne, impelled by functional considerations, was the first to perform internal fixation by means of small screws and plates. His results in 17 cases were published in 1958. Stable internal fixation and plaster-free postoperative treatment of the hand looked very promising, since prolonged immobilization often results in ankylosis.

In 1959 ASIF developed the so-called "scaphoid screw" for cancellous bone. Later it was altered and renamed "small cancellous screw" because of its wider application. In the case of the scaphoid fracture, however, its use is restricted to certain situations. Yet in order to cope with the smaller and variable proportions of the peripheral skeleton, a complete instrument set with the largest possible diversification seemed to be desirable. Here the credit is due to Robert Mathys of Bettlach, who developed this set. The early types of small cortical screws with unthreaded necks allowed interfragmentary compression, but their removal could be almost impossible. The year 1964 brought about the completion of the instrument set for small fragments, which was assembled into a standard set and then approved for clinical testing. New plate types have since been developed and the lengths were meanwhile altered.

In response to the urgent demand of several hand surgeons, the "mini cortex screws" and the appropriate plates were developed in 1970 and tested in the meantime.

The small fragment set of ASIF (hereafter abbreviated to SFS) has been developed in the field and partly in accordance with the principles of the Swiss watch industry. It represents as it were their "treasure chest". All instruments and implants are delicate and their fine-

1

ness suggests that their handling calls primarily for skill rather than force. In fact, the screws have considerable strength and provide remarkable stability, but they nevertheless have their limitations. They should never be applied in places where, for mechanical and anatomical reasons, implants of standard sizes are required. The existence of such small implants should never induce the surgeon to endanger rigidity. Errors of the past, when many failures in operative fracture treatment were due to too short or too weak implants, must be avoided in the future. The small screws and plates should not be used to obtain a makeshift hold in an open reduction but they should, like the standard set, set the stage for functional post-operative treatment. To emphasize this aim is one of the purposes of this book.

The basic problems of the indications for the techniques of internal fixation have been solved for most fractures and pseudarthroses, as a result of animal experiments and clinical studies. The SFS enables the surgeon to treat skeletal parts of hand and foot as well as small fragments according to the basic principles of rigid internal fixation.

The Manual of Internal Fixation, 1970, already contained various illustrations of small implants, particularly the small cancellous screws, the 3.5 mm cortex screws, as well as the small semi-tubular plates. Several papers on internal fixation in hand surgery have recently been published (Burri, Durband, Heim, Koob, Pannike, Rüedi, Segmüller, Simonetta, and Wilhelm). These individual authors, however, supply relatively few results, and so far statistics are scarcely available. There are still noticeable gaps with regard to techniques. The lack of differential indication has been repeatedly a subject of criticism, and the uncertainties about peripheral approaches have been very obvious.

As experience has been collected over a sufficient length of time, it is felt that a systematic presentation of the SFS and its diverse range of applications will therefore meet a widespread need. The following account is derived from clinical studies and primarily intended to serve operative practice.

General Section

II. Implants and Instruments of the SFS

Experience has shown that the diversity of the implants leads to confusion and mistakes. For this reason it seemed to be imperative to furnish figures of their actual size and to indicate the special instruments in this section.

1. The SFS Screws (Fig. 1)

The SFS contains four different types of screw:

a) The Small Cancellous Screw

The outer diameter of the thread is 4.0 mm, the shaft diameter between head and thread is 2.3 mm, the thread core is 1.8 mm. The length of thread rises in proportion to the increasing screw length from 5 to 15 mm. Screw lengths begin at 10 mm and then increase by 2 mm stages up to 30 mm, and thereafter they are 35, 40, 45, 50 mm in length.

Application (Fig. 2): Screw fixation needs a drill bit of 2.0 mm with a drill guide, and a tap of 3.5 mm with a tap sleeve.

Properties: Very good hold in cancellous bone due to the broad thread. The screw can also be used in small semi-tubular plates and in special plates. It has partly replaced the so-called malleolar screw.

b) The 3.5 mm Cortex Screw

Outer diameter thread 3.5 mm, diameter of thread core 2.0 mm. Full length thread in each screw. Lengths begin at 10 mm and then increase by stages of 2 mm up to 28 mm, after which they are 32, 36, 40 mm in length.

Application (Fig. 2b): Screw fixation is with a drill bit of 2.0 mm with a drill guide, a tap

of 3.5 mm with a tap sleeve. The drill bit of 3.6 mm is used for obtaining a gliding hole. When using this screw with a plate, the drill bit of 2.0 mm with a drill guide is used, and a tap of 3.5 mm with tap sleeve.

Properties: The small cortex screw of 3.5 mm has a broad thread and a slim core so that it provides a very good hold. It is suitable for cortical bone as well as for strong cancellous bone, and fixes the small semi-tubular plate as well as some of the small plates used in hand and foot surgery.

c) The 2.7 mm Cortex Screw

Outer diameter of thread is 2.7 mm, the diameter of the core is 2.0 mm, and each screw is fully threaded. Lengths begin at 6.0 mm increasing by stages of 2 mm to 24 mm.

Application (Fig. 2c): Screw fixation with a drill bit of 2.0 mm with drill guide. A tap of 2.7 mm with tap sleeve, and the drill bit of 2.7 mm for the gliding hole.
Plate insertion is with a drill bit of 2.0 mm with drill guide, and a tap of 2.7 mm with tap sleeve.

Properties: The 2.7 mm cortex screw is only suitable for strong cortical bone of metacarpals and metatarsal and for the proximal phalanges. Exceptionally it may be used in small semi-tubular plates and in mini-plates.

d) The Small 2.0 mm Cortex Screw (So-Called Mini-Screw)

The outer diameter of the thread is 2.0 mm, the diameter of the thread core is 1.4 mm, and each screw is threaded throughout. The lengths begin at 6 mm, increasing by stages of 2 mm up to 20 mm.

Application (Fig. 2d): Screw fixation is with a drill bit of 1.4 mm with drill guide, the tap of 2.0 mm (set in small chuck, Fig. 10), a drill bit of 2.0 mm for the gliding hole. Plate insertion is with the drill bit of 1.4 mm with a drill guide, and a tap of 2.0 mm.

Properties: The small 2.0 mm cortex screw is suitable for cortical bone of the peripheral hand skeleton (proximal and middle phalanges, fragile metacarpals on occasions). It is specially designed for fixing the small plates (the so-called mini-plate).

e) The Screw Head (Fig. 3)

A matching socket fits the Phillips screw-driver. It is proposed for the future to equip the small screws with hexagonal socket *heads* like those in the standard screws. The *lower surface* of the head is congruous to the plate hole with an angle of 120°. Thus the screw ensures a satisfactory hold even in thin cortical bone. For the hexagonal socket head a lower surface of spherical shape is provided, which will improve the seat in the plate. The above mentioned screw-driver with sleeve (Fig. 4) can be used for all screws with Phillips heads. A special screw-driver for the small screws with hexagonal socket heads is also provided.
The following technical figures only show screw heads with Phillips sockets.

2. The SFS Plates

These plates are of several shapes because they have to fit at special sites. They are slightly concave, are flexible, and they may be shortened and their shapes altered with the help of the bending pliers (Fig. 10) or the cutting forceps (Fig. 10).

a) The Standard Plates

The Small Semi-Tubular Plate (Fig. 5a): This slightly concave plate of 10 mm width is available in lengths of 26 mm (2 holes) to 97 mm (8 holes) and is the most widely used implant of the SFS. The oval drill-holes allow eccentric drilling to place the plate under tension, giving axial compression of the fragments (Fig. 18). The holes are designed for the use of the 3.5 mm cortex or the 4.0 mm cancellous screw.

The Small Plates for Hand and Foot Surgery (plates for Phalanges, metacarpals and metatarsals [Fig. 5b]): Slightly concave small plates of 7 mm width are available in the following shapes:

— Straight plates 25 mm long (three holes), 35 mm long with four holes, 65 mm with eight holes.
— L-shaped plates, left and right, 3,5 mm long with five holes.
— T-Plates, 35 mm long with five holes.
— Multiple fragment plates (of serpentine shape).

The screw holes are round though somewhat wider than the diameter of the appropriate screws (small cortex screws of 2.7 mm and occasionally 3.5 mm).

The Mini-Plates (Fig. 5c): These are 25 mm long. Their shapes are identical with those of the small plates for hand and foot surgery. The screw holes are round, slightly wider than the ones for the small cortex screw of 2 mm. They also allow the use of the small cortex screw of 2.7 mm.

b) The Special Plates

The *small T-shaped plates* for the lower radius and olecranon (Fig. 6a). These are 10 mm wide and 50 mm and 57 mm in length, with round screw holes and with 3 and 4 holes respectively. They are suitable for small cortex screws of 3.5 mm, or the small cancellous screw of 4.0 mm on occasions.

The Cloverleaf Plate (Fig. 6b): This plate is for the combined application of screws of the standard instrument set and small screws. It is especially designed for comminuted fractures of the lower tibial epiphysis, but it can also be used in other locations. It is flexible and the individual leaves may be cut off with the cutting forceps to make it fit at the appropriate site.

The small implants are assembled in a separate *metal case* (Fig. 7), which contains a complete set of all SFS screws (small cancellous screws of 4.0 mm, small cortex screws of 3.5, 2.7 and 2.0 mm). A calibrated groove in the front of the tray inside the case enables screw lengths to be checked. The screw forceps (Fig. 10, numbered 28) fits into a depression. This tray can be taken out of the case.

Separate trays underneath contain the standard plates of the SFS, the washers and the thin cerclage wires for tension wiring. Kirschner wires of various gauges are in a separate tray in the instrument case (Fig. 8). Thus the entire SFS equipment is clearly arranged and easily accessible.

3. The Instruments of SFS

Special instruments have been developed for the application of small implants, some of which are smaller copies of those in the standard set (drill bits, drill guides, small Hohmann retractors etc.). Another group of instruments (reduction forceps, cutting forceps, small chuck etc.) have been designed and are used for their individual functions.

The number of instruments and implants have increased considerably during recent years so that it became impossible to have them all in a single case. They were therefore divided up and arranged in two separate boxes, one of which is reserved for instruments alone (Fig. 8).

The individual groups of instruments are shown and described according to their functions. To clarify its individual function, each instrument is numbered. The instrument numbers are identical with those in the technical and functional drawings of the instruments.

The instrument case contains:	Functional presentation fig.:
Instruments for Reductions and Temporary Fixation (Fig. 9)	
— Reduction forceps (No. 1) with pointed ends ("towel forceps").	16
— Reduction forceps (No. 2) ("small ASIF forceps").	15
— Bone forceps for small finger plates (No. 3): for reduction of fractures and temporary fixation of small plates.	19, 20, 24, 29
— Small Hohmann retractors (No. 4).	
Drill Bits (Fig. 9)	
— Drill bit of 3.6 mm (No. 5): for drilling the gliding hole for a small cortex screw of 3.5 mm used as a lag screw.	2b, 15
— Drill bit of 2.7 mm (No. 6): for drilling the gliding hole for small cortex screw of 2.7 mm used as lag screw.	2c, 16
— Drill bit of 2.0 mm (No. 7): for drilling the thread hole for all small screws (4 mm cancellous and 3.5 mm cortex and 2.7 mm cortex) as lag screws as well as for plate insertion. For drilling gliding hole for small cortex screw of 2.0 mm.	2a–d, 14, 15, 16, 18, 19
— Drill bit 1.4 mm (No. 8): for drilling the thread hole for small cortex screw of 2.0 mm.	2d
Drill Guides (Fig. 9)	
Drill bits must always be used together with drill guides and drill sleeves as follows:	
— The triple drill guide for the 2.0 mm drill bit (No. 9).	2a, 14, 18, 19
— Drill guide for central plate-holes; for drill bit 2.0 (No. 10).	2b, 19
— Double drill guide for drill bits 1.4 and 2.0 mm for use with small cortex screws of 2.0 mm (No. 11).	2c, d

The instrument case contains:	Functional presentation fig.:
— Drill sleeve. This has an outside diameter of 3.5 mm, and an inside diameter 2.0 mm, and is used inside the gliding hole of 3.6 mm and guides the drill bit 2.0 mm, for a thread hole (No. 12). The appropriate instrument is the small pointed drill guide.	15

Taps (Fig. 10)

— A 3.5 mm tap is used for cancellous screws of 4.0 mm and the cortex screw 3.5 mm (No. 13).	2a, b, 14, 15
— The 2.7 mm tap (No. 14) cuts the thread for cortex screws of 2.7 mm.	2c, 16
— The 2.0 mm tap (No. 15) cuts the thread for the small cortex screw of 2.0 mm. It needs to be mounted in the small chuck (No. 23).	2d
— Tap sleeve (No. 16) should always be used with the 3.5 mm and 2.7 mm taps.	2a, 14, 15

Screwdrivers (Fig. 10)

— The Phillips screwdriver (No. 17) is the universal one for all screws with Phillips heads	4, 14–16
— Screwdriver for screws with hexagonal socket heads (No. 18).	
— There is a special sleeve for this screwdriver (No. 19).	4

Other Instruments (Fig. 10)

— The scale (No. 20) for accurate measurement of screw lengths.	15
— A countersink tool for 3.5 and 2.7 mm cortex screws (No. 21).	15
— A countersink tool for cortex screws of 2.0 mm (which needs to be mounted in the small chuck) (No. 22).	
— Small chuck (No. 23). This holds the Kirschner wires of all sizes, the 2.0 mm tap and the small countersink tool.	
— Bending iron (No. 24): for bending Kirschner wire ends.	24
— Bending pliers (No. 25): for bending small plates.	20
— Bending iron (No. 26): for bending small plates.	20
— Cutting forceps (No. 27): for altering the length and shape of the small plates as well as for nipping off Kirschner wires.	
— Screw forceps (No. 28): for lifting screws out of the rack. This is included in the screw case.	7
— Open-ended wrench (No. 29). This is the size that fits all ASIF nuts.	

Fig. 1 **The small ASIF screws,** scale 2:1 ▷

    — Screw heads with Phillips socket
    — The shortest and longest screw of different types
    — The core and thread of the screws
    — Detail of thread (scale 20:1)

  a   Small cancellous screw of 4.0 mm

  b   Small cortex screw of 3.5 mm

  c   Small cortex screw of 2.7 mm

  d   Small cortex screw of 2.0 mm

  e   Washers for small screws

	a	b	c	d
Thread	$\varnothing$ 4,0	3,5	2,7	2,0 mm
Core	$\varnothing$ 1,8	2,0	2,0	1,4 mm
Shaft	$\varnothing$ 2,3 mm			

SW 2,5

10 5

50

15

10

40

6

24

7   e

6

20

2:1

20:1

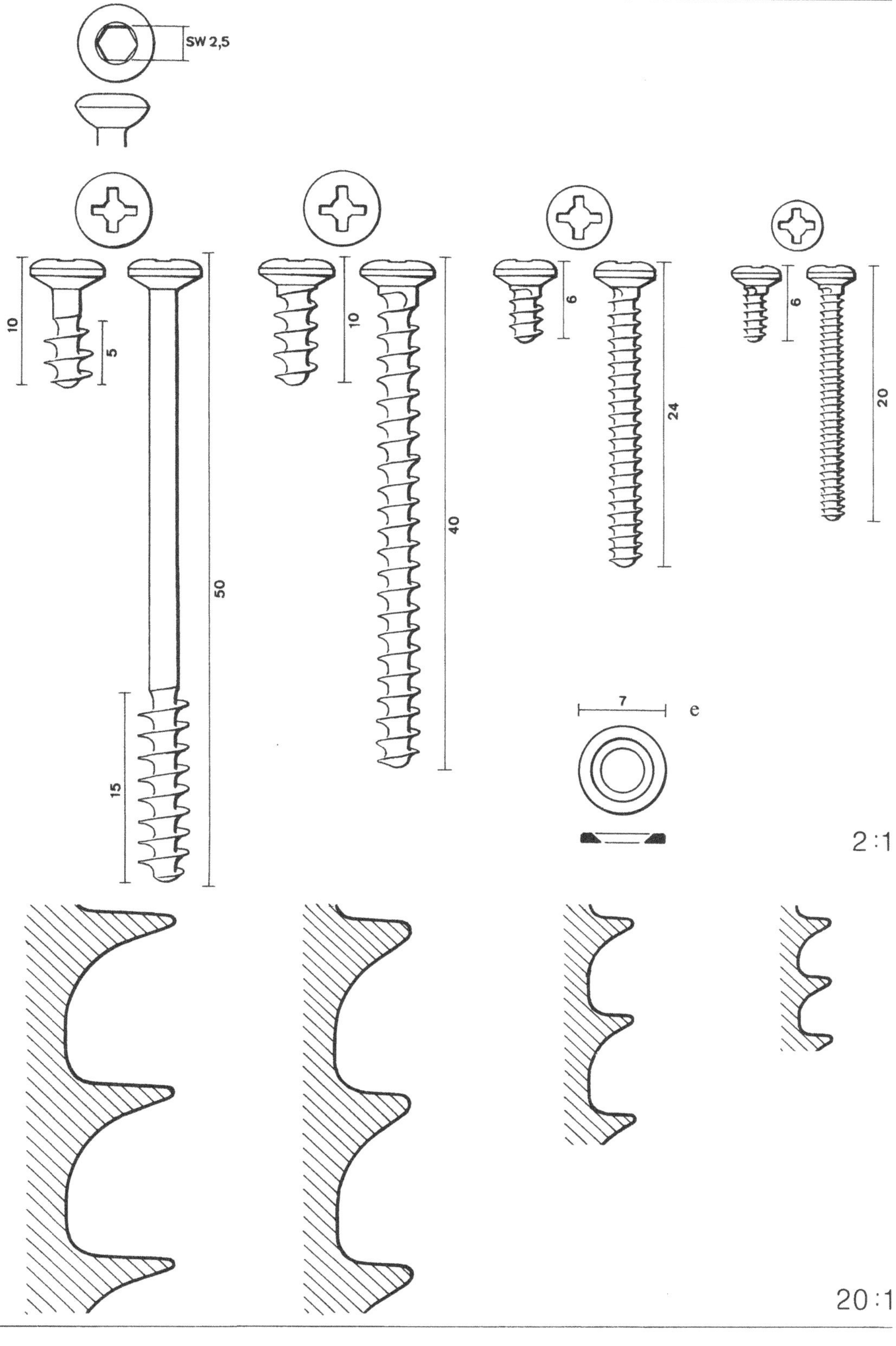

Fig. 2   **The range of small ASIF screws** shown at full size **together with the appropriate instruments**

The four small ASIF screws (details shown in Fig. 1 a–d) with the appropriate instruments (drill guides, drill bits, taps, tap sleeves) shown at full size. These instruments are shown in detail in Figs. 9 and 10 and are numbered accordingly

	a	b	c	d
Thread ⌀	4,0	3,5	2,7	2,0 mm
Core ⌀	1,8	2,0	2,0	1,4 mm
Shaft ⌀	2,3 mm			

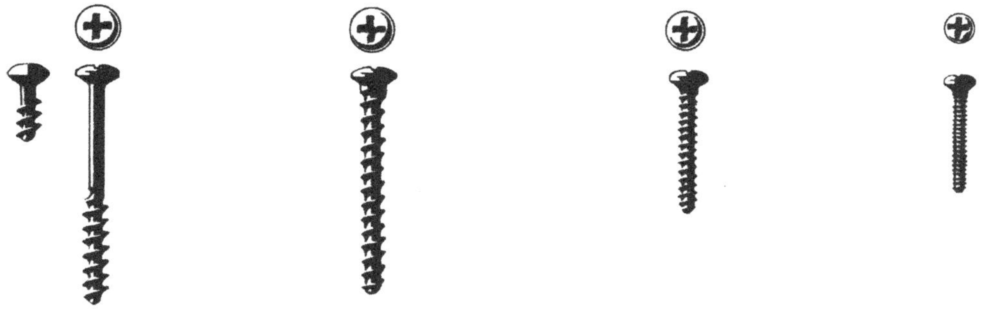

1:1

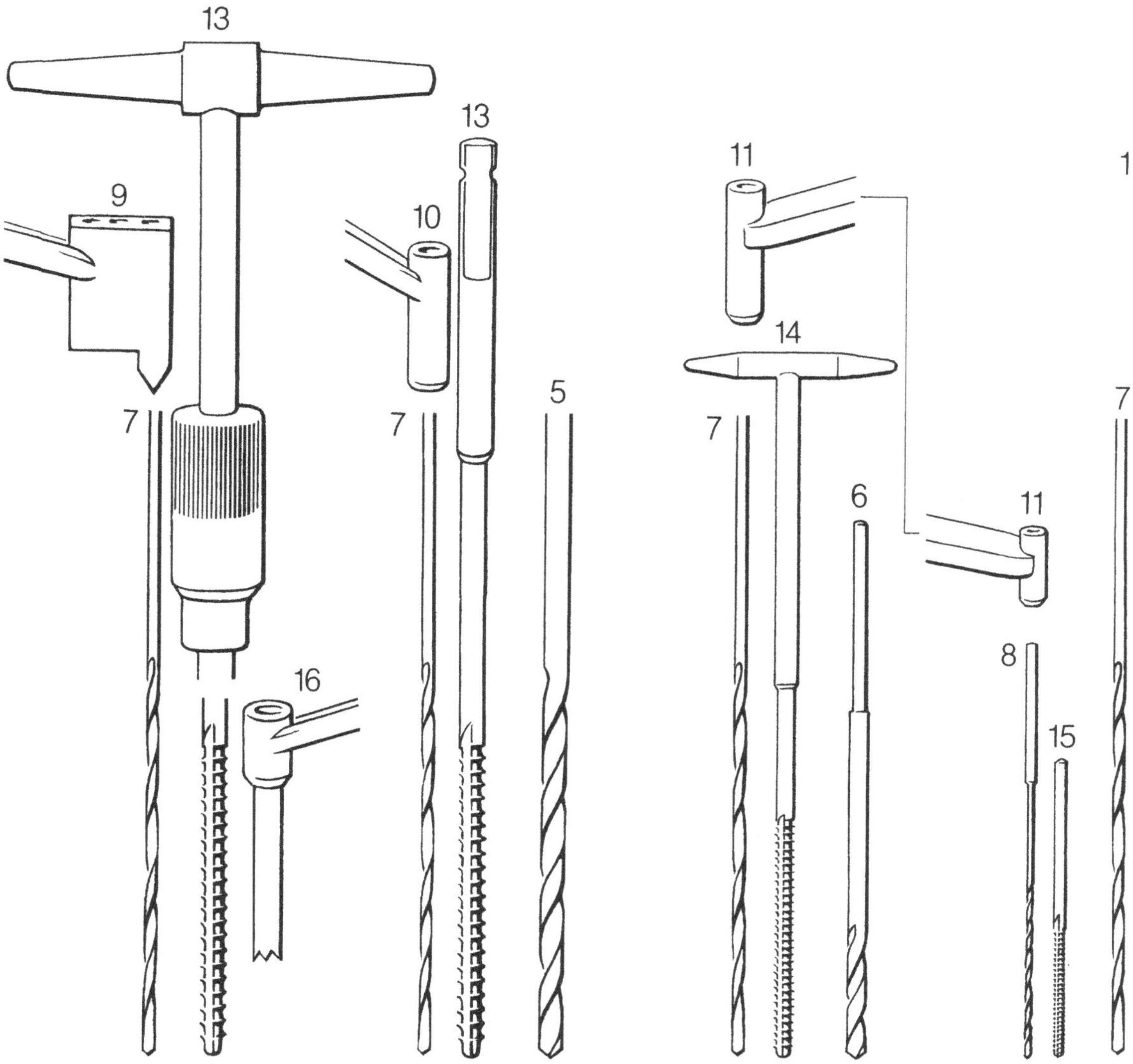

1:1

| ⌀ | 2,0 | 3,5 | | 2,0 | 3,5 | 3,6 | | 2,0 | 2,7 | 2,7 | | 1,4 | 2,0 | 2,0 |

		a	b	c	d
Head	Ø	6,0	6,0	5,0	4,0 mm
Thread	Ø	4,0	3,5	2,7	2,0 mm

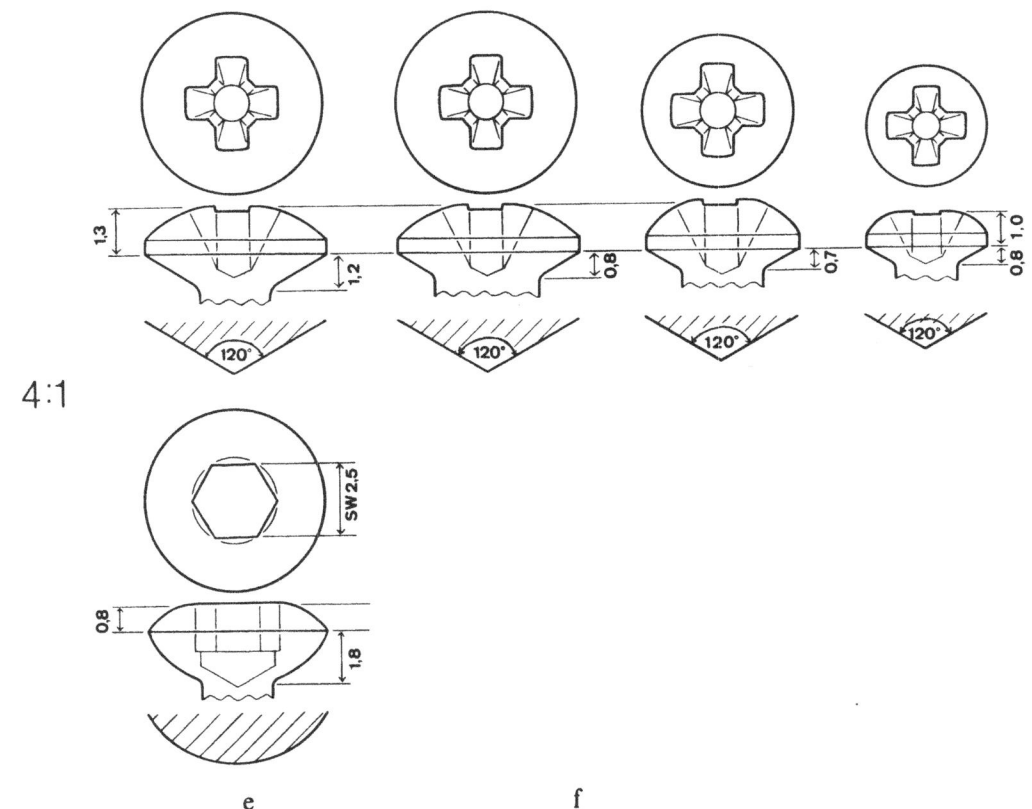

4:1

		e	f
Head	Ø	8,0	8,0 mm
Thread	Ø	4,5+6,5	4,5 mm

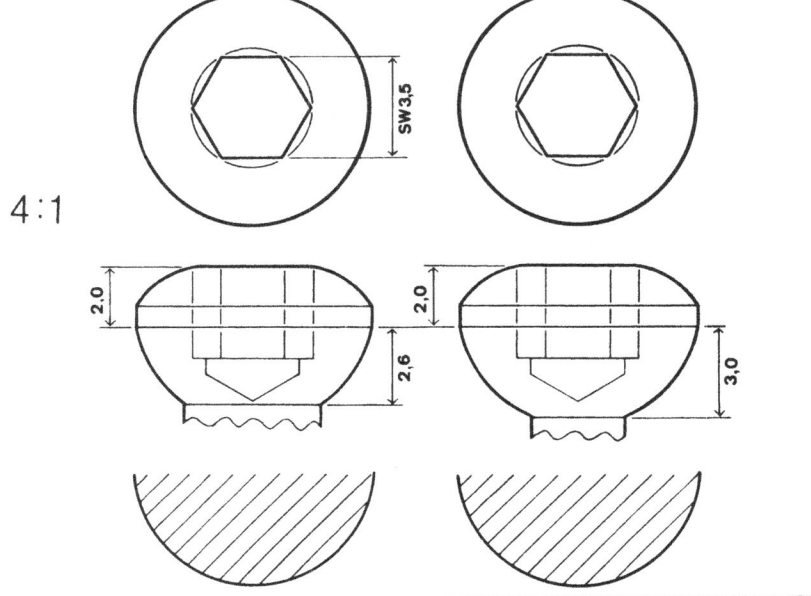

4:1

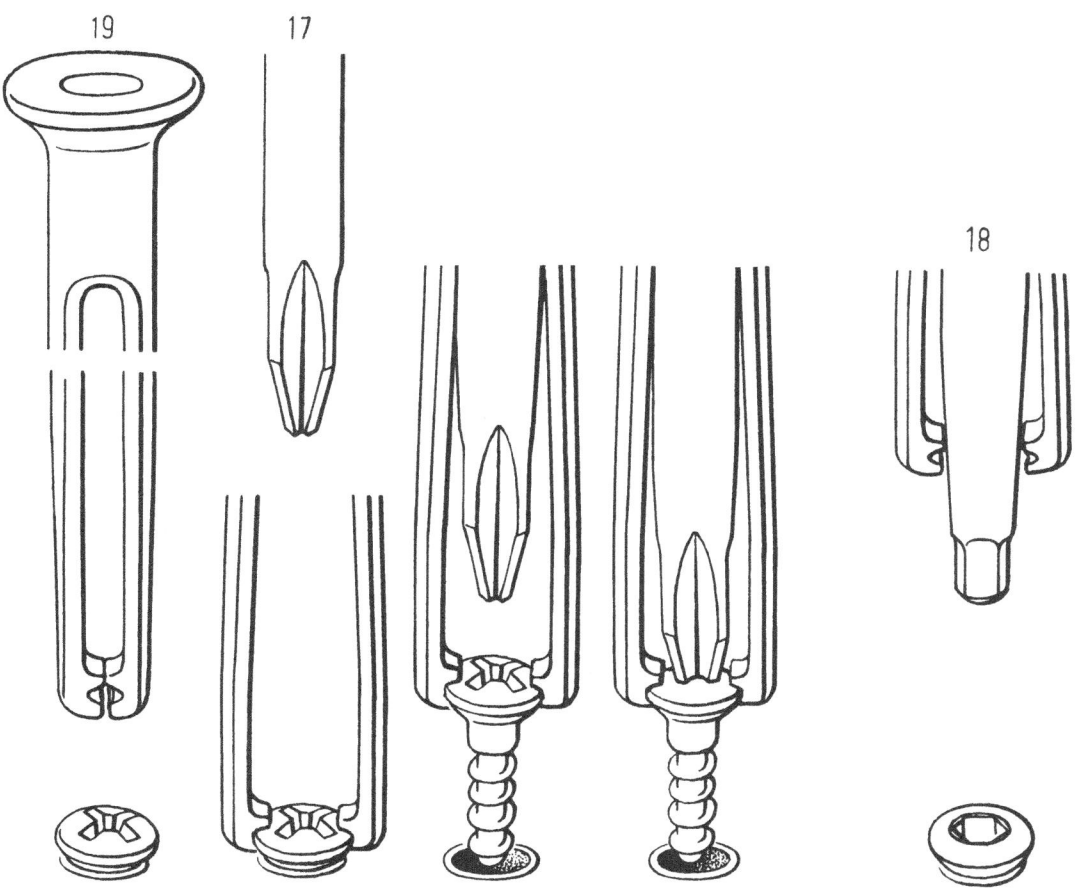

Fig. 4   Screwdriver with sleeve

Screwdriver for screws with Phillips heads (No. 17)
Screwdriver for screws with hexagonal socket heads (No. 18)
A screw is lifted from the rack with the aid of the sleeve (No. 19), and then the end of the screwdriver engages the screw head

◁

Fig. 3   Details of the ASIF screw heads, scale 4:1

a–d   Upper half: The screw heads of SFS (a–d) with Phillips sockets and conical necks (120°). Below the small cancellous screw its hexagonal socket head is shown

Lower half: Heads of the large screws

e   ASIF standard screw with its spherical neck (cortex screw of 4.5 mm and cancellous screw of 6.5 mm)

f   Malleolar screw

Fig. 5 **The standard SFS plates** shown at full size

    a   Small semi-tubular plates of various lengths with the appropriate screws (3.5 and 4.0 mm)

    b   Small plates for hand and foot surgery (straight plates, multiple fragment plates, oblique angled finger plates, L- and T-plates angled for fingers with the appropriate screws of 2.7 and 3.5 mm)

    c   "Mini-plates" of various shapes with their respective screws of 2.0 mm and occasionally of 2.7 mm

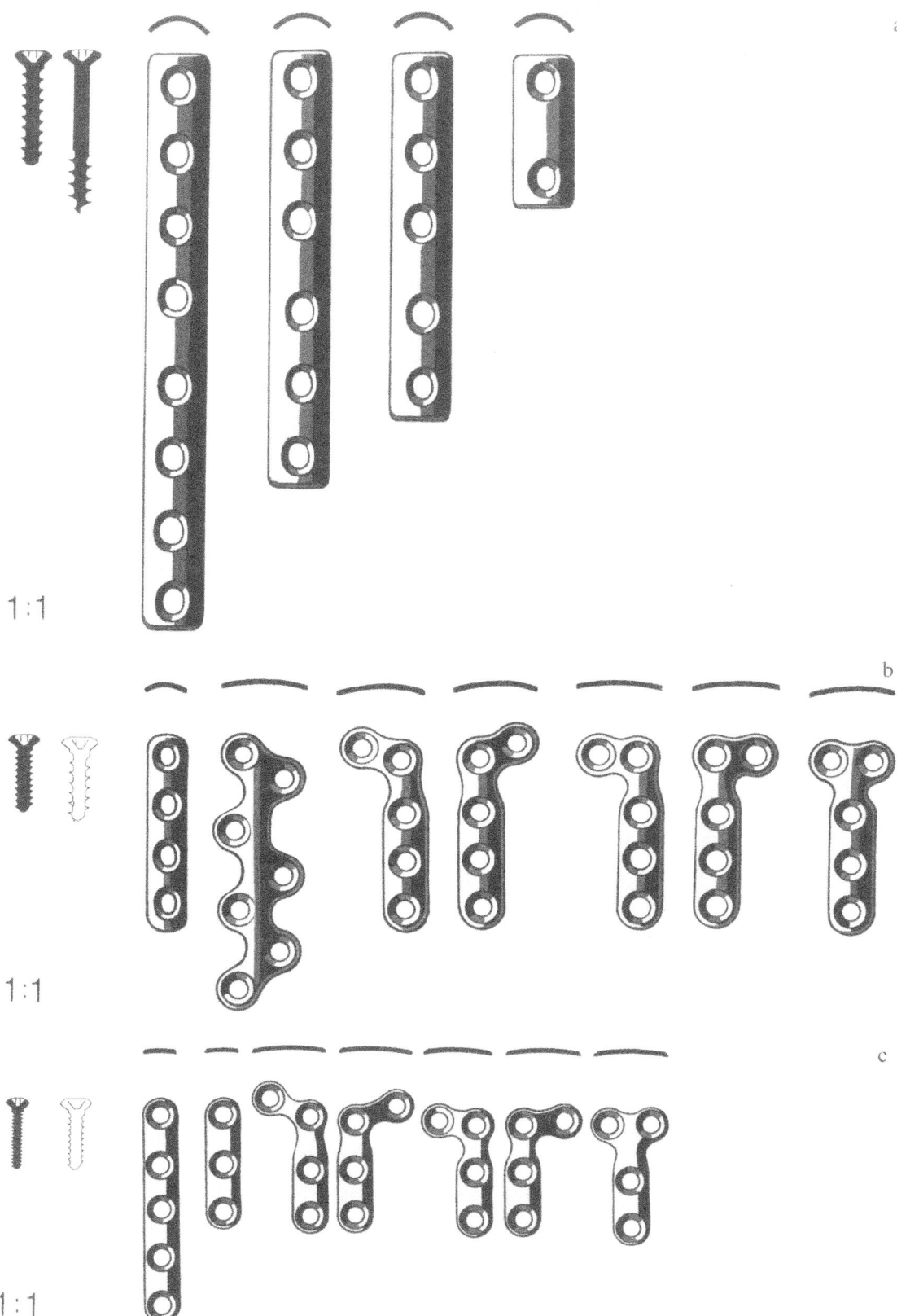

a

1:1

b

1:1

c

1:1

15

Fig. 6 **The special plates of SFS** shown at full size

a   The plates for the lower radius with their appropriate screws of 4.0 and 3.5 mm

b   The cloverleaf plate with its screws which are of 4.0, 3.5, and 4.5 mm

Shown on a smaller scale are the adaptations that may be made to a plate with the help of the cutting forceps—the side leaves or end leaf may be removed and the whole plate may be shortened.

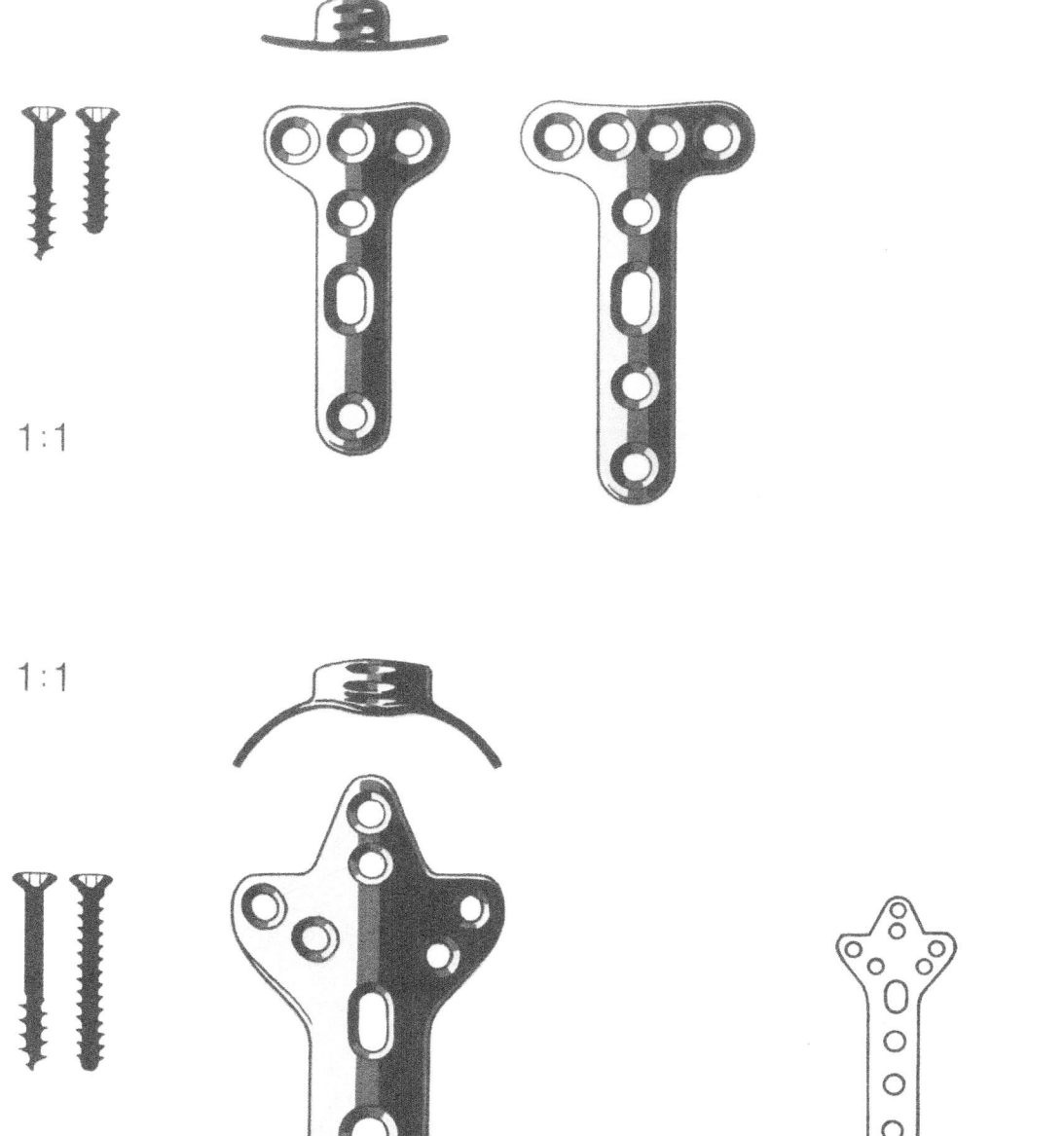

1:1

1:1

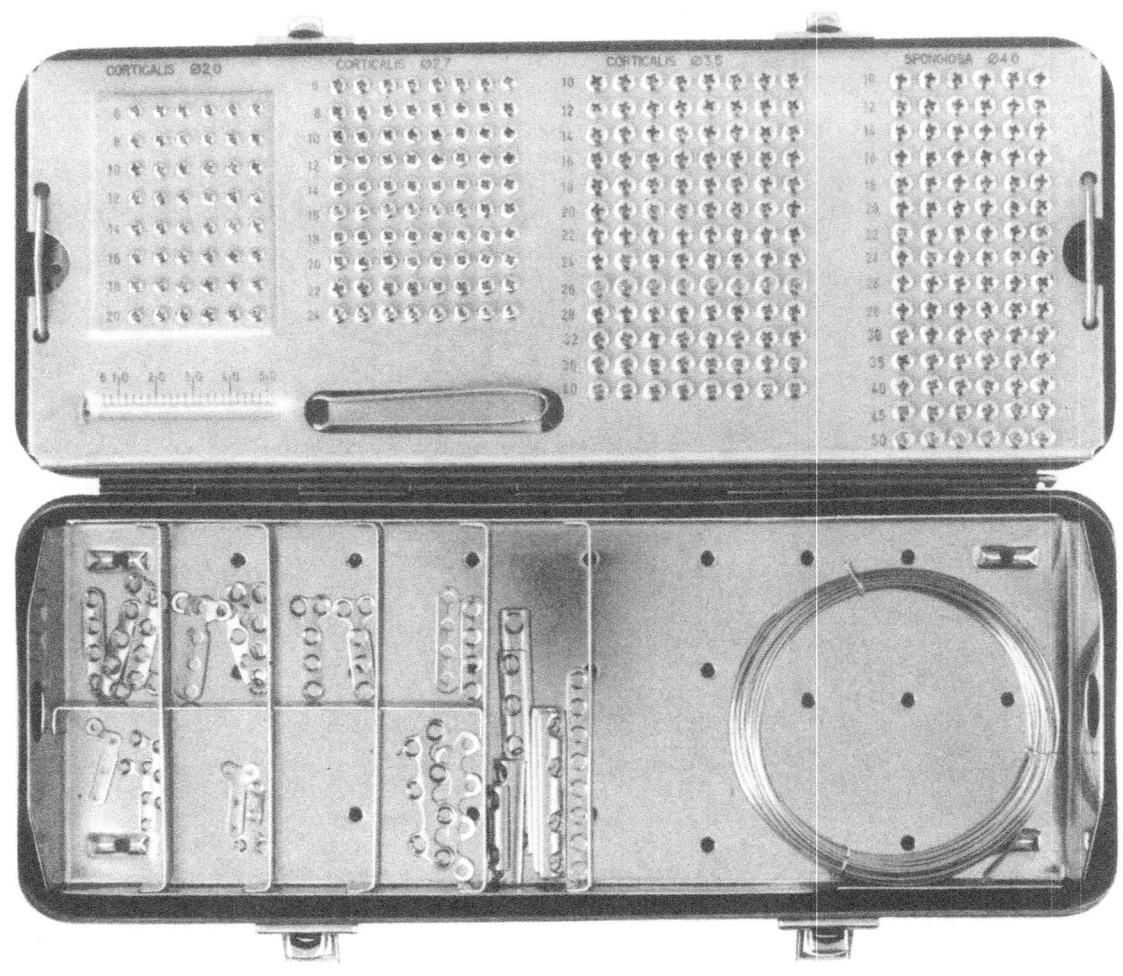

Fig. 7   The case for the small implants

Upper tray: Container with complete set of SFS screws, the measuring scale in its groove and the screw forceps (No. 28)

Lower tray: Container for small plates, and thin cerclage wire

18

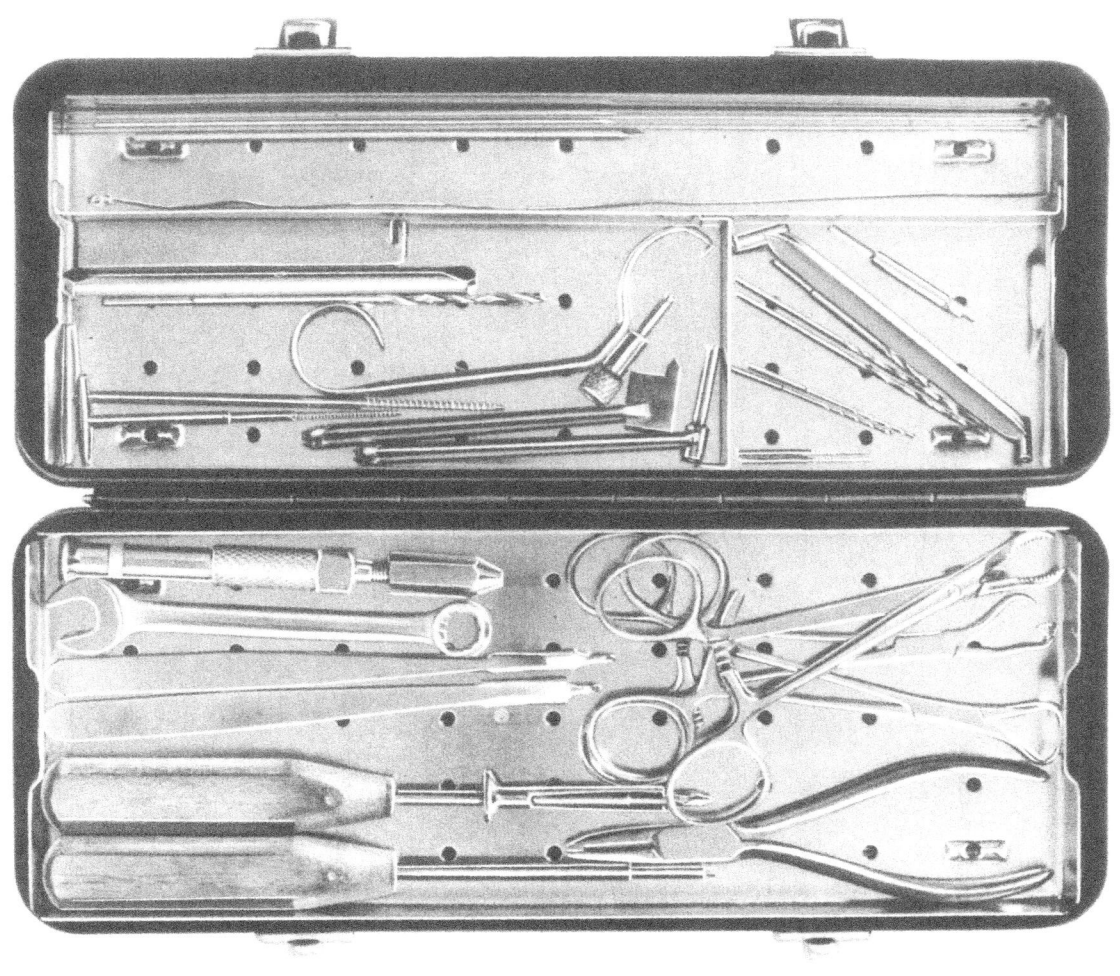

Fig. 8   Case for the SFS instruments

Two divided trays containing the instruments, of which the details are shown and the numbers given in Figs. 9 and 10. The lower tray also holds thin Kirschner wires

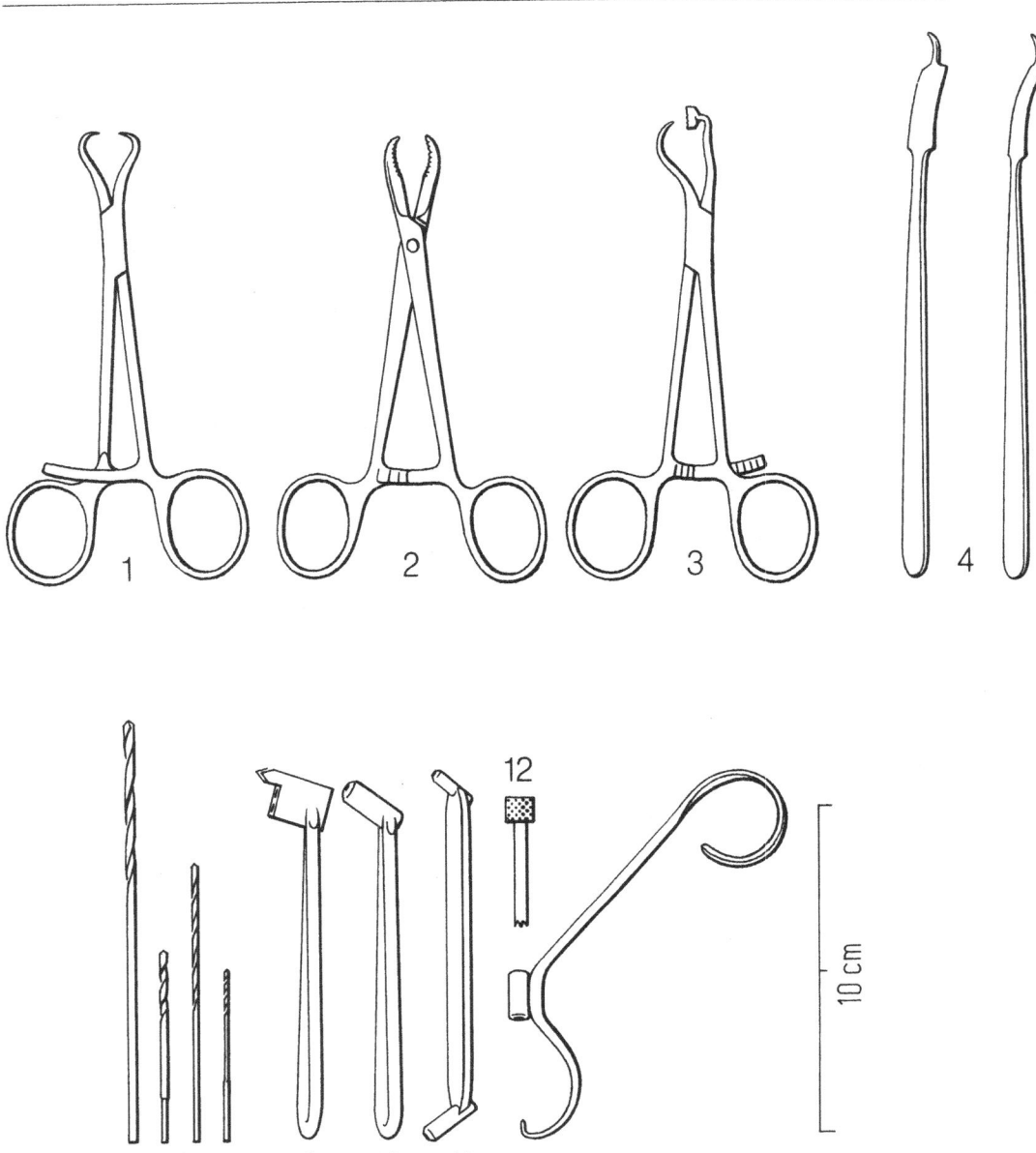

Fig. 9 **SFS instruments** (first series)

Instruments for reduction (Nos. 1–4), drill bits (Nos. 5–8), drill guides and small pointed drill guides (Nos. 9–12). For details of these see the text

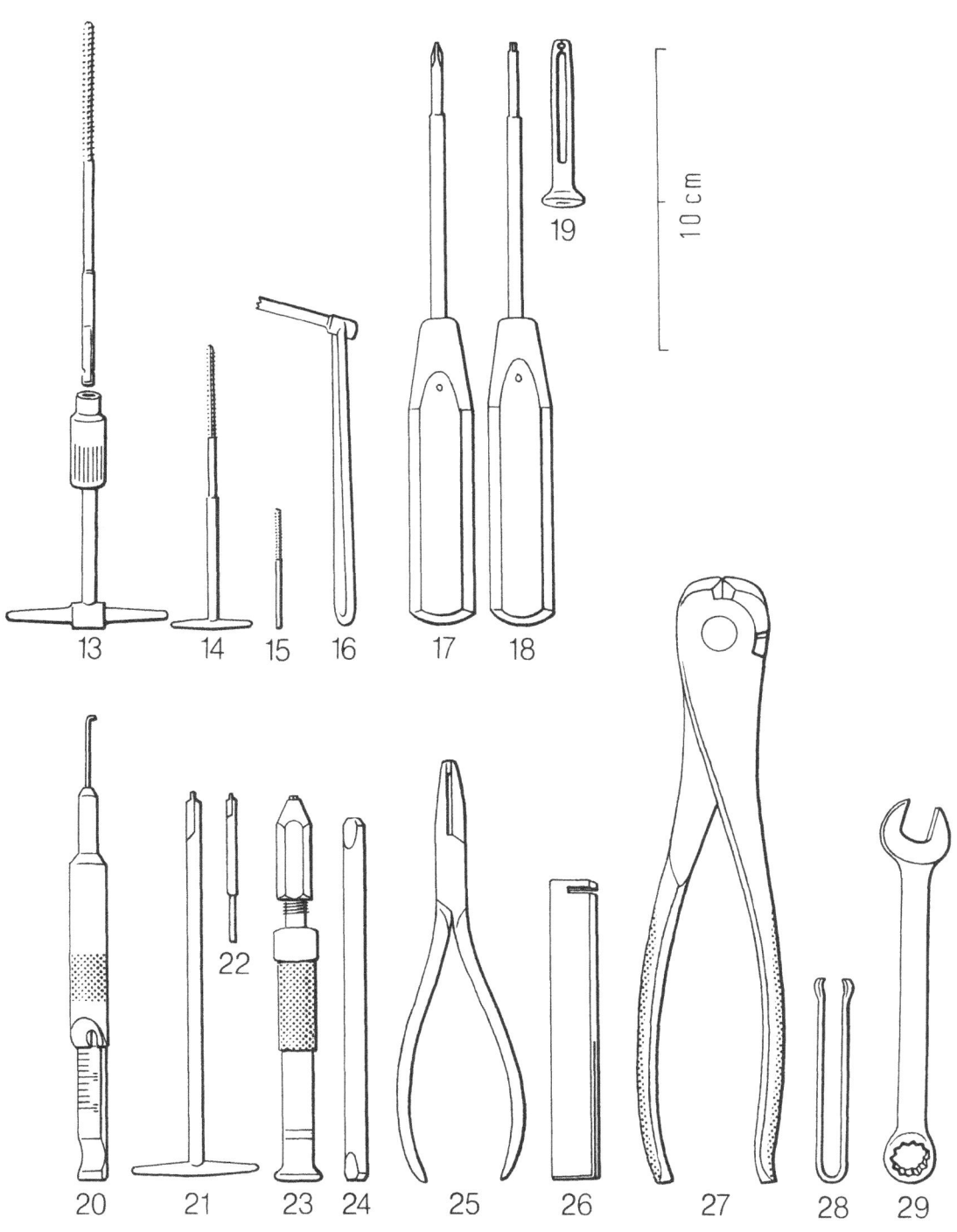

Fig. 10   SFS instruments (second series)

Taps (Nos. 13–15), tap sleeve (No. 16), screwdriver (No. 17, 18), with sleeve (No. 19) depth gauge (No. 20), countersink tools (No. 21 and 22), small chuck (No. 23), bending iron (No. 24). Bending pliers (No. 25). Second bending iron (No. 26). Cutting forceps (No. 27), screws forceps (No. 28) and open ended wrench (No. 29)

III. General Techniques of Internal Fixation Using the SFS

1. Fundamental Principles

The fundamental techniques of ASIF are laid down in detail in the Manual of Internal Fixation (Müller *et al.*, 1969). Since these provide the basis for the use of the SFS, extracts of this book are given here:

Rigid internal fixation is the prerequisite for rapid and economic fracture healing, as well as for functional postoperative treatment. Rigid internal fixation can be achieved by either compression or intra-medullary nailing.

Interfragmentary compression can be applied in long oblique fractures and is then achieved by means of the lag screw, while axial compression is used for transverse and short oblique fractures. The latter is produced by applying tension to the plate with the tension device.

Interfragmentary compression using the lag screw principle is only obtainable when the screw pulls the "far" fragment toward the "near" fragment in which a hole must be drilled which is thread-free so that the screw can glide. Consequently the screw threads must only engage the far fragment. All the cancellous screws having thread-free long necks must act lag-wise (Fig. 11a). With an ordinary cortex screw, the drill hole in the near cortex must be wider than the outer diameter of the screw, thus providing a gliding hole (Fig. 11b).

Larger metaphysial and epiphysial fractures as well as long diaphysial oblique and spiral fractures can be fixed by screws only. In the former group cancellous screws are used while in the latter cortex lag screws. The placing of the screws in relation to the fracture line must be biomechanically correct. The entire fracture interface should be uniformly compressed to achieve maximal rigidity. This rigidity serves to counteract shearing and bending stresses.

Screws should, therefore, be inserted in different rather than parallel directions (Fig. 11c). At least one of the screws should be placed at right angles to the shaft of the bone; the other screws are inserted so that they bisect the angles between the perpendicular to the long axis of the shaft and the perpendicular to the fracture plane.

Rigidity is improved by *axial compression*, applied wherever possible according to the tension band principle defined by Pauwels. Here one must be familiar with the tensile forces of muscles as well as with the leverage and bending effects which may influence one side of the fracture. The plate acts like an external beam which is first placed under tension in order to counteract tensile forces and to convert them into symmetrical compressive forces. Classic occasions for the use of the *tension wire* are in transverse fractures of the patella and olecranon where the wire is applied under tension (Fig. 12b). When applying *tensionband internal fixation with a plate*, compression of the fragments is either obtained with the help of the tension device (Fig. 12c), by eccentric drilling, or by the special shape of the screw head and the plate hole (Perren *et al.*, 1969; Allgöwer *et al.*, 1970). Many complex fractures, however, are not amenable to either of these methods. Two further techniques are at our disposal, however.

The Neutralization Plate: In cases where interfragmentary compression can be applied, but where torsional and leverage effects are great, the latter must be counteracted or neutralized by an additional plate. This holds true for all short oblique fractures of the shaft (femur and humerus) as well as for any comminuted fracture. The neutralization plate provides a firm bridge between the main fragments (Fig. 13a). Wherever possible it should be placed under axial tension.

In suitable situations this plate may effect interfragmentary compression when individual screws are inserted as lag-screws in the plate through a gliding hole in the near cortex (Fig. 13b). The neutralization plate must often be contoured to fit the bone involved, by bending and twisting.

The Buttress Plate: Application of a plate may prove to be necessary to improve interfragmentary compression. Its action may be compared to an external scaffold, and comes to the rescue when reconstitution of the loadbearing capacity of bone is insufficient, which might result in depression (articular or metaphysical comminuted fractures together with cancellous bone defects) or where an internal fixation is exposed to slowly progressive deforming forces (Fig. 13c).

2. Interfragmentary Compression by Means of the SFS

a) Fixation Using the Small Cancellous Screws

The deep cut thread and flat broad head provides substantial compression between fragments. The thread should only engage the "far" fragment using the 2.0 mm drill and the 3.5 mm tap. The rather narrow thread cut presents no inconvenience and is hardly noticed when the screw with a larger 4.0 mm thread is driven in.

Example: Oblique fracture of medial malleolus (Fig. 14).

b) Fixation with the Small Cortex Screws

In a relatively wide cylindrical bone, this fixation is performed using the standard ASIF technique, though with the smaller gauge, The gliding hole in the near cortex is drilled with the 3.6 mm drill bit. The 3.5 mm drill guide is inserted. The thread hole is drilled with the 2.0 mm drill bit in the "far" cortex, tapping the thread in this hole with the 3.5 mm tap (Fig. 15) using the tap sleeve.

Example: Oblique and spiral fractures of the distal fibula. Insertion of individual small screws in the combined internal fixation of long cylindrical bones.

In the case of *small cylindrical bones,* both cortices are first drilled with a 2.0 mm drill bit and tapped with the corresponding tap (3.5 and 2.7 mm respectively).
The gliding hole is then made by over-drilling the near cortex with 3.6 and 2.7 mm drill bits respectively. Where the distance between both cortices is small, the screw easily engages the far threaded hole (Fig. 16).

Example: Long oblique fracture of metacarpal.

Analogous procedure with the 2.0 mm miniscrew, the 1.4 mm drill bit, the 2.0 mm tap and the 2.0 mm drill for the gliding hole.

Example: Small articular fractures and spiral fractures of phalanges.

c) Stabilization Rule 1: Screw Fixation Rule

The following rule applies to the rigidity of screw fixation:

Fixation of spiral and long oblique fractures is accomplished with two screws placed in different planes. The resistance against tensile and shearing forces of *two* screws fixing the fragment ends is considerably higher than that of a *single* large screw placed in the centre.
Where the fragment is too small, two screws of the next smaller diameter should be used instead of a single broad screw. This rule applies in the descending order to all gauges (Fig. 17a and b).

Guiding principle: *"Two small screws obtain a better fixation than a single large one".*

Exception: Perfect stabilization of articular fractures with indented fracture lines can be achieved with a single lag screw (Fig. 17c).

3. Axial Compression by Means of SFS

a) Tension-Band Principle

This very important biomechanical principle (Pauwels) is often applied in peripheral bones with the help of SFS. Internal fixation using this method is almost always done by means of plates.

Axial compression of fragments with the small semi-tubular plate is accomplished in the following manner: after reduction of the fracture and contouring of the plate, drill holes are made eccentrically. The drill bit is placed at the end of each hole that is farthest from the fracture. The first drilling is made in the plate holes that overlie the fragment that is nearest to the fracture. As the screws are tightened, the conical or spherical heads of the screws will push the plate away from the fracture, as it were, so that the fragments are compressed together (Fig. 18).

For axial compression only the nearest screw on each side of the fracture needs to be inserted eccentrically, and the other ones should be inserted right in the centre of their holes. Otherwise the compression force of the first two screws may be eliminated by the following ones.

It is rather more difficult to obtain *axial compression with small plates in the hand or foot,* particulary with the angled finger plate. This is for two reasons: first the fact that a reduction is quite feasible, while temporary fixation with a thin oblique Kirschner wire is difficult; secondly the plate covers so much of the bone that it prevents visual control of the reduction.

As a rule we adopt the following procedure (Fig. 19):

— Open reduction while the assistant temporarily maintains the correction achieved.

— The plate is then bent, accurately contouring it to the skeleton, which is of special importance in hands and feet.

— Selection of the first drill-hole in the long axis of the bone.

— Fixation of a plate to the distal fragment with the first screw, the accurate position of which is decisive.

— Due to its grip on the distal fragment the plate can now be used as an auxiliary instrument which is fixed proximally with the reduction forceps, thus reducing the fracture.

— Checking the axial alignment which can still be corrected.

— Insertion of the second screw in the distal fragment. Control of rotation which may still be correctable by changing the position of the plate on the proximal fragment.

— Drilling the eccentric tension hole in the proximal fragment. Removal of the reduction forceps. Axial compression is obtained by tightening the screws.

— Insertion of the remaining proximal screws.

The purpose of this procedure is to avoid *two of the most frequent faults* of this type of internal fixation, namely:

— *Malposition of the axes* when angled finger T-plates are applied: This malposition is produced by eccentric tensile forces when the fracture is exposed to compression before insertion of both peripheral screws (Fig. 20a).

— *Rotational deformities* when an angled L- or oblique plate is used: this plate will compress the peripheral fragment and then displace the finger (Fig. b).

b) Neutralization and Buttress Plates

Are frequently used in hands and feet. Wherever possible they should be fixed according to the procedure outlined above (Fig. 21). In badly comminuted fractures and bony defects, an initial filling in with autogenous cancellous bone is occasionally indicated (see below).

Examples: Comminuted fracture of the lateral malleolus.
Transverse and oblique fractures of metatarsals.

c) Stabilization Rule 2: Rule of Number of Threads

Where internal fixation with plates is applied, the screws should fix the main fragment with several threads. As bending and shearing forces increase with body weight, the number of threads required for effective stabilization increases from the peripheral to the proximal parts of the skeleton. In phalanges, three threads in each cortex are sufficient, in metacarpals and metatarsals four threads in each cortex should be placed in each fragment. Where oblique fractures in more proximal areas are concerned, five cortex threads per fragment should be inserted, whereas transverse fractures require six cortex threads as they are exposed to higher shearing forces (Fig. 22).

Guiding Principle: "*Distal 3–4, proximal 5–6 cortex threads*".

4. Combined Internal Fixation with Small and Large Implants

The transitional zone between "large" and "small" parts of the skeleton often calls for the simultaneous use of various operative techniques and different implants (distal tibia, malleoli, elbow, or distal forearm). According to the circumstances, the SFS can be the chief means or only a supplement for the performance of the internal fixation. For typical examples refer to the special section.

5. Multiple Fractures

Multiple fractures occur frequently in the peripheral parts of the skeleton. They are either mechanically independent from each other (we call them "autonomous fractures") or there is a mechanical interdependence of such fractures. Then one fracture is predominant and we call it the "*dominant fracture*"; the other one is in the background, less conspicuous and depends on the first for its position and stability. It lies more or less protected and we have labelled it the "*vassal fracture*". The dependence is chiefly found in fractures of the metacarpals 2–5, in the forefoot, in the malleoli, and in the distal forearm. It also holds true for certain segmental fractures. A classical example in the larger skeleton is the oblique fracture of the distal fibula which may occur together with a spiral fracture of the lower leg. (Fig. 23). Treatment should be concentrated on the dominant fracture as removal of all stress is for practical reasons imperative in the treatment of multiple fractures. The time factor (interruption of blood supply, infection, and protection of soft parts) plays an important role in this type of internal fixation, the technical performance of which is often rather difficult. This leads us to the

Stabilization Rule 3: The So-Called "Vassal Rule"

In the presence of mechanical dependence between two fractures, the types of internal fixation should be differentiated. The dominant fracture should be the first to be reduced after which the "vassal" fracture will either reduce spontaneously or can easily be reduced. Stabilization of the dominant fracture is obtained by a "load bearing beam", which also prevents any secondary displacement of the vassal fracture. Its fixation can be achieved by the most simple means, for instance an isolated screw or single Kirschner wire, and sometimes even this fixation proves to be unnecessary (Fig. 24).

Guiding principle: "*Only the dominant fracture requires a plate*".

26

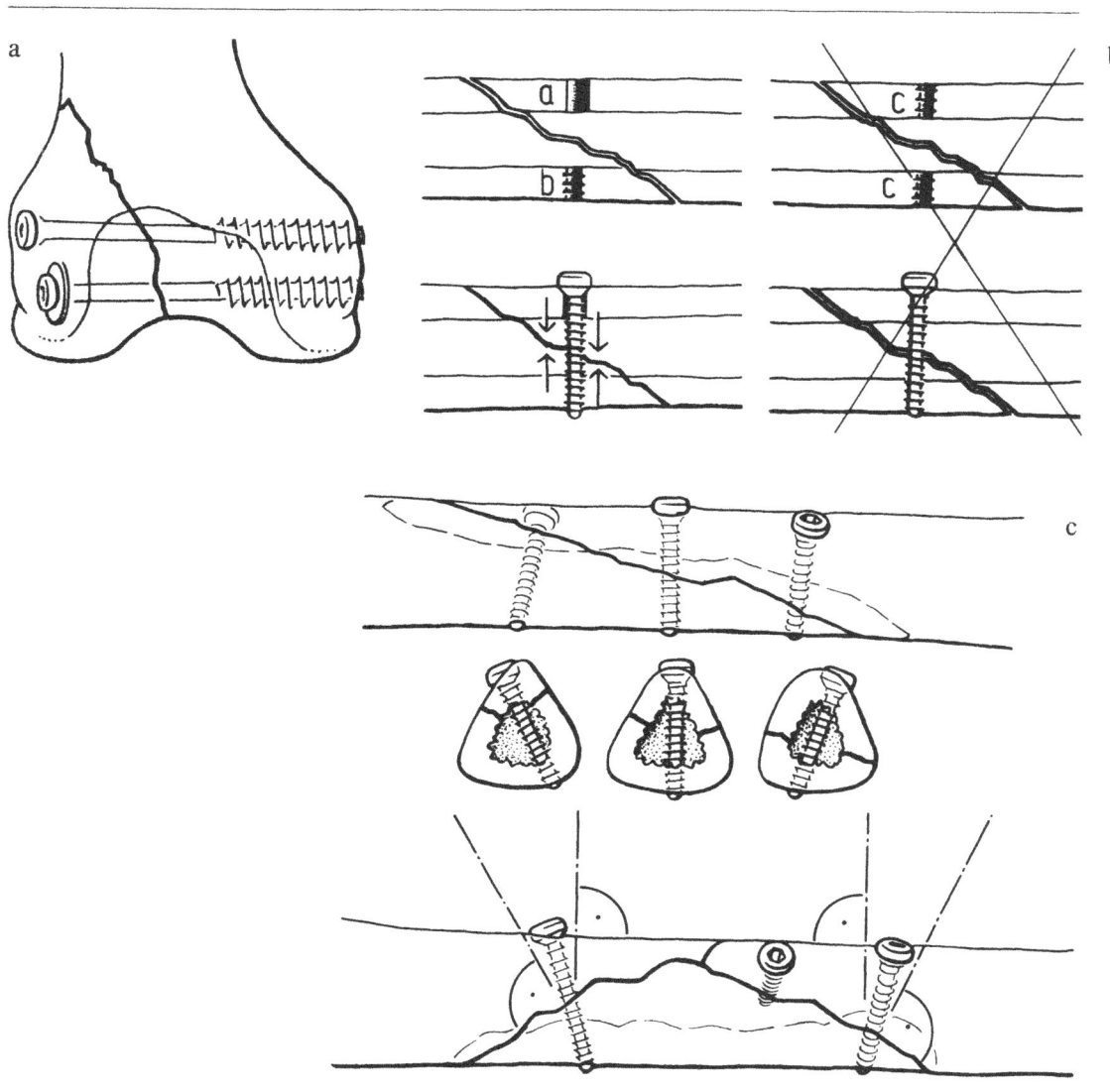

Fig. 11   Basic technical principles: Interfragmentary compression

a   Fixation with cancellous screws: Simple fracture of lateral femoral condyle. One cancellous screw must be fitted with a washer in order to prevent the screw head sinking into the thin cortical bone. Principle: When using a screw with a threadfree neck the threaded part should always reach beyond the fracture line (see also Müller *et al.*, Manual of Internal Fixation, 1970, Fig. 13)

b   Fixation with cortex screws: The hole in the cortex nearest to the screw head (gliding hole) must be as wide as the outer diameter of the screw thread. The hole in the far cortex is tapped (thread hole). Tightening the screw produces interfragmentary compression (see also Müller *et al.*, Manual of Internal Fixation, 1970, Fig. 17)

c   Accurate direction of screws: Long spiral fracture of the shaft. Interfragmentary compression must exert an even effect upon the entire length of the fracture. Screws, therefore, have to be inserted in different planes. The central screw is placed at right angles to the shaft of the bone, the remaining screws are inserted so that they bisect the angle between a perpendicular to the long axis of the shaft and a perpendicular to the fracture plane (see also Müller *et al.*, Manual of Internal Fixation, 1970, Fig. 24)

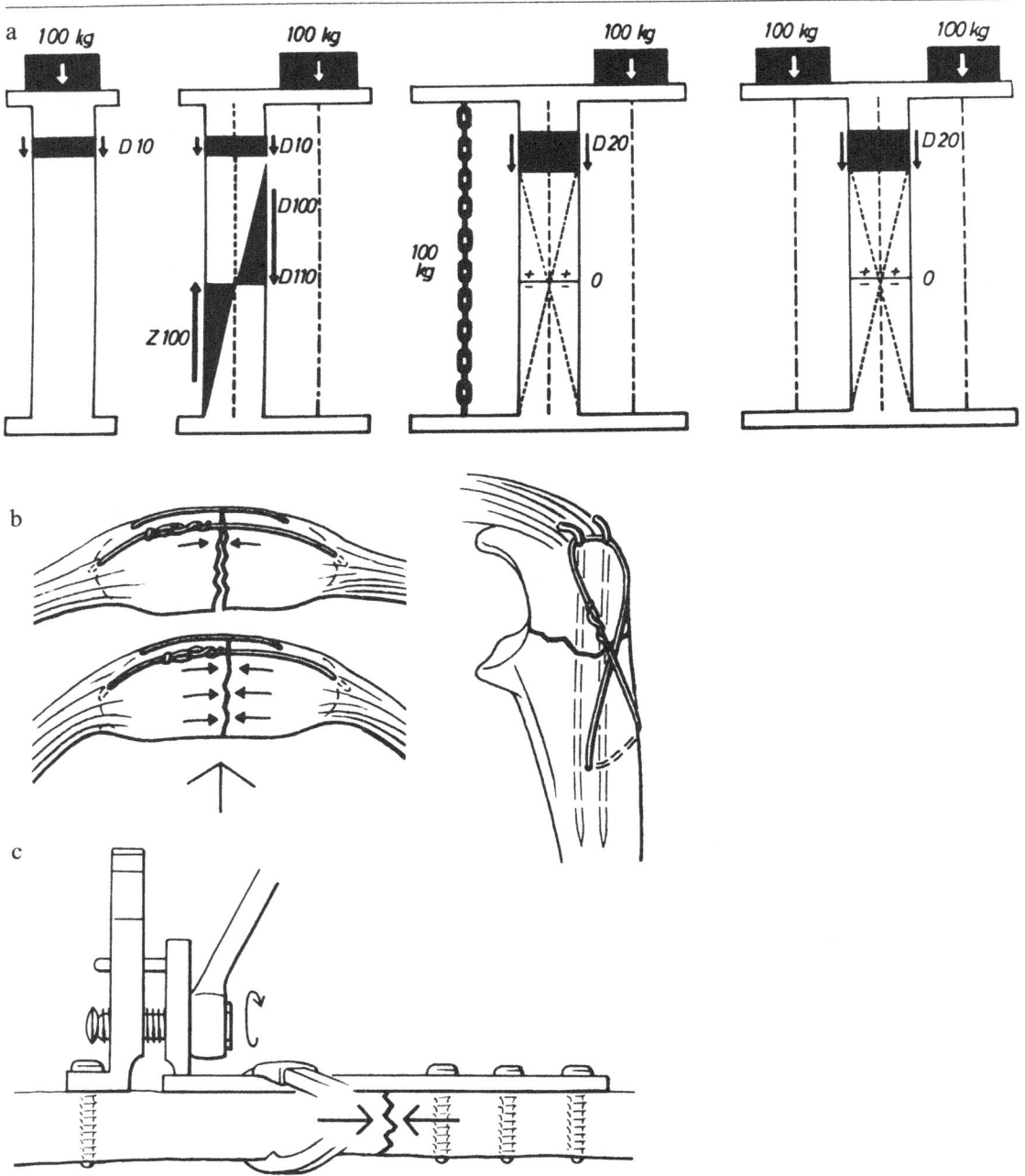

Fig. 12   Basic technical principles: Tension-band principles

   a   Model of the loaded T-beam after Pauwels: where the weight is placed eccentrically, it creates equal and opposite tensile stresses in the interior of the column. These can be neutralized by a chain or weight applied to the opposite side and converted into symmetrical axial compressive forces (see also Müller *et al.*, Manual of Internal Fixation, 1970, Fig. 26)

   b   Tension-wiring of olecranon and patella: The wire is fixed on the side opposite to the muscular tensile force (triceps on the olecranon) or to the compressive tensile force (femoral condyle on patella) and placed under tension (see also Müller *et al.*, Manual of Internal Fixation, 1970, Figs. 28 and 30)

   c   Tension-band fixation using a plate: The plate is placed under tension by the ASIF tension device on the side on which tensile forces would fall (see Müller *et al.*, Manual of Internal Fixation, 1970, Fig. 32)

28

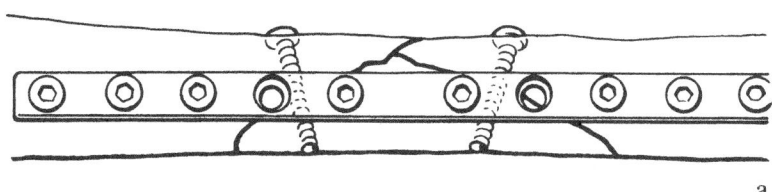

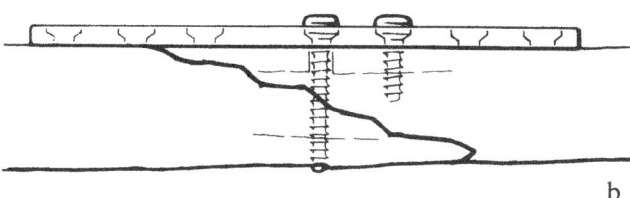

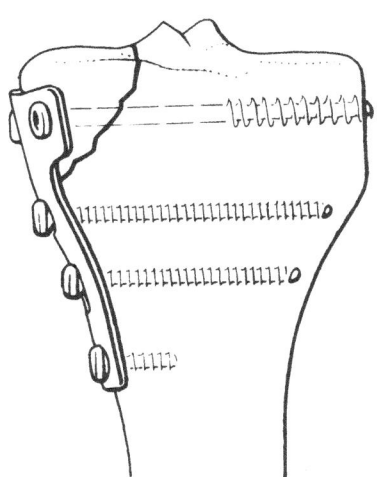

Fig. 13   Basic technical principles: Neutralization and support

  a   Screw fixation of long spiral fracture with butterfly fragment. The shearing forces affecting the fracture surface are neutralized by a plate which joins the main fragments (see also Müller *et al.*, Manual of Internal Fixation, 1970, Fig. 48)

  b   Combination of neutralization plate and lag screws. In an oblique fracture, interfragmentary compression can be obtained using a plate, as long as the drill hole in the near cortex under the plate is drilled wide enough to provide a gliding hole. Thus the far fragment is drawn up towards the plate so that the near fragment is compressed between the far fragment and the plate (see also Müller *et al.*, Manual of Internal Fixation, 1970, Fig. 47)

  c   Supporting a fracture of the tibial plateau by the use of a T-plate (see Müller *et al.*, Manual of Internal Fixation, 1970, Fig. 54)

29

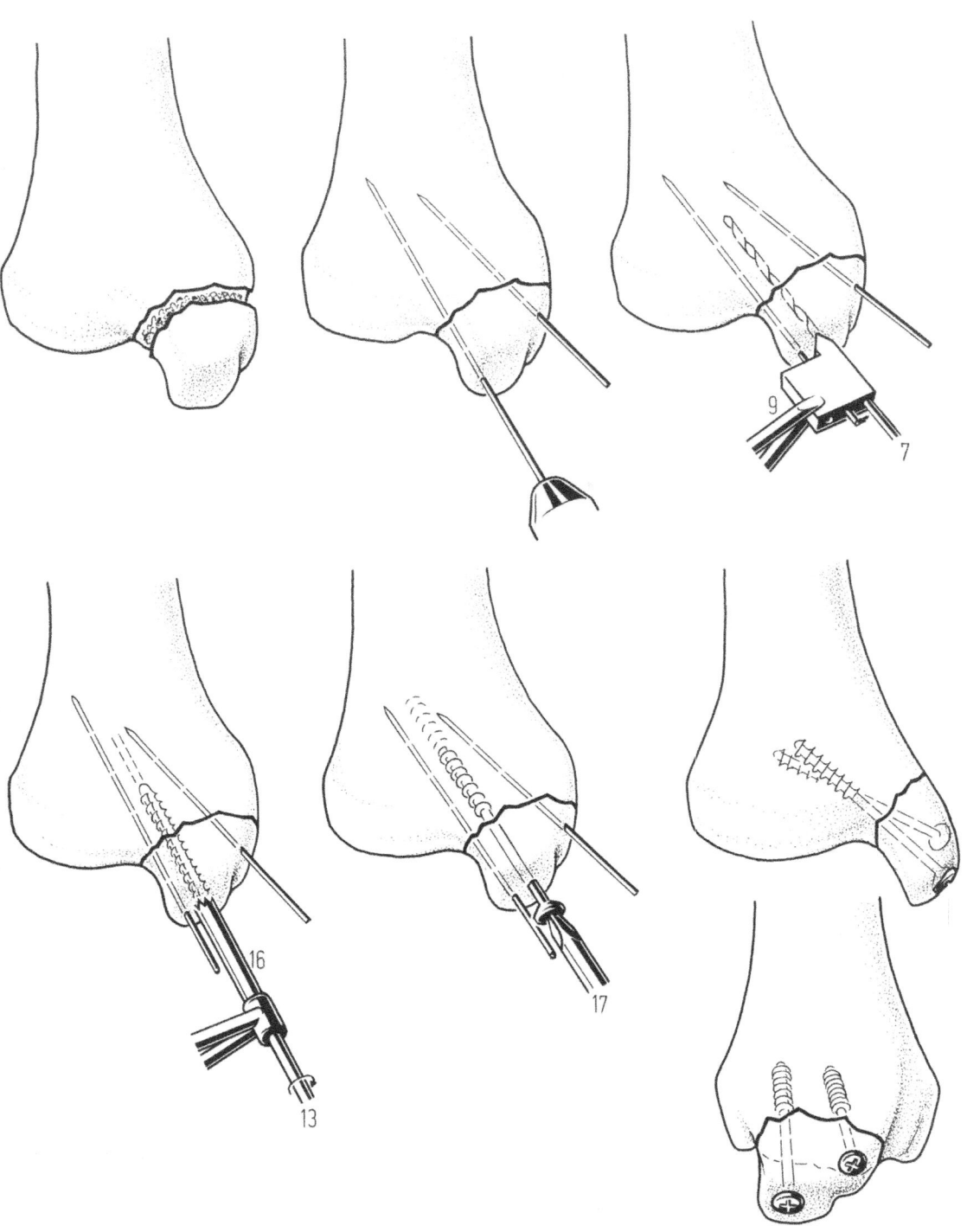

Fig. 14   Screw fixation with small cancellous screws

Oblique fracture of medial malleolus. Reduction and temporary fixation with thin Kirschner wires. A parallel drill hole is made with the drill guide and 2.0 mm drill bit. The thread is cut with the 3.5 mm tap and tap sleeve. The first screw is inserted. The identical procedure is carried out with the second screw. The Kirschner wires are then removed before final tightening of the screws

30

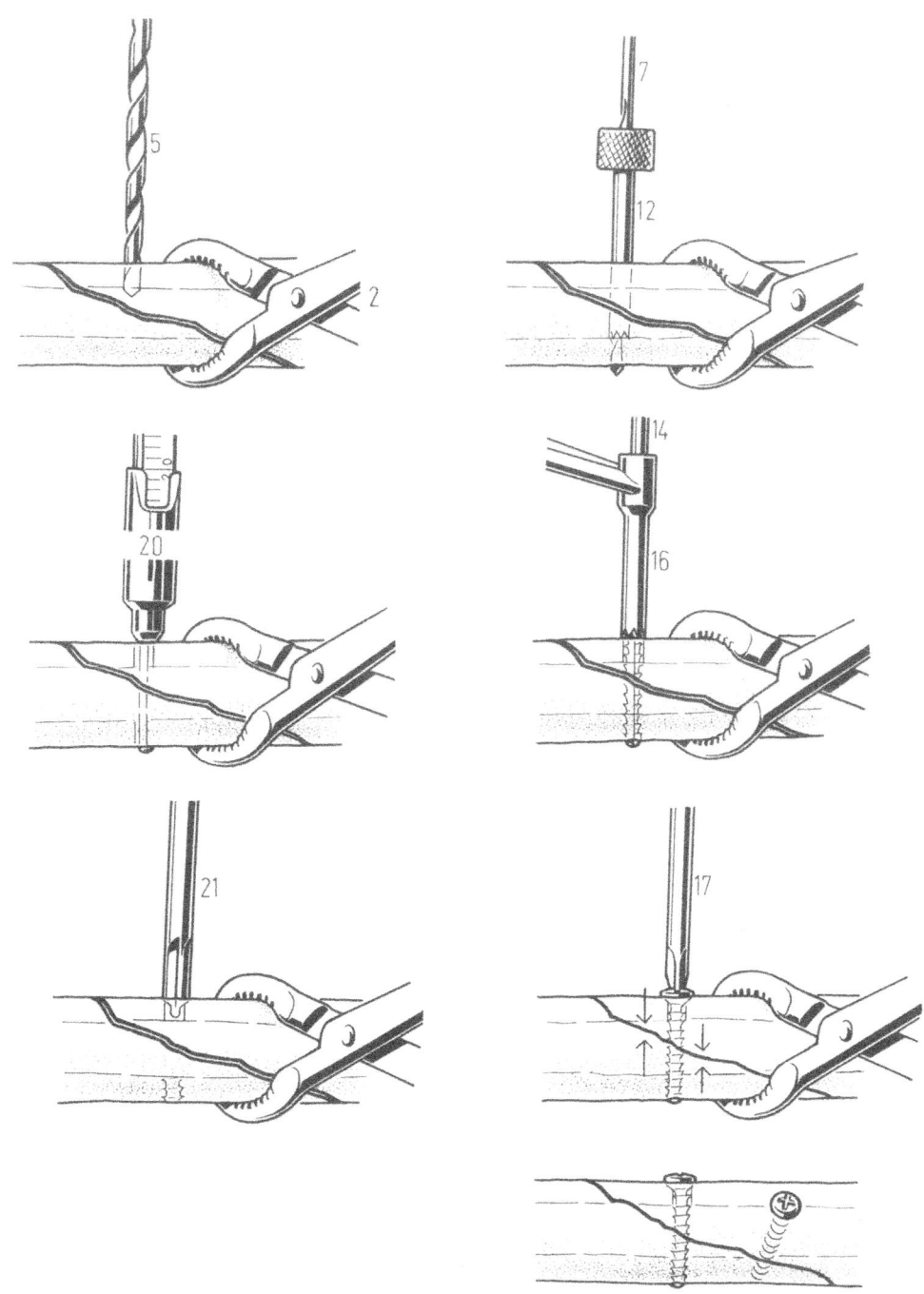

Fig. 15   Screw fixation with small cortex screws in large cylindrical bones

Diaphysial fracture of the shaft. Reduction and temporary fixation with the reduction forceps. At first a gliding hole is made in the near cortex with the 3.6 mm drill bit. The drill sleeve is inserted. The hole in the far cortex is drilled with the 2.0 mm bit, then the depth gauge is used to measure the required screw length. Tapping the hole with the 3.5 mm tap and the tap sleeve. Countersinking the hole for the screw thread. After insertion of the first screw, the reduction clamp is replaced by a second screw

31

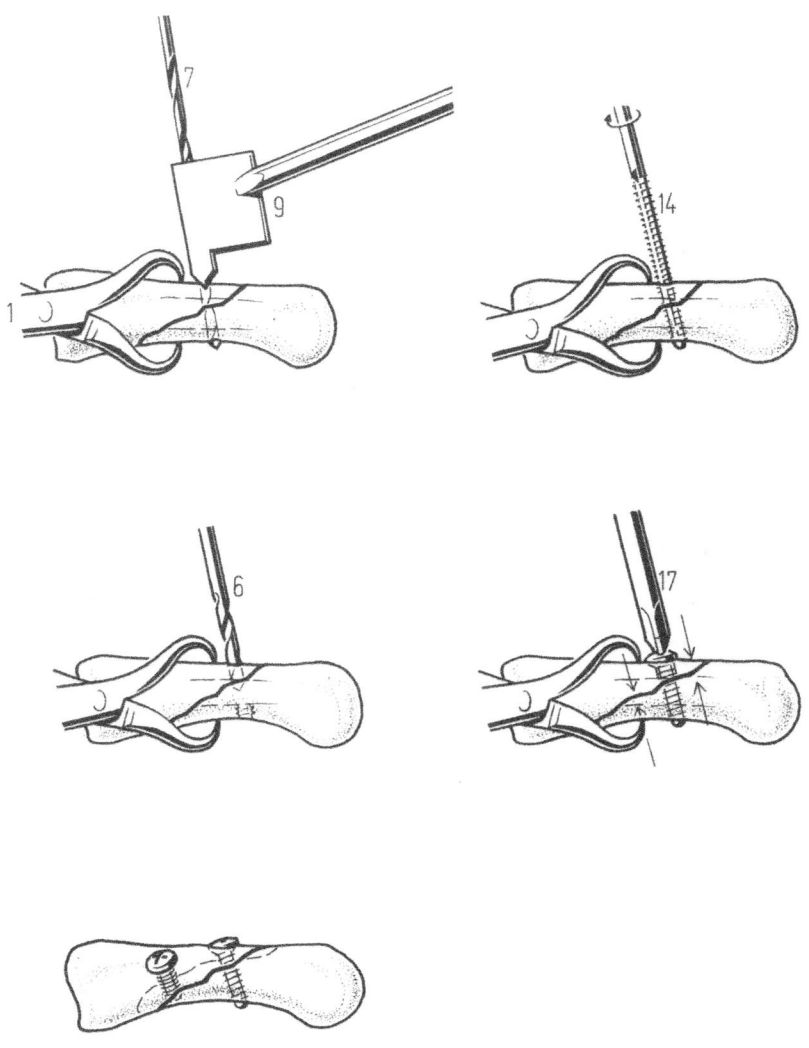

Fig. 16   Fixation with cortex screws in a narrow tubular bone

Long oblique diaphysial fracture. Reduction and temporary fixation with reduction forceps. Both cortices drilled with the 2.0 mm drill bit and drill guide. Both cortices tapped with the 2.7 mm or sometimes the 3.5 mm tap. A gliding hole is now provided by drilling the near cortex with a 2.7 mm or sometimes a 3.5 mm drill bit. First screw inserted. A second screw is inserted in a different direction and when this is tightened the reduction clamp can be removed

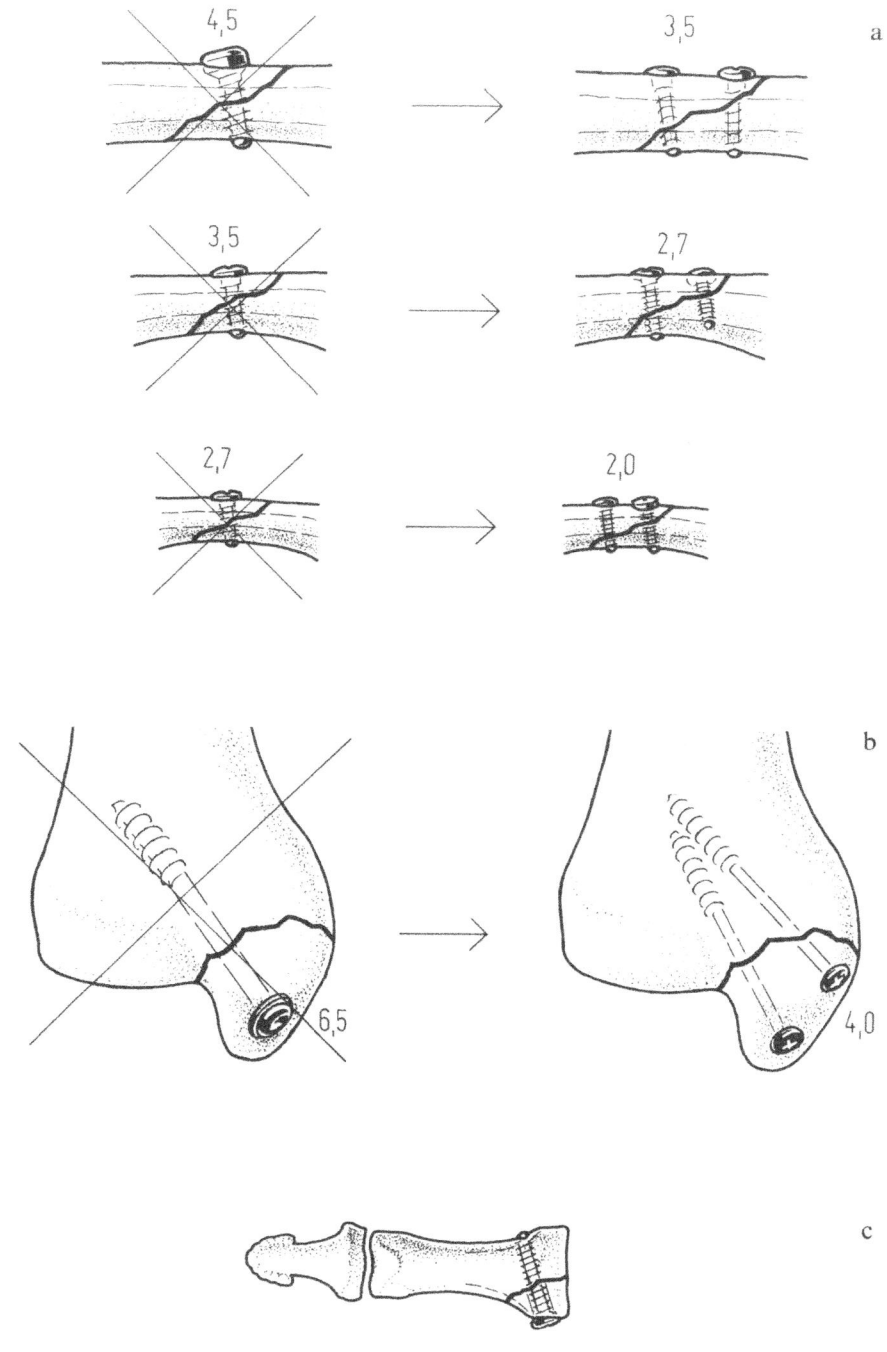

Fig. 17   **Stabilization rule 1: The screw fixation rule**

a, b   To provide stability two smaller screws are inserted near the ends of the fracture line rather than a single large central screw. The gauge of the two small screws is determined by the size of the fragment. This rule applies to cortical (a) and cancellous fractures (b)

c   Exception: An indented articular fracture can be fixed with a single lag screw

33

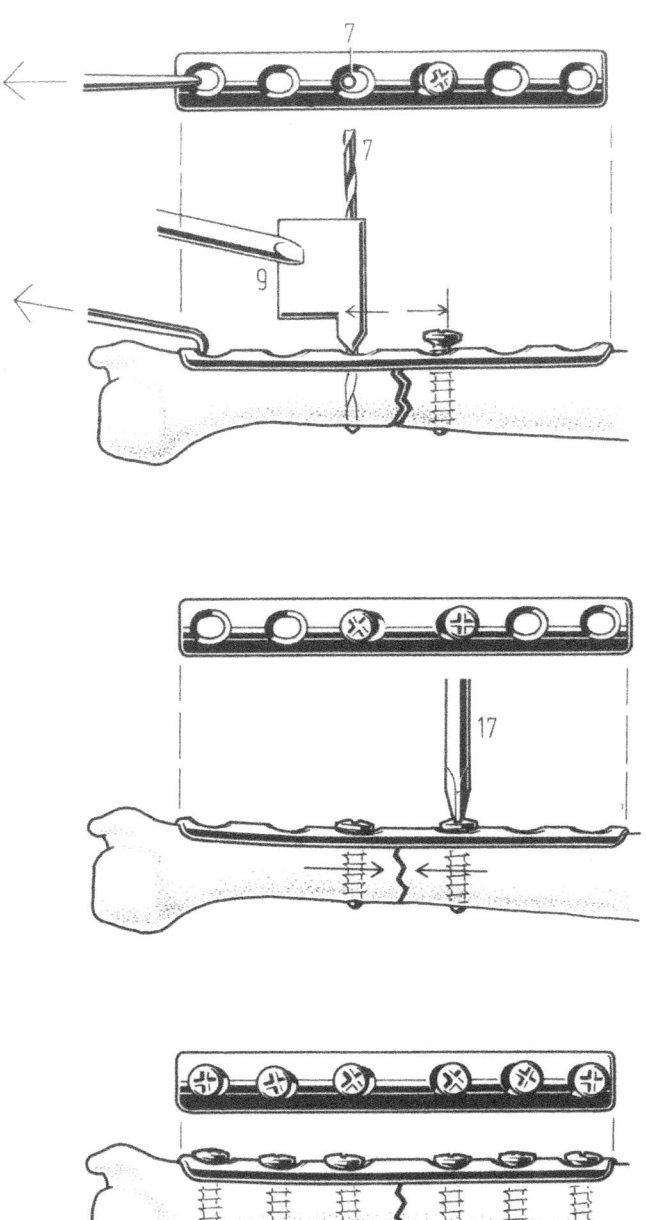

Fig. 18 Axial compression with the small semi-tubular plate

Narrow transverse fracture: the bone is first drilled through the holes in the plate that are nearest to the fracture line, one on each side. These holes are eccentrically drilled, putting in the drill guide at a point in each hole farthest from the fracture. While the second screw is drilled, a hook is used to pull the plate away from the first screw. When the screws are tightened, the screw neck will put the plate under tension and the fracture is thus compressed. The remaining screws are then inserted, each in the centre of the plate hole

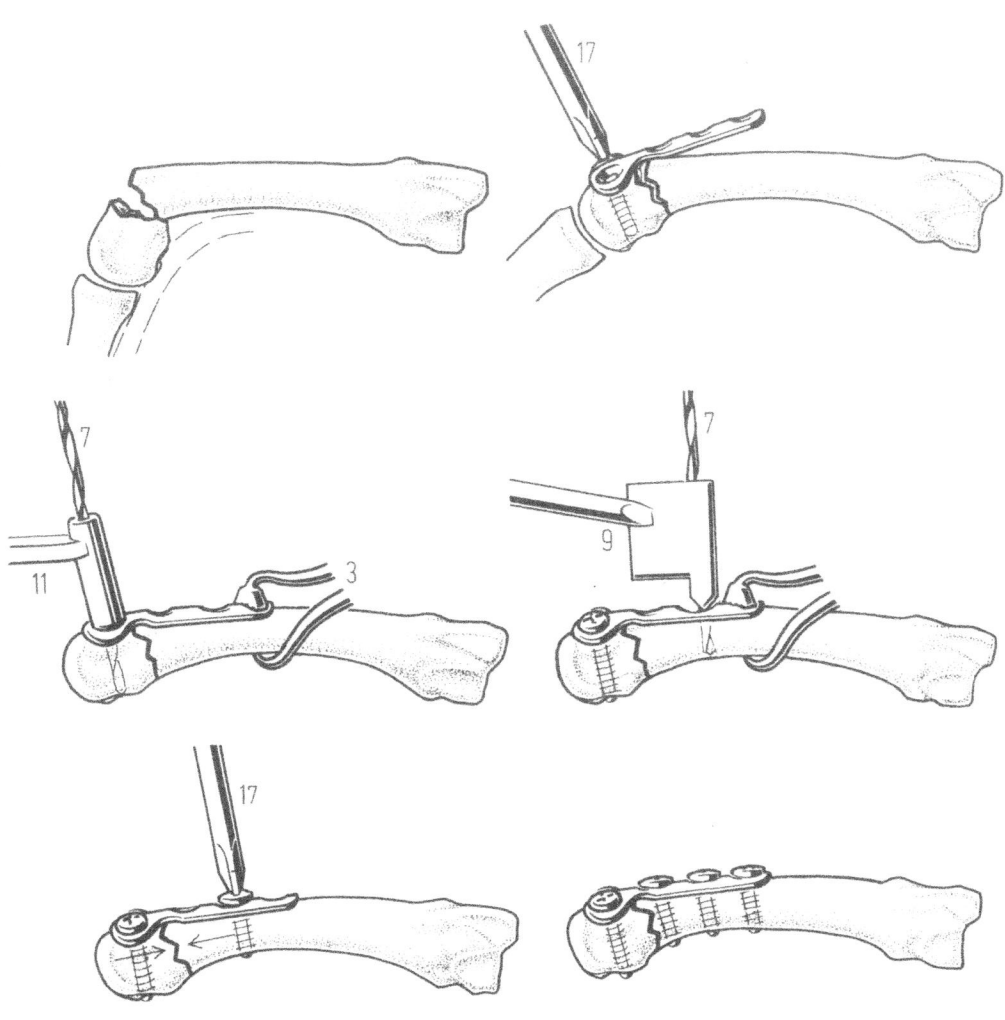

Fig. 19   Axial compression with small plate

Transverse fracture of neck of metacarpal. Screw fixation of the plate on the peripheral fragment while maintaining alignment. Reduction of the fracture with the help of the plate which is already screwed to the head fragment and with the bone forceps. Checking rotation. Eccentric drilling of the proximal fragment and insertion of one screw. Tightening this screw compresses the fragment axially

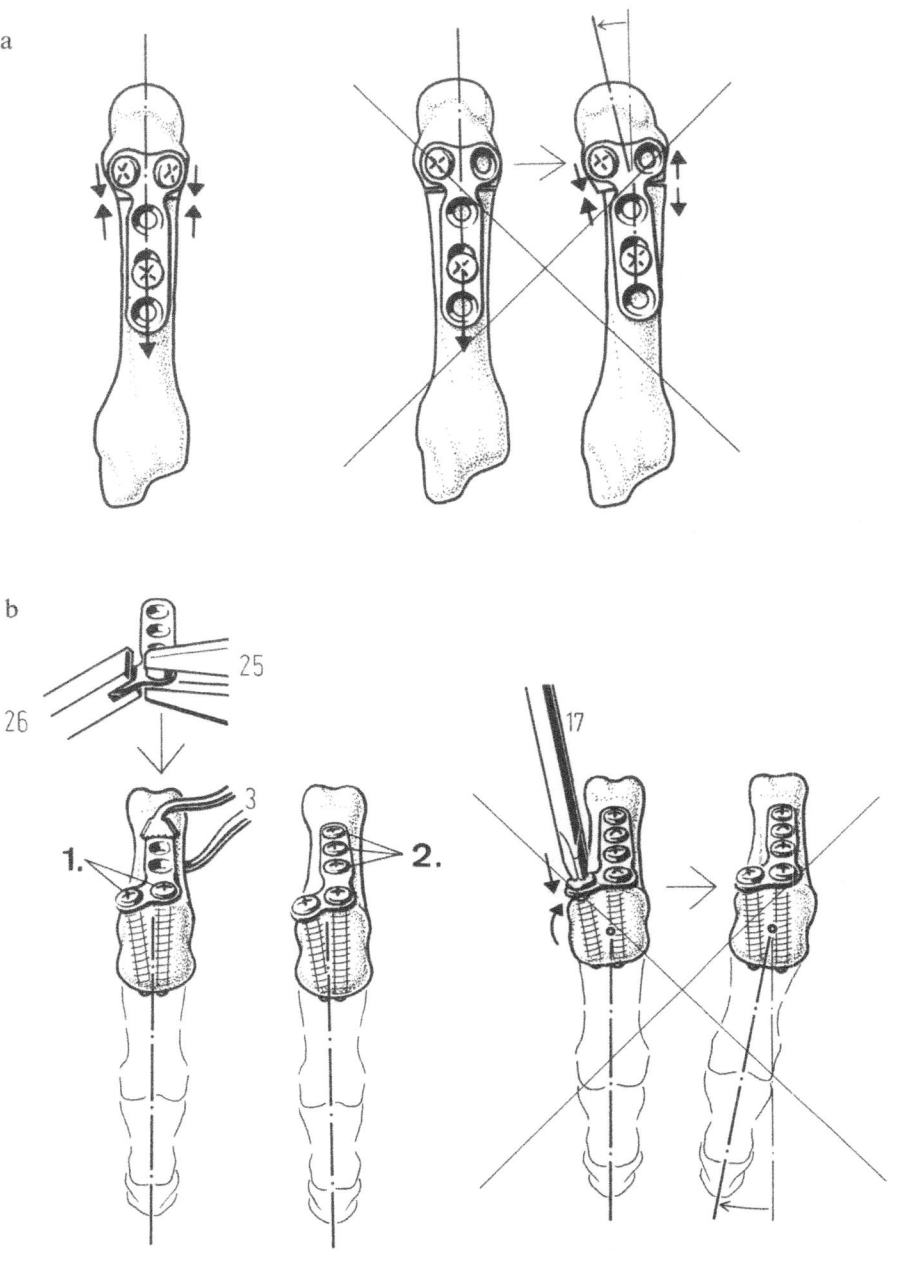

Fig. 20   Two faults in applying the small plate for the hand and foot

a   Angled T-plate: Before axial compression can take effect, both screws must be inserted in the distal fragment. Otherwise the eccentric tensile effect produces mal-alignment

b   Angled L-Plate: The plate must be accurately contoured to the surface of the bone using bending pliers and a bending iron. Both distal screws have to be inserted (*1*) before the final reduction, after which the proximal screws are driven in (*2*). If the procedure is reversed, the lateral distal screw produces an eccentric tensile effect which twists the fracture

36

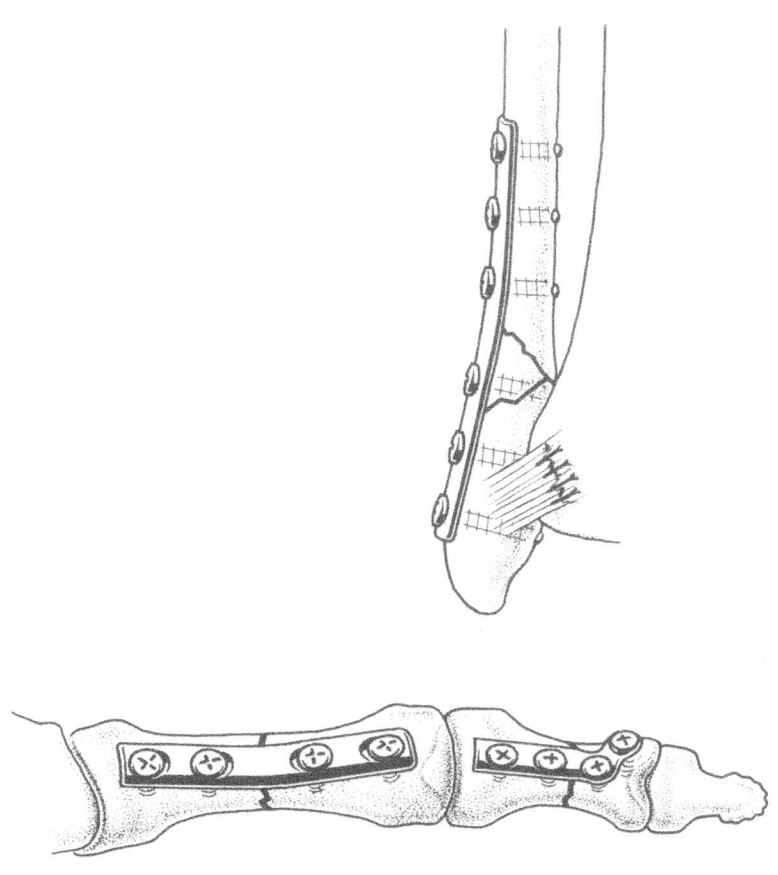

Fig. 21   Small fragment plates used as neutralization plates,

as in a malleolar fracture of the C-type, a transverse fracture of the first metatarsal, and the proximal phalanx of the hallux

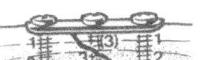

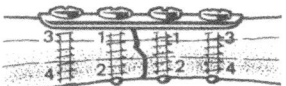

Fig. 22　Stabilization rule 2: The number of threads for internal fixation with plates

In phalanges, three cortex threads are required per fragment, in metacarpals and metatarsals four threads. This number increases to five or six according to the type of fracture. The numbers in the drawing show the sequence of tapping and of placing the screws

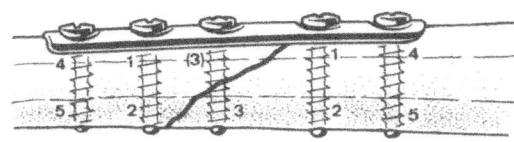

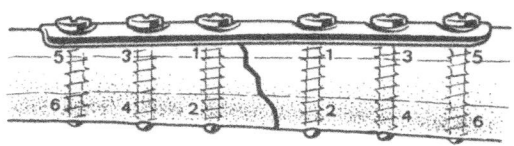

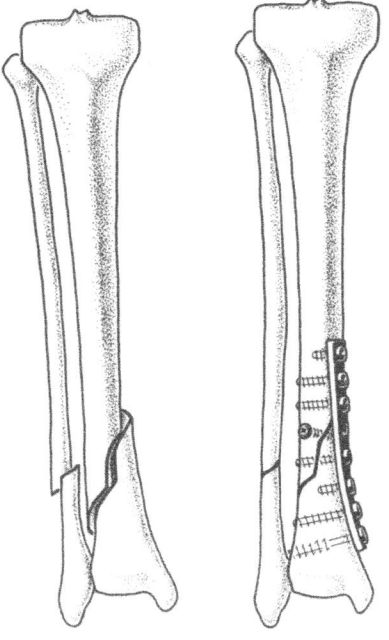

Fig. 23　Typical example of a "vassal" fracture in the larger skeleton

In the case of a spiral fracture of the lower leg, the fracture of the fibula represents the vassal. Reduction of the tibia usually results in spontaneous reduction of the fibula which therefore does not require any further treatment

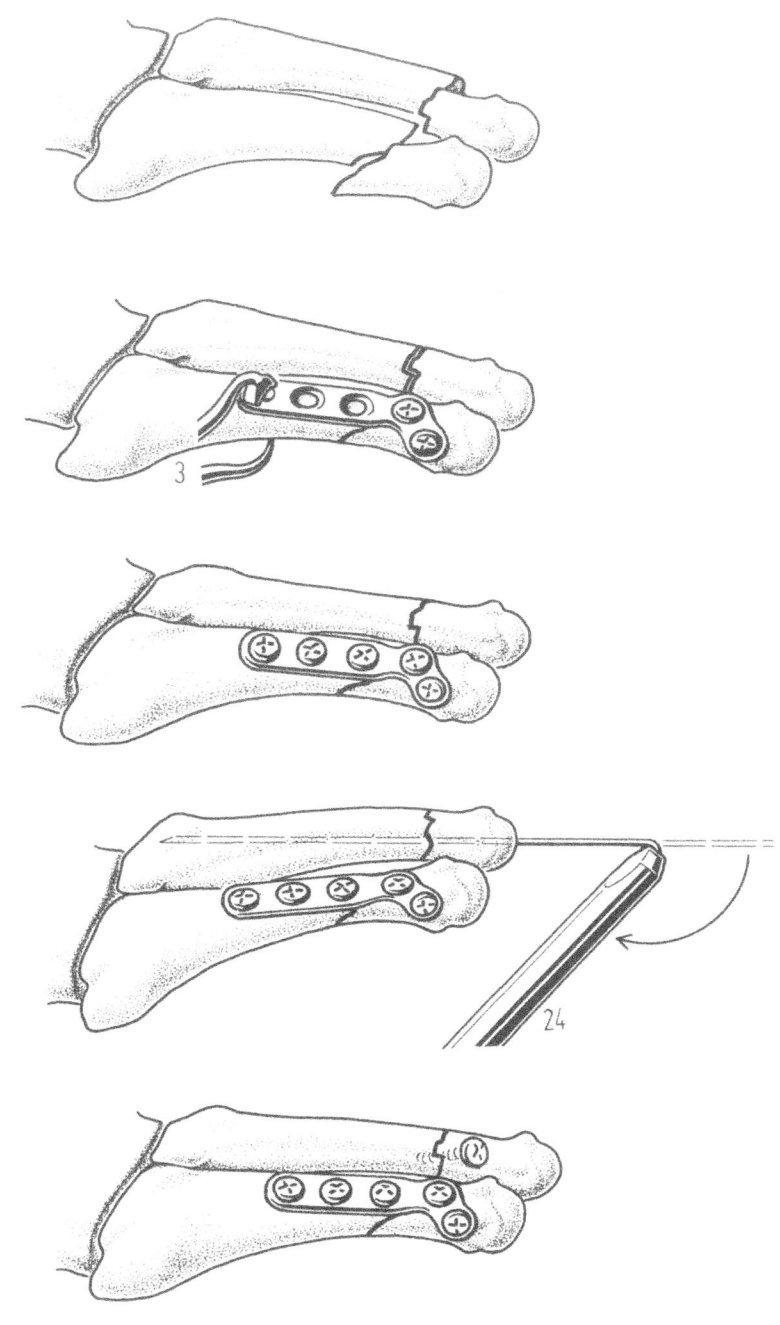

Fig. 24   Stabilization rule 3: Vassal rule

Mechanical interdependence of multiple fractures. The dominant fracture (metatarsal V) is being stabilized by an angled L-plate, while the vassal fracture (metatarsal IV) reduces spontaneously. It is either left alone or fixed with an axial Kirschner wire or a single screw

IV. Pre-Operative, Operative, and Post-Operative Guide Lines

There is a high tendency towards *post-traumatic swelling* of the hand and foot, which must be considered in the timing of the operation. Operation must either be carried out immediately, or after swelling has decreased, which means a delay of some days. Where operation is postponed, the skin of the operation site should on the eve of the intervention be *disinfected* with a sterile alcohol dressing which should, however, not entail a moist enclosure. Close attention must be paid to asepsis. Because of their shapes, disinfection of the hand and foot is difficult and unreliable. The use of a pressure gun which forces the disinfectant into the skin has proved to be most suitable for these parts. (Herold and Heim). This is of special importance since an adhesive plastic drape cannot be used on the hand. The movement of fingers, above all in flexion, must be constantly checked during the operation to avoid any *rotational deformities*. A bloodless field is provided by a *pneumatic tourniquet*; it should not be left in place for longer than two hours in younger patients.

The peripheral skeleton is surrounded by a thin, delicate soft-tissue layer which does not stretch easily. Careful protection of these soft-tissues is even more important than in proximal areas, and the skin too must be protected from damage due to pressure or stretching. To obtain such protection can be difficult, as approaches are often limited and extending incisions may be impossible.

Problems of scarring also play a significant part. On the one hand, scars on the outside of the upper limb are so conspicuous that cosmetic considerations may substantially influence indications. On the other hand, badly placed skin incisions can result in hypertrophic scars or even scar contractures.

The position of incisions in the foot must be orientated towards walking comfort and footwear. Appropriate details are given in the special sections.

Reduction and the temporary holding of a fracture can be rather complicated. Here we use the special clamps or very fine Kirschner wire, particularly on the apophyses. Wherever possible, cerclage wire should be avoided as this can involve nerve or tendon injuries. Yet in some cases all these devices are inapplicable which compels us to perform "freehand" reductions. Stabilizations is then achieved with small plates for hand and foot fractures, according to the technique indicated for axial compression.

Skin is closed with Donati's sutures or Allgöwer's modification of this where the suture is partly subcuticular. The vascularity of a precarious flap can thus be maintained. Donati's sutures are, however, unsuitable for the thick skin on the flexor aspect of hand and foot. Here we prefer accurate adaption of skin edges with fine, simple interrupted sutures made of non-absorbable synthetic material such as monofilament nylon. These sutures should not be removed before the twelfth to fourteenth day. The Redon *suction drain* (small gauge) and its modifications (Manovac etc.) prevent post-operative haematoma formation. They can, however, not be applied where the wound has not been made completely water-tight by the sutures. Therefore a large *compression bandage* together with limited conventional drainage not exceeding 24 hours, is often used in the hand.

Post-operative elevation should be maintained as long as there is swelling.

Active movement within the range permitted by the bandage may be begun immediately. *After operation* the patient should be prevented from *stressing the limb unduly*. This is easy where the leg is concerned, but difficult in the case of the upper limb where every movement produces some stress. Thus most internal fixations in arm and hand have to withstand considerable mechanical load. The time when active stress can be allowed should be determined at the *four week X-ray check*. Bony consolidation of shaft fractures ensues as a rule between the eighth and the twelfth week, but active use of the injured limb need not be delayed for so long.

The period between the fourth and the sixth post-operative month has proved to be the most appropriate time for the *removal of metal* implants from small fragments. Particularly in the hand, the implant may represent a relatively large foreign body which may interfere with extensor movements. After removal of metal implants, we often find an obvious improvement of extension and flexion.

Removal of the small cancellous screws should not be delayed, since the narrow thread-free screw neck invokes substantial periostosis. Here the resistance to the withdrawal of the screw may lead to breakage of the screw neck.

The appropriate time for removal of small screws in combined internal fixation with larger implants is usually determined by the removal of the metal from the main fracture. Removal of metal implants may sometimes prove to be totally unnecessary, and this is chiefly in symptom-free cases where screws only have been used. When removing plates, technical difficulties and the need for a second operation, as well as the age of the patient have to be taken into consideration. Metal removal is not so vital when using the SFS, as corrosion occurs very rarely since contact surfaces between straight plates and screws are small. Moreover, the adverse effects of plates on tibial and femoral shaft fractures which involve the change of cortical into cancellous bone, and re-fracture due to stress protection, never appear in the peripheral skeleton, including the upper limb.

V. Autogenous Bone Graft Combined with the Use of SFS

Grafts, especially of cancellous bone and sometimes of cortico-cancellous chips are frequently indicated in the peripheral skeleton. While smaller defects, as on the volar side of metacarpal necks, heal up rapidly with the help of simple metal fixation, larger *defects and comminuted areas* (distal radius, talus, comminuted fractures of the lower end of the tibia, the first metatarsal, etc.) should be filled with primary *autogenous cancellous bone*. Such bone grafting is often needed at the time of secondary internal fixation for delayed consolidation or mal-alignment and in certain cases of pseudarthrosis and arthrodesis.

The combination of autogenous cancellous bone grafting with exterior metal fixation is *biologically a more effective procedure*. Grafting often improves the stability of the bony structure as a whole, whether by a supporting effect or by the better hold provided for screws in grafted bones.

The following considerations apply to the donor site. Only biologically optimal bone should be obtained and the graft volume should not be larger than is absolutely necessary. To keep the operation time short and to reduce the chance of sepsis, it is better to remove bone from a single site. A bone graft should preferably be obtained from the neighbourhood of the defect, but proximal to it where there is a good independant blood supply. These three requirements can sometimes not be met, when choosing a site for operation on the larger skeleton. Besides the standard areas like the iliac crest, the iliac fossa and greater trochanter, there are the olecranon, the lower radial epiphysis, the head of the tibia and the distal tibial epiphysis. Suitable combinations of donor site and recipient area are shown in Fig. 25. Where juveniles are concerned, such selection is considerably curtailed when epiphysial cartilages are still open.

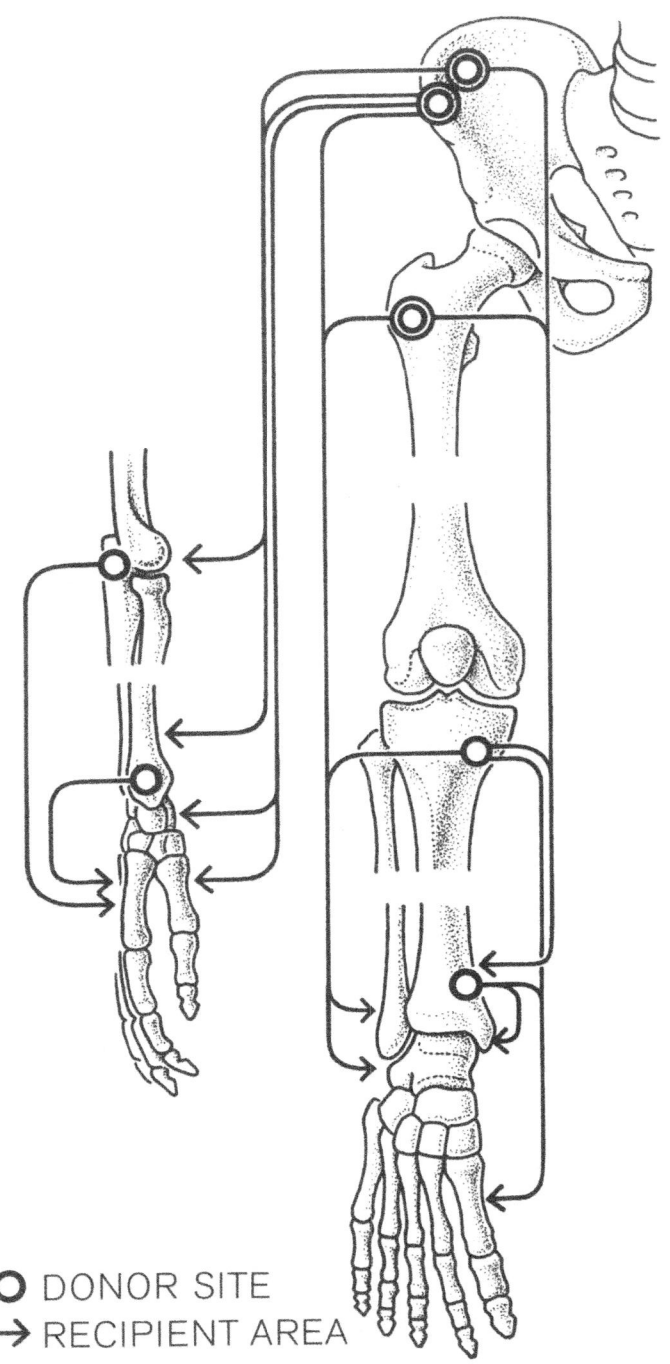

O DONOR SITE
→ RECIPIENT AREA

Fig. 25   Autogenous bone grafting

Donor sites and recipient areas in peripheral internal fixation:
Main donor sites: Iliac crest, iliac fossa, greater trochanter
Occasional donor sites: Olecranon, epiphysis of lower radius, head of tibia, epiphysis of lower tibia

44

VI. The Use of the SFS for Reconstructive Bone Surgery

There are many indications for secondary operations on the peripheral skeleton. Most peripheral fractures are less conspicuous and, therefore, either primarily overlooked or their functional significance underestimated. The approved methods of conservative treatment, especially in the hand, seem to have met with too little recognition. Malpositions of rotation, angulation and shortening call more frequently for operation than do pseudarthroses. Painful post-traumatic arthrosis as well as congenital or rheumatic affections of joints can be either corrected or at least relieved from pain by arthrodesis. Here fixation with small plates has proved to be very useful, and has largely replaced the application of Kirschner wires. The stability achieved is good enough to make external fixation by plaster almost always unnecessary. Intensive mobilization of neighbouring joints and immediate full weight bearing achieves surprisingly good functional results. In our experience the combination of autogenous bone grafting with metal fixation is the safest procedure. In many cases, however, reliable arthrodesis can be carried out without any bone grafting. The requirements, therefore, are good vascularity, broad contact surfaces and faultless compression. Six different operations are available from which the one most suitable for the specific situation can be selected.

1. Bone Pegging Combined with a Plate

This method is particularly indicated for osteotomy and for a mobile pseudarthrosis, though less often for arthrodesis. The fracture must be mobilized and the medullary canal in each fragment opened up and drilled through. The openings are filled with a spindle-shaped cortico-cancellous bone peg which holds the frag-

ments together with partial stabilization of the axis, while rotation can still be corrected, if necessary. The osteotomy is finally stabilised by a tension-band plate, longer than the graft, placed dorsally and fixed at both ends with screws (Fig. 26 a). Shortening of the bone may also be corrected by pegging (Fig. 26 b).

2. Graft Interposition Combined with a Plate

In either a primary or secondary operation, the defect is filled with cortico-cancellous bone graft which spans the entire width of the long bone and is also fixed by a posterior tension-band plate (Fig. 27).

This method, recommended by Pannike, is indicated for bridging larger defects in primary as well as secondary fixations. The plate should be relatively long.

3. Compressed Bridging Graft Combined with a Plate

This technique is applied in pseudarthrosis and osteotomy when pegging cannot be carried out because of restricted mobility of the fragments, or in arthrodesis in an area with reduced blood supply; the dorsal cortex is opened and a deep bed drilled in both fragments (in arthrodesis in the metaphysis bordering the joint).

Either a fine osteotome or a reamer is used. Here alignment and rotation must be checked first, since they cannot be corrected later. The prepared cortico-cancellous bone graft is embedded in the groove which must be slightly smaller than the graft. The tension-band plate is then fixed with screws, compressing the graft which organises rapidly (Fig. 28 a and b).

In some pseudarthroses, compression can be obtained by tension-band wiring as in the medial malleolus (Fig. 28c). Peg-grafting and a compressed bridging graft may also be combined (Fig. 28 d).

4. Bone Pegging with Screw Fixation

This is particularly indicated for arthrodesis in extension or with flexion of less than 10 degrees, e.g. in the terminal joint of the fingers:
A concave opening is made in the medullary canal of the middle phalanx from the dorsal aspect. A tunnel is reamed through the joint into the medullary canal of the distal phalanx with maximal flexion. The prepared cortico-cancellous bone peg is driven in a distal direction. It must obtain a tight fit in the distal site. Its proximal end is pressed into the trough in the proximal phalanx with the small reduction forceps. The joint is now realigned and the proximal end of the graft is fixed to the palmar cortex by a 2.0 mm cortex screw inserted obliquely (Fig. 29). It is unnecessary to excise the joint which is an appreciable advantage in treating the fragile distal phalanx. Stability is reliable and no external fixation is needed.

5. Excision of Joint and Subsequent Fixation with a Tension-Band Plate

This is indicated for arthrodesis in a slightly flexed position when a degree of shortening has no detrimental effect, e.g. in the metacarpo-phalangeal joint of the thumb. A standard excision of the joint is carried out, correcting the position, and fixation is then obtained with a dorsally applied tension-band plate (Fig. 30).

6. Excision of the Joint Followed by Screw Fixation

At a Proximal Site: This technique is indicated for arthrodesis in moderate flexion (20 degrees or more) e.g. in the middle joints of the fingers. A standard arthrectomy is performed with correction of the position. A channel is drilled with the 2.0 mm bit and the thread tapped. The screw must be long enough to grip the distal fragment and this may be done with the 4.0 mm cancellous screw (Fig. 31 a). In some cases the small cortex screws of 3.5 and 2.7 mm are better, as removal is easier. This, however, requires a gliding hole to be drilled in the proximal cortex (Fig. 31 b) (Pfeiffer, Segmüller).
If there is previous axis deviation, this method may be difficult. The tightening of the screw may produce increased flexion or mal-alignment, while the protruding screw head may jeopardize the skin. Plate fixation may, therefore, sometimes be preferred to this simple operative technique.

At a Distal Site: This in indicated for arthrodesis of the thumb and the interphalangeal joint of the big toe in extension: standard excision of the joint and correction of position first. A channel is drilled with the 2.0 mm bit in a distal direction, after which the drill bit is reversed and driven proximally. The thread is tapped in the proximal phalanx. The incision across the tip of the thumb and big toe lies transversely 2 mm below the nail. Burying the screw-head presents no difficulty as skin closure can be achieved without tension. Tactile and prehensile surfaces are beyond the scar, and removal of the screw is simple (Fig. 31 c).

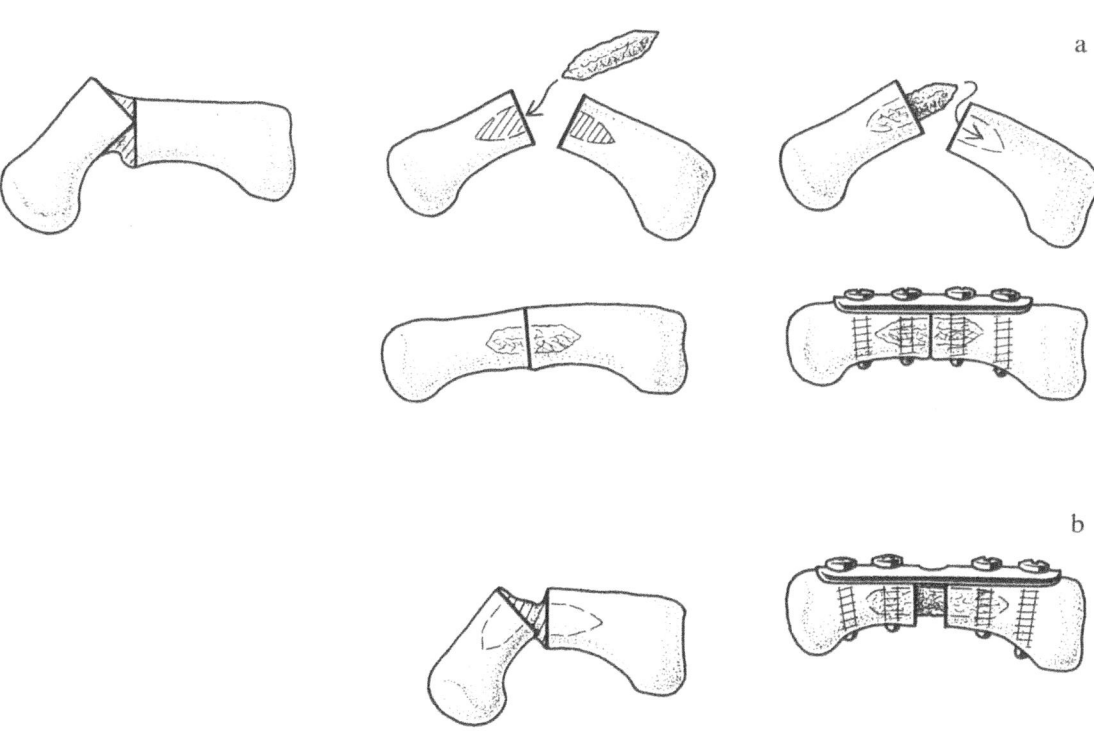

Fig. 26 **Bone pegging combined with a plate**

   a   Indicated for osteotomy and a mobile pseudarthrosis: Mobilization of the pseudarthrosis, drilling through both medullary canals, insertion of a bone peg. Screw fixation of a tension-band plate which must be anchored beyond both ends of the graft

   b   In pseudarthroses with bone defect: Bone pegging with an elongation effect

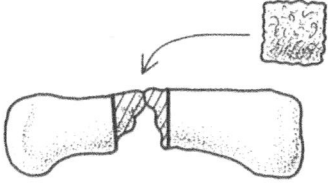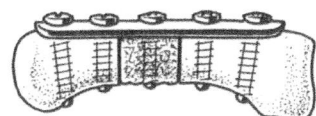

Fig. 27 Graft interposition

In shortened pseudarthrosis, the defect is filled with a cancellous bone graft, replacing the entire width of the bone. Two screws on each side guarantee plate fixation of the main fragments. The plate also stabilizes the interposed cancellous graft

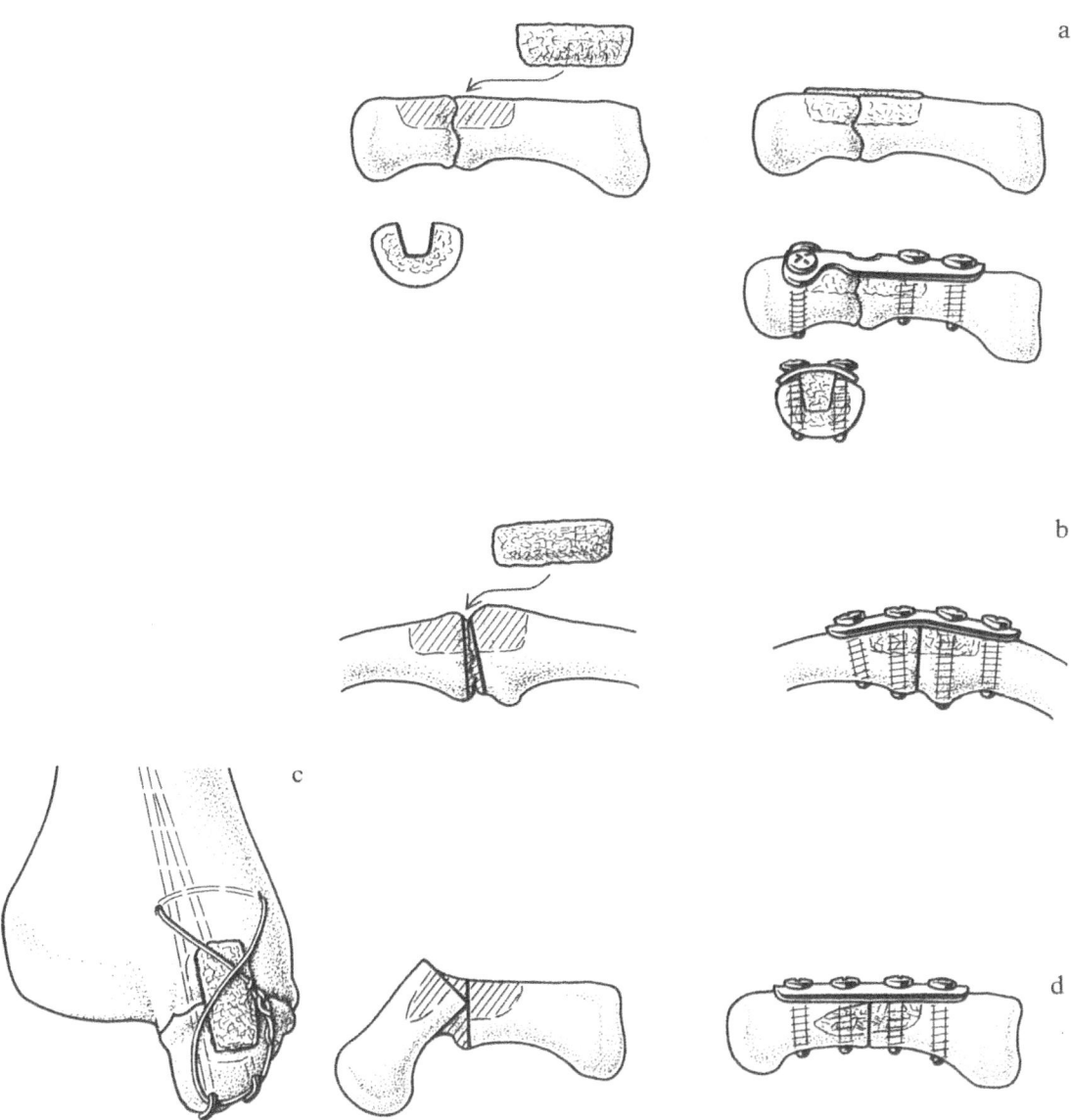

Fig. 28   Compressed bridging graft

a   In pseudarthrosis: Opening of dorsal cortex and drilling a bed in both fragments. Insertion of graft which is slightly larger than the bed. Screw fixation of plate, which must be longer than the graft. The graft is thus compressed in its bed

b   In arthrodesis: A similar procedure to (a). A dorsal bed is drilled in both metaphyses. In most cases excision of the joint is unnecessary

c   Example of graft compression with cerclage wire in pseudarthrosis of the medial malleolus

d   Combination of bone pegging and compressed bridging graft: A distal hole is drilled to accommodate the peg, while proximally a bed is drilled in the dorsal cortex. Compression is obtained with a plate which is longer than the graft at both ends

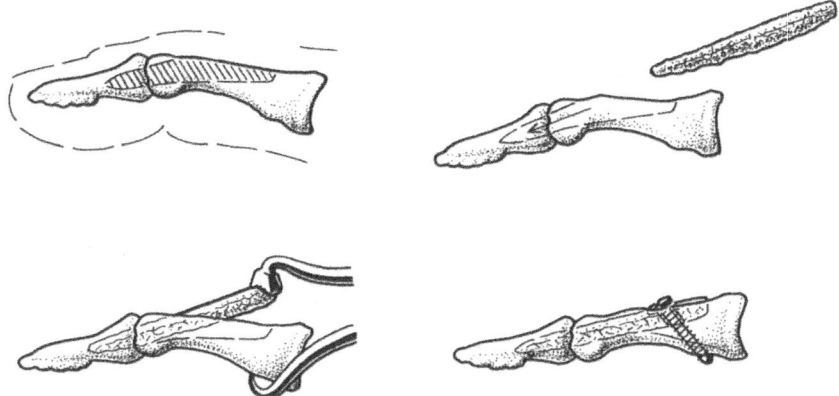

Fig. 29   **Bone pegging with screw fixation**

Arthrodesis of the distal phalanx of a finger: The graft bed is drilled in the distal part of the middle phalanx and continued into the distal phalanx while the joint is held flexed. The joint is straightened which impacts the graft. A small cortex screw of 2.0 mm is then inserted obliquely in the proximal palmar cortex. This fixes the joint position as well as the graft in its bed

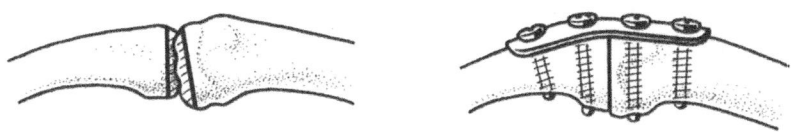

Fig. 30   **Excision of joint followed by fixation with a tension-band plate**

Example of arthrodesis without cancellous grafting. Here excision of the joint is obligatory and some shortening must follow

▷

Fig. 31   **Excision of the joint with screw fixation**

a   A moderately flexion position. Middle joint of long finger. Small cancellous screw: Excision of joint, drill bit of 2.0 mm used through both phalanges followed by tapping of the thread and insertion of the screw

b   Resection of the distal joint, with fixation by cortex screws. In order to obtain interfragmentary compression, the drill hole in the proximal phalanx must be converted into a gliding hole

c   Arthrodesis by screw fixation in a disto-proximal direction. This is done in the interphalangeal joint of thumb or big toe. A dorsal incision is made over the joint and another 2 mm below the nail. The distal phalanx is drilled in a distal direction with the 2.0 mm bit. The drill is then reversed and drilled into the proximal phalanx. In order to obtain interfragmentary compression, the cancellous screw must be long enough

50

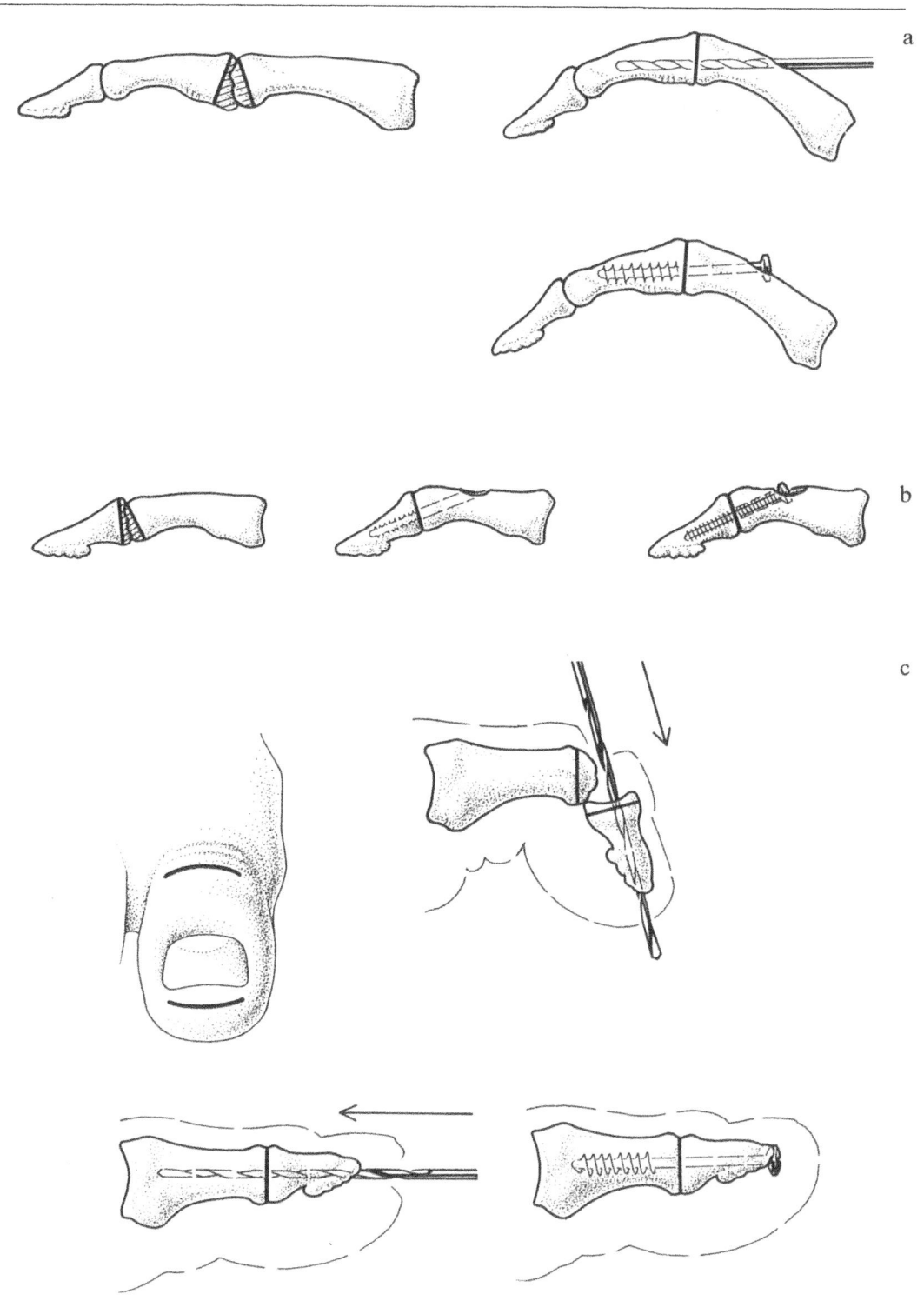

Special Section

VII. Introduction and Summary

Fractures of the distal bones of a limb and related articular fractures are regular indications for the use of the SFS. Therefore injuries in these areas are described in a systematic way. Since small implants can also be applied to every other part of the skeleton, a number of typical examples from more proximal areas are added.

There are however some distal internal fixations which cannot be carried out with small screws and plates. Thus the semi-tubular plate is frequently used in sites where small implants are more often used. Tension-band fixation with cerclage wire is also used in the olecranon, malleolus, etc., where it achieves excellent results.

Repetition of subjects and figures already published in the Manual of Internal Fixation could not be avoided in our presentation. Figures taken from this volume have been adapted to our purposes, and problemes of positioning, approach and post-operative treatment are only dealt with as far as they require solutions which differ from those indicated in the Manual as a result of the use of the small implants.

It has become evident that there is a special need for precise descriptions of approaches and operative techniques. Therefore considerable space has been devoted to semi-schematic drawings to show typical situations.

Furthermore, it seemed to be imperative to include the essential case material. For this reason, a series of clinical X-ray examples was added to each chapter. They are intended to exhibit the variability of the individual case and the scope of practice compared with the classical examples shown in the drawings. In addition to our own cases, the extensive material of the AO/ASIF Documentation Centre was also used, and for this we express our gratitude. The large number of these records make it difficult to standardize figures from the size and informative points of view.

Here we have chosen two different types of presentation:

Clinical examples are fully described in extracts from the case histories which particularly emphasize the final results.

Technical examples are X-rays of the fracture and its operative treatment. This model was especially chosen for malleolar fractures. Here the problems of indication and the functional results achievable by internal fixation have been solved by the clinical investigations of Weber and Willenegger. Thus the sole purpose of this volume is to describe the use of small ASIF implants.

Furthermore, the chapters dealing with hand surgery were supplemented by the specific statistics kept on our own patients. These comprise our entire operative experience in hand surgery using small implants. They have enabled us to assemble for the first time a large number of results obtained in this field. The functional results clearly differentiate between the cases where ASIF implants may successfully be used, and those in which indications should be reconsidered. Indications for methods of reconstructive bone surgery are given in addition to the description of the essentials internal fixation.

Five chapters deal with the standard areas for the application of the SFS:

Upper limb:	The elbow	VIII
	The wrist joint	IX
	The hand	X
Lower limb:	The ankle joint	XI
	The forefoot	XII

Uncommon applications are dealt with in two additional chapters:

| | Special locations | XIII |
| | Special indications | XIV |

VIII. The Elbow

Fractures of the elbow are unstable and most cases cannot be accurately reduced by conservative means. Inadequate treatment often leads to malposition of fragments and eventual arthrosis so that internal fixation is frequently indicated. The slender bony components are as a rule untreatable by standard implants so that the SFS is often used. As many operative procedures have only recently been tried out, they are here described in detail.

1. Lower End of Humerus

a) Fracture of the Condyles and Avulsion Fractures of the Epicondyles

These fractures, frequently occurring in adolescents and children, must be accurately reduced in order to prevent later malposition (Baumann). Strong muscular bony insertions in adults may also cause considerable displacement. Bone fragments can be displaced and enter the joint. Indication for operation is then absolutely clear. *Access* is obtained by a lateral incision. The first step is then to isolate and protect the ulnar nerve. In children sufficient fixation is obtained by parallel Kirschner wires which are removed after three to four weeks as the epiphyseal cartilages are still open (Fig. 32). Screw fixation with a small cancellous screw, or sometimes a small cortical screw of 3.5 mm is carried out in the adult (Fig. 36).

b) Intra-Articular Fracture of the Lower End of the Humerus

Internal fixation is undisputedly indicated for these fractures which are of two different types:

The *simple "Y" fracture* with slight displacement: A bilateral approach and stabilization with lag screws alone is often enough for this fracture. The best method is the combination of small cancellous screws for the trochlea with long malleolar screws to fix the articular fragment and the humeral shaft (Fig. 34).

The *complex comminuted fracture* with displacement of trochlear fragments: Reduction of these fractures can be extremely difficult. As a rule reduction can be accurately achieved, provided that a systematic operative procedure is complied with. Guiding rules are laid down on page 126 of the Manual of Internal Fixation. They are repeated here with the slight modifications required when using small implants.

Anaesthesia: Inhalation anaesthesia with an endotracheal tube. The *prone position* is used. The forearm hangs at the side of the operating table. The angle of the elbow is supported by an accurately adjusted well-padded roller. A pneumatic tourniquet is used. Mobility and flexion of the joint have to be provided for (Fig. 35a).

Incision: The length of the incision is 25–30 cm and it is slightly curved, preferably on the radial side, in order to avoid the olecranon. The exposure must provide a full view of the posterior aspect of the joint (Fig. 35b).

Ulnar Nerve: This nerve must be identified and protected by retraction with a tape (Fig. 35c).

Osteotomy of the Olecranon: This is recommended to provide a perfect exposure. Our experience is that it heals rapidly in the well vascularized area of the elbow.
First a hole is drilled from the tip of the olecranon into the ulnar medullary canal. This hole is tapped for the large cancellous screw of 8–9 cm (Fig. 36a). The olecranon is then osteotomized perpendicular to the axis of the tro-

chlea, using a narrow osteotome or an oscillating saw. Now the olecranon and triceps together are turned up proximally (Fig. 36b). Thus a complete exposure of the lower end of the humerus and the comminuted trochlea can be obtained.

The later reduction of the osteotomized olecranon is carried out with a cancellous screw and a washer. The olecranon should always be fixed with an additional tension-band wire, since even long cancellous screws do not obtain a perfect grip in the wide ulnar medullary canal. Moreover, the triceps exerts a bending stress on the screw itself.

A Second Approach is possible without osteotomy of the olecranon: A tongue-shaped incision of the triceps aponeurosis is made with a broad base distally (Fig. 37). In this procedure, complete exposure of the trochlea is only obtained if the elbow can be flexed to 40 degrees during the operation. Because of the local anatomy, the positioning technique, and local swelling, this is seldom possible.

Reconstruction of the Trochlea: The most important step of internal fixation is the strictly accurate reconstruction of the trochlea. Fragments of the humerus are often considerably displaced. Devitalized, completely detached fragments should not be removed, but accurately replaced. Major defects are rare and when they occur, must be filled in with autogenous cancellous bone graft.

We use Kirschner wires for reduction and provisional fixation. The first wire serves as a guide and its exact placement is decisive. It pierces the radial fragment from the side of the fracture, which means from the ulnar side. We apply it as a lever for the reduction and drill. it through the central trochlear fragment or fragments, and then back into the ulnar fragment (Fig. 38a and b). After reduction, a hole parallel to the guiding wire is made with the triple drill guide (Fig. 38c). A small cancellous screw of sufficient length is inserted into this hole for interfragmentary compression. Then the Kirschner wire is replaced by a second small cancellous screw for rotational stability (Fig. 38d).

Connecting the Trochlea and Metaphysis of the Humerus: After stabilization of the trochlea, the connection between the articular fragments and the metaphysis of the humerus is established. Here the use of long narrow semi-tubular plates with 5–7 holes is indicated and they have to be accurately fitted, i.e. they have to be bent considerably. Implants must be kept clear of the olecranon fossa and the coronoid fossa. Moreover, the plates should not have any immediate contact with the ulnar nerve, and at the radial side should not impede extension of the elbow. It is better not to have the proximal plate ends crossing each other, but to fix them laterally on to the humeral shaft. This facilitates the internal fixation as well as the subsequent plate removal. Plates are fixed with small cortex screws of 3.5 mm and on occasions a small cancellous screw can be used (Fig. 39). In simpler fractures, the second plate can be replaced by a long screw such as the small cancellous or malleolar screw (Fig. 39d).

Internal Fixation of the Olecranon: The olecranon is now reconstructed according to the method described above.

Closure: Adequate Redon suction drainage is established, followed by simple closure of the wound with skin sutures, and elevation of the arm.

Post-Operative Treatment: This is determined by the stability achieved. A removable plaster splint, with the elbow flexed to about 120 degrees, is often applied for several weeks. Consolidation of a comminuted fracture may take 12 or more weeks. Recovery of flexion is always more rapid than that of extension.

Only after secure consolidation can metal be removed. First a thorough clinical and possibly an electromyographical check of the ulnar nerve must be performed. In the presence of irritation and paresis, the removal of a plate is combined with anterior transposition of the ulnar nerve (Mumenthaler). The nerve must always be re-identified and isolated when an implant is removed from the ulnar side.

58

2. Radial Head

The principle treatment of displaced fractures of the radial head is by operation, since closed reduction is never feasible. In children, open reduction and transfixion with a single Kirschner wire has proved to be the best method.

In adults we have three different types of fracture:

a) Comminuted Fracture

Comminuted fractures which preclude any type of reconstructive measure (Fig. 40a). Here the primary removal of loose fragments and resection of the head to an extent of about 1 cm is recommended as prophylaxis against arthrosis. Although this shortening of the upper radius is far from being ideal, it is the lesser evil.

b) Fissure Fractures

In this fracture the head remains uninjured while a sharp edge fragment is split off and displaced to a greater or lesser degree. The anular ligament may be intact. Operation is recommended even if the X-ray only shows a fissure fracture. The extent of displacement is always considerable (Fig. 40b).

c) The Cap-Over-Ear Depressed Fracture

These depressed fractures of the joint surface are often hardly discernible on the X-rays. Most of these fractures can be completely replaced by open reduction (Fig. 40c).

d) Approach and Internal Fixation

A slightly 'S'-shaped incision at the back beginning at the lateral epicondyle (Fig. 40d). Division of a few muscle fibres of the extensors. The situation of the delicate deep radial nerve must be taken into consideration. It lies 2–3 finger-breadths distal to the radial head. Therefore the use of Hohmann retractors for the identification of the fracture should be avoided as they compress the muscles too strongly. The articular capsule is opened from the epicondyle in a distal direction. Rotation of the forearm will bring the radial head into view. In pronation, the depressed parts lie as a rule adjacent to the incision while uninjured areas are on the ulnar side. After reduction of the articular surface with an elevator, a provisional fixation is obtained with Kirschner wires. Firm fixation is achieved with a screw. In most cases a single screw is sufficient (Fig. 40e). Where the articular surface is depressed, 2 small cortex screws inserted in different planes and lying parallel to the articular surface as supports, may be an advantage.

Post-Operative Treatment: Immobilization in a dorsal plaster splint for three weeks, followed by active mobilization. Removal of the metal after 4 months.

3. Olecranon

Most fractures of the olecranon can be primarily fixed with a tension-band wire, followed by functional postoperative treatment. We refer to the Manual of Internal Fixation, pages 130–132. The use of the SFS is restricted to three special conditions:

a) Oblique Fracture of the Olecranon

In addition to the tension-band wire inserted like a figure of 8, a screw is often recommended to counteract shearing forces (Fig. 41a and b). Wide fissures can sometimes be closed with a single screw.

b) Fracture of the Coronoid Process

This must be joined to the main fragment by screw fixation (Fig. 41c). Here a small cancellous screw has proved to be most useful.

c) Comminuted Fractures

Simple tension-band wiring is sometimes insufficient for the reduction of such fractures. In certain cases, internal fixation with a small semi-tubular plate should be preferred. If possible the plate should be positioned as a tension-band plate and put under tension from its distal end (Fig. 41 d).

4. Secondary Operations on the Elbow

In pseudarthrosis in the region of the olecranon, compression is obtained with a tensionband wire as a standard procedure. To get enough stability, juxta-articular osteotomies and arthrodeses in adults are performed with implants of the standard size.

5. Clinical X-Ray Examples
Figs. 42–46, pages 75–83

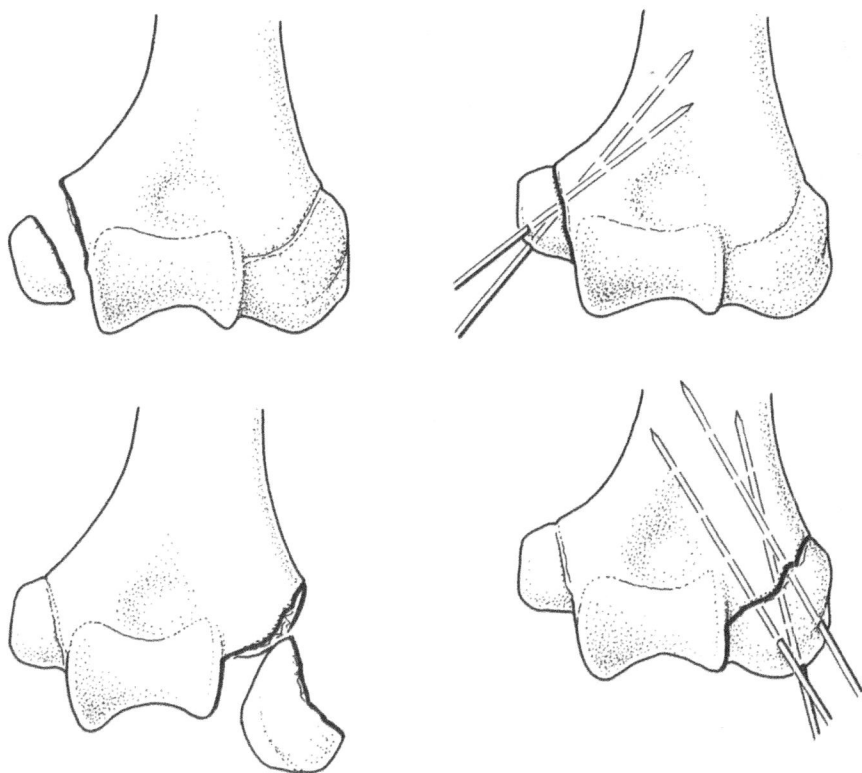

Fig. 32   Fractures of epicondyles and condyles in children

Internal fixation with Kirschner wires (see Müller *et al.*, Manual of Internal Fixation, 1970, Figs. 220 and 221)

60

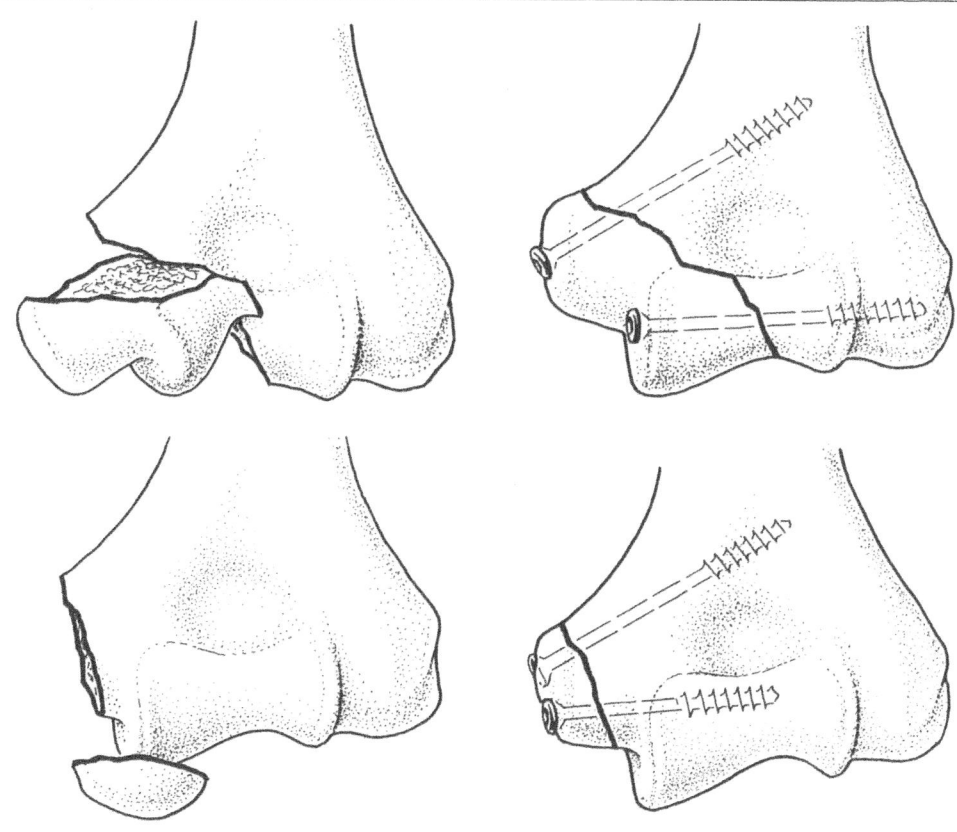

Fig. 33 Fractures of condyles and epicondyles in adults

Internal fixation with small cancellous screws

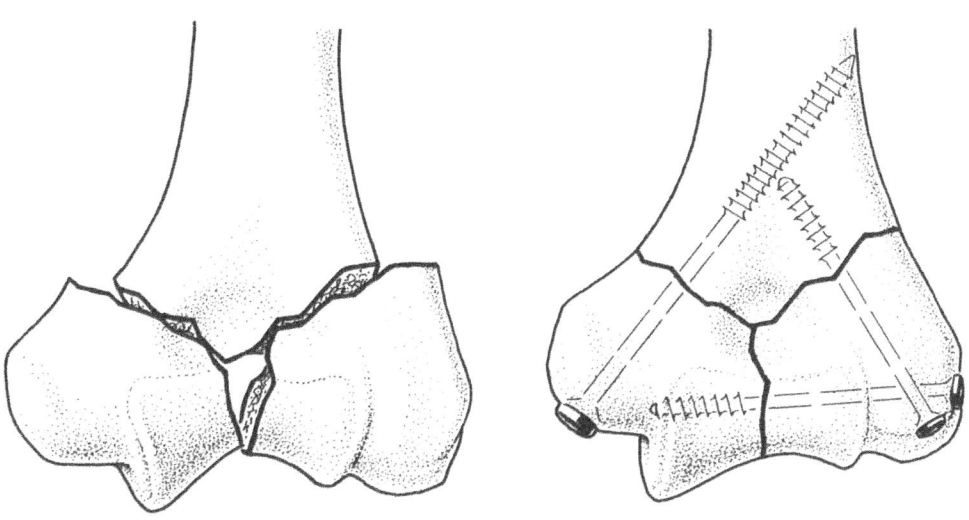

Fig. 34 Articular Y-fracture of the lower humerus with slight displacement

Combined internal fixation with small cancellous screws and malleolar screw

61

Fig. 35   Comminuted intra-articular fracture of the lower humerus

    a   Anaesthesia, positioning of patient

    b   Incision

    c   Access to olecranon, retraction of the ulnar nerve

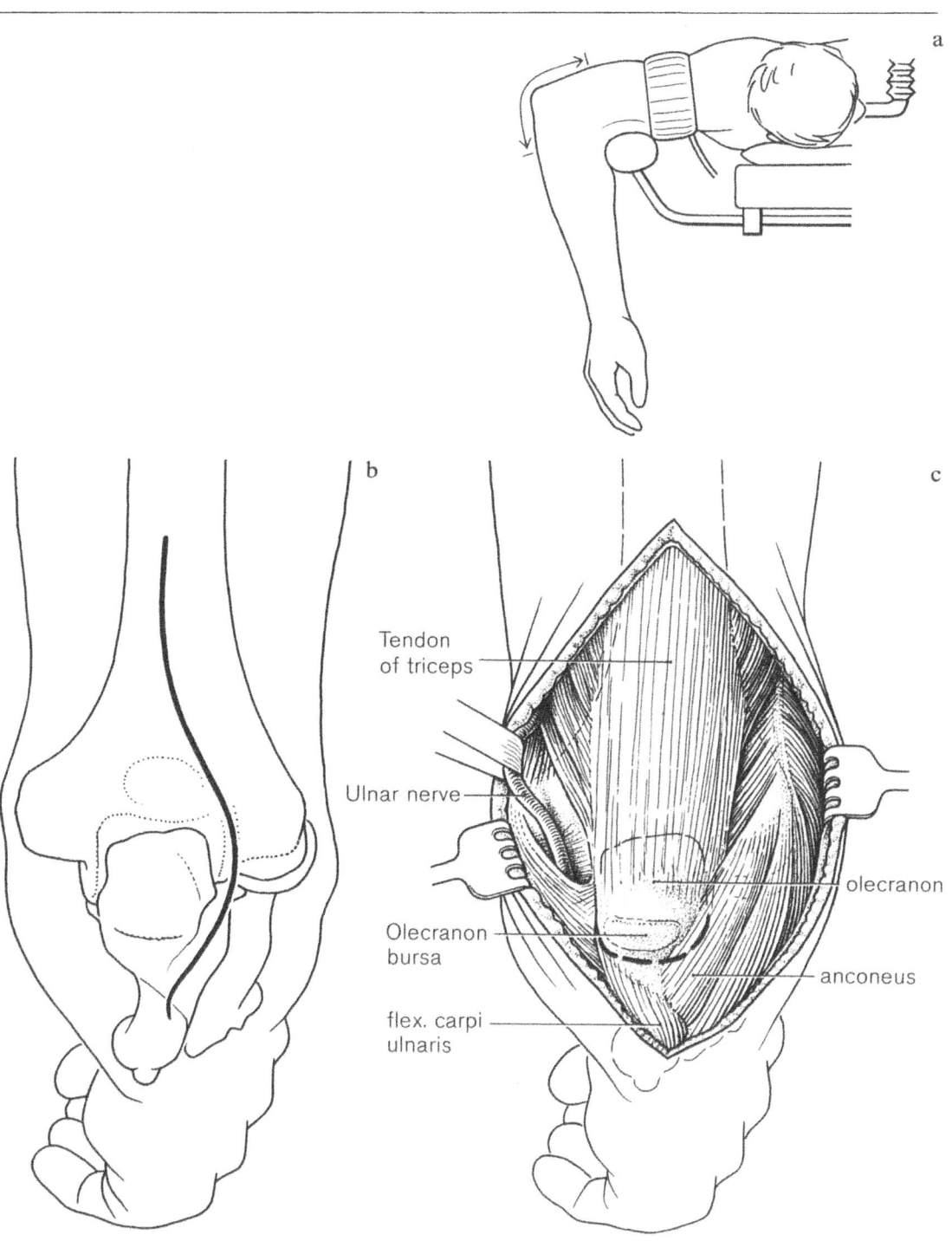

Tendon
of triceps

Ulnar nerve

Olecranon
bursa

flex. carpi
ulnaris

olecranon

anconeus

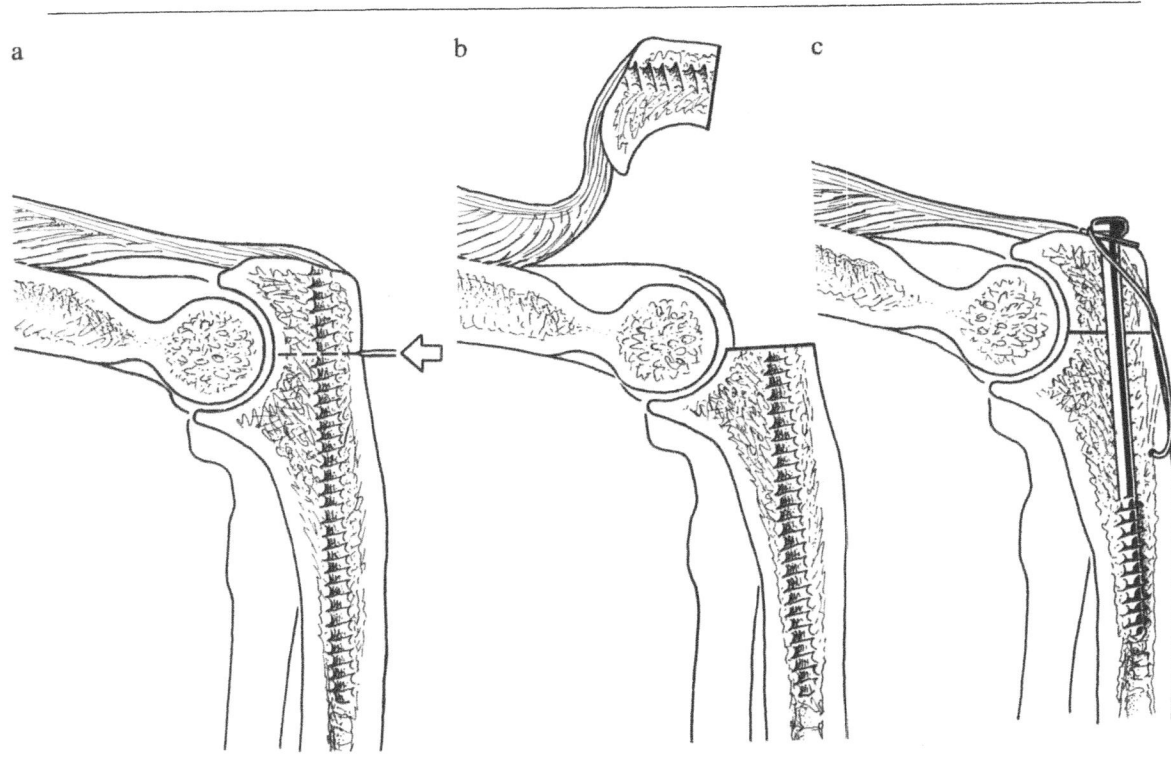

Fig. 36   Comminuted intra-articular fracture of the lower humerus, access: osteotomy of the Olecranon

   a   Pre-drilling and tapping of the olecranon for the long large cancellous screw, osteotomy in a direction perpendicular to the trochlea

   b   Turning up of the osteotomized olecranon together with the triceps

   c   Replacement of the olecranon with a long cancellous screw, a washer and a figure-of-8 tension-band wire

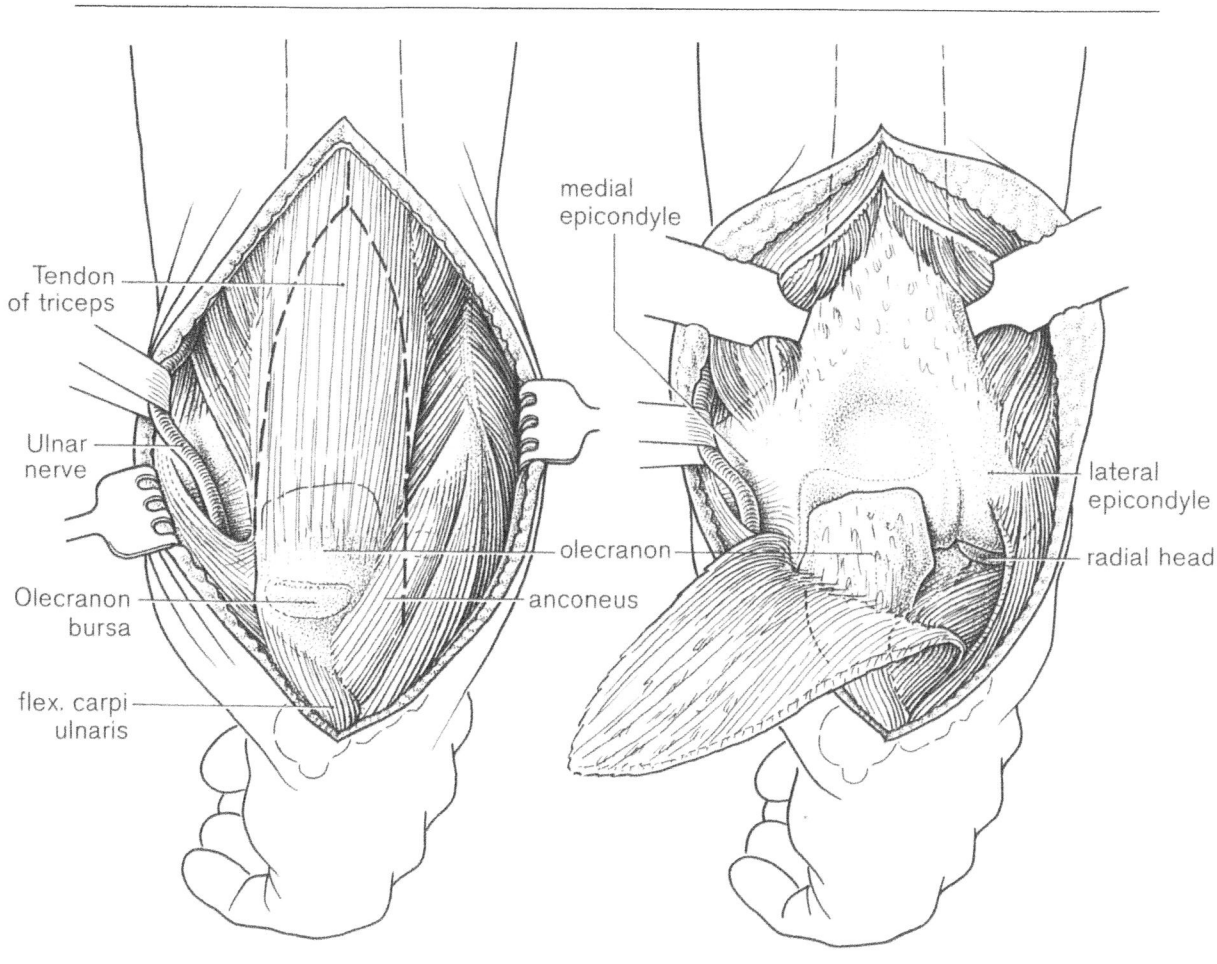

Fig. 37   Intra-articular fracture of the lower humerus, second approach

Tongue-shaped incision of the triceps aponeurosis and turning down of this tongue in a distal direction

Fig. 38   Intra-articular fracture of the lower humerus, internal fixation: reconstruction of the trochlea

a   Insertion of guide-wire into the radial fragment from the ulnar side

b   Drilling back of the guide-wire to the ulnar side: the wire used as a lever: reduction of the trochlear fragments

c   Drilling of a hole parallel to the guide-wire with the help of the triple drill-guide. Insertion of the first small cancellous screw

d   Replacement of the guide-wire by a second small cancellous screw

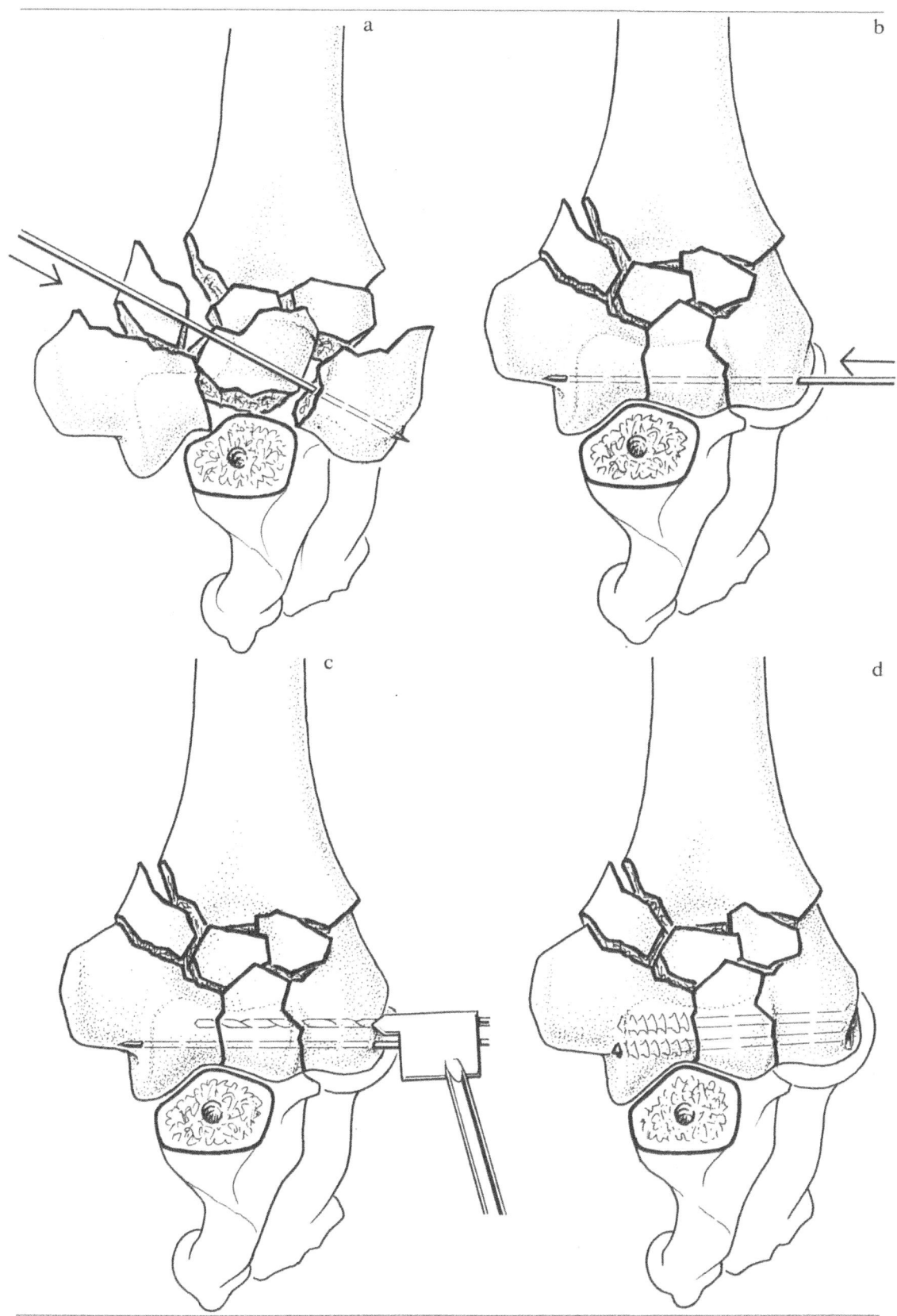

Fig. 39 **Intra-articular comminuted fracture of the lower humerus, internal fixation: The trochlea joined to the humeral metaphysis**

a Reduction and temporary fixation with Kirschner wires

b Placing of small semi-tubular plate on the ulnar side

c Internal fixation with two small semi-tubular plates

d One small cancellous screw on the radial side is sufficient in simpler fractures

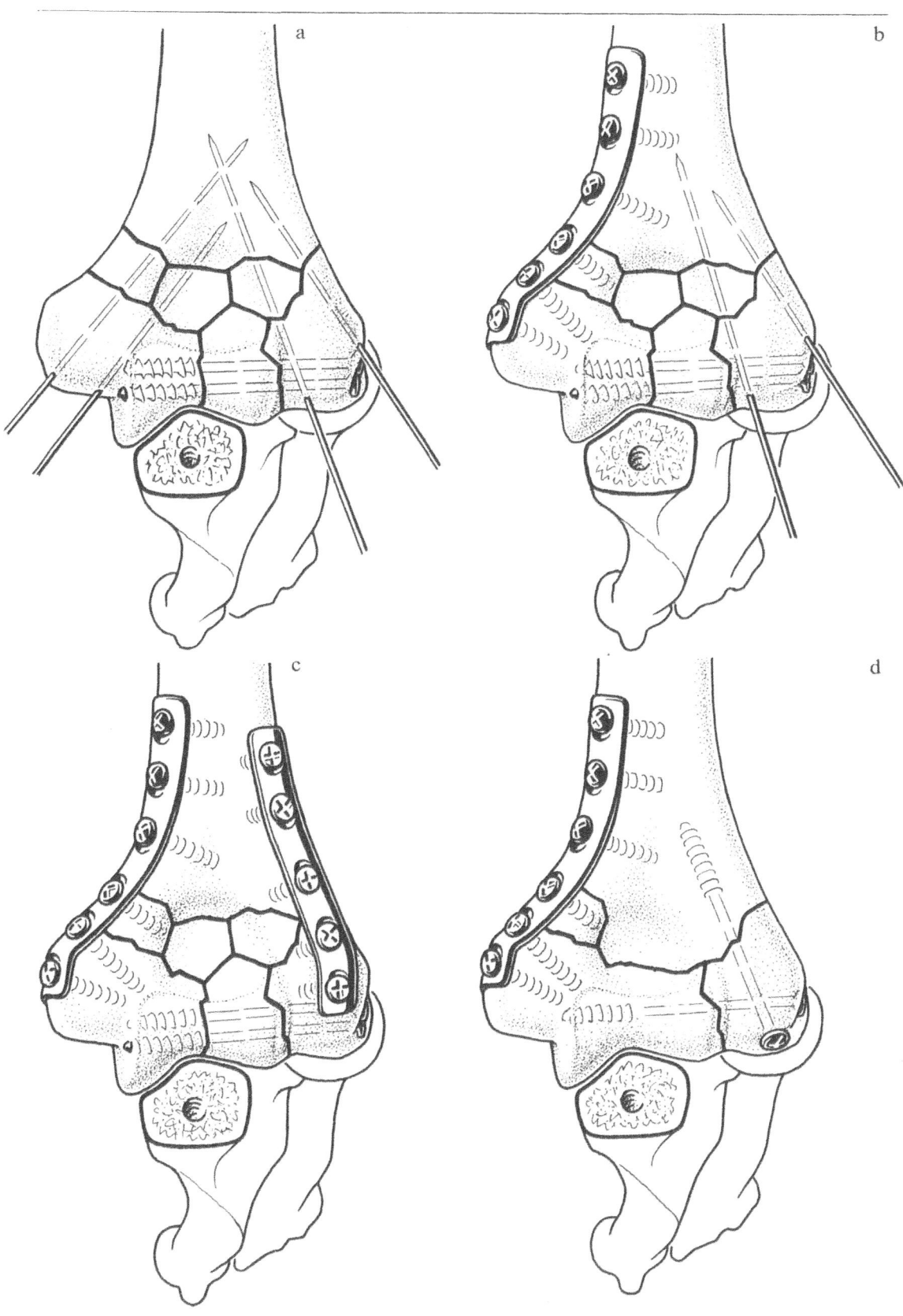

Fig. 40 **Radial head: Fractures and internal fixation**

    a   Comminuted fracture

    b   Fissure fracture

    c   Impacted fracture

    d   Incision and approach to the radial head

    e   Internal fixation from b and c with one or two small screws

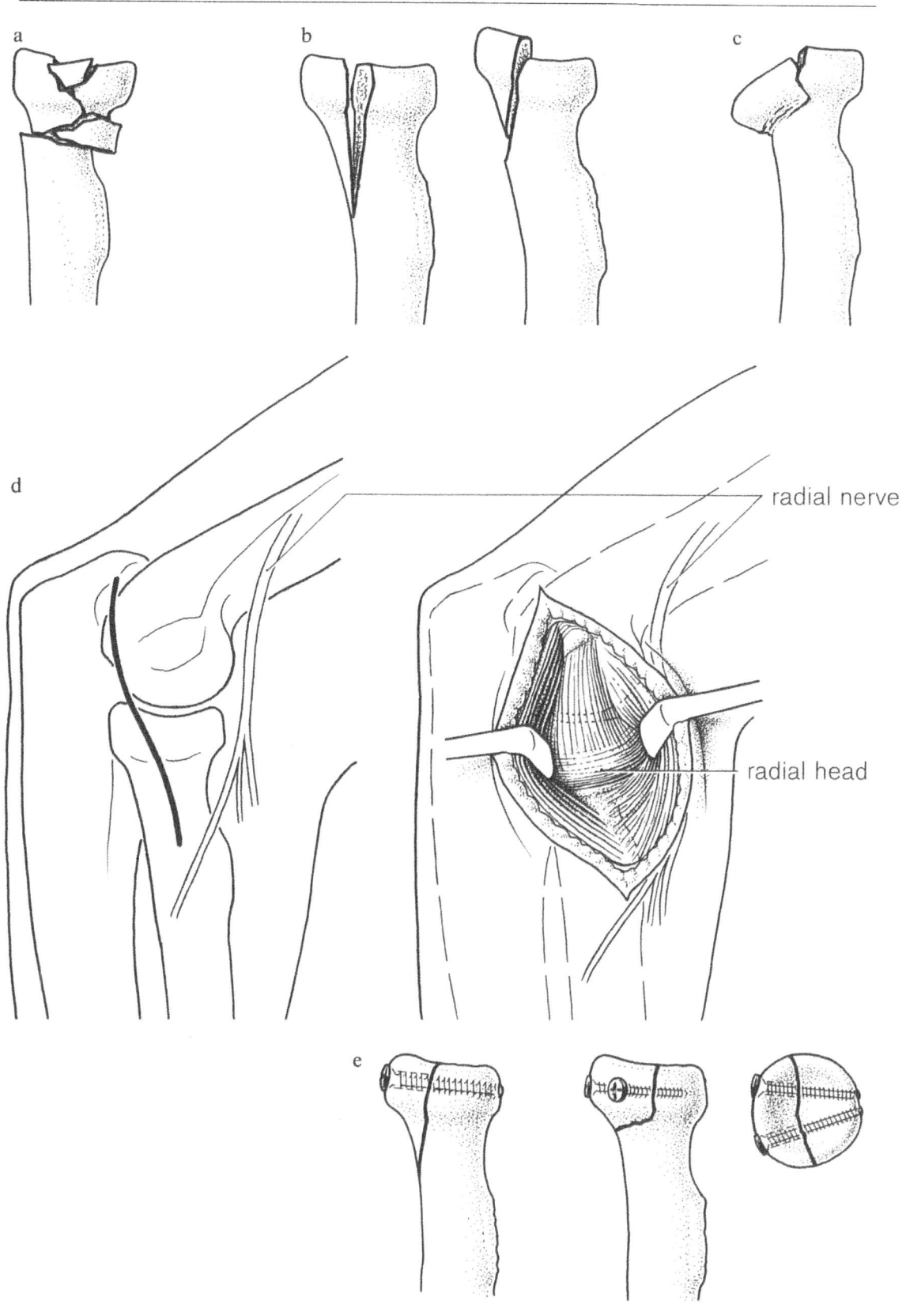

radial nerve

radial head

Fig. 41   Olecranon: Internal fixation with SFS

a, b   Oblique fracture, combined fixation with a tension-band wire and screw

c   Fracture of the coronoid process, screw fixation

d   Comminuted fracture, internal fixation with a long small semi-tubular plate placed as a tension-band

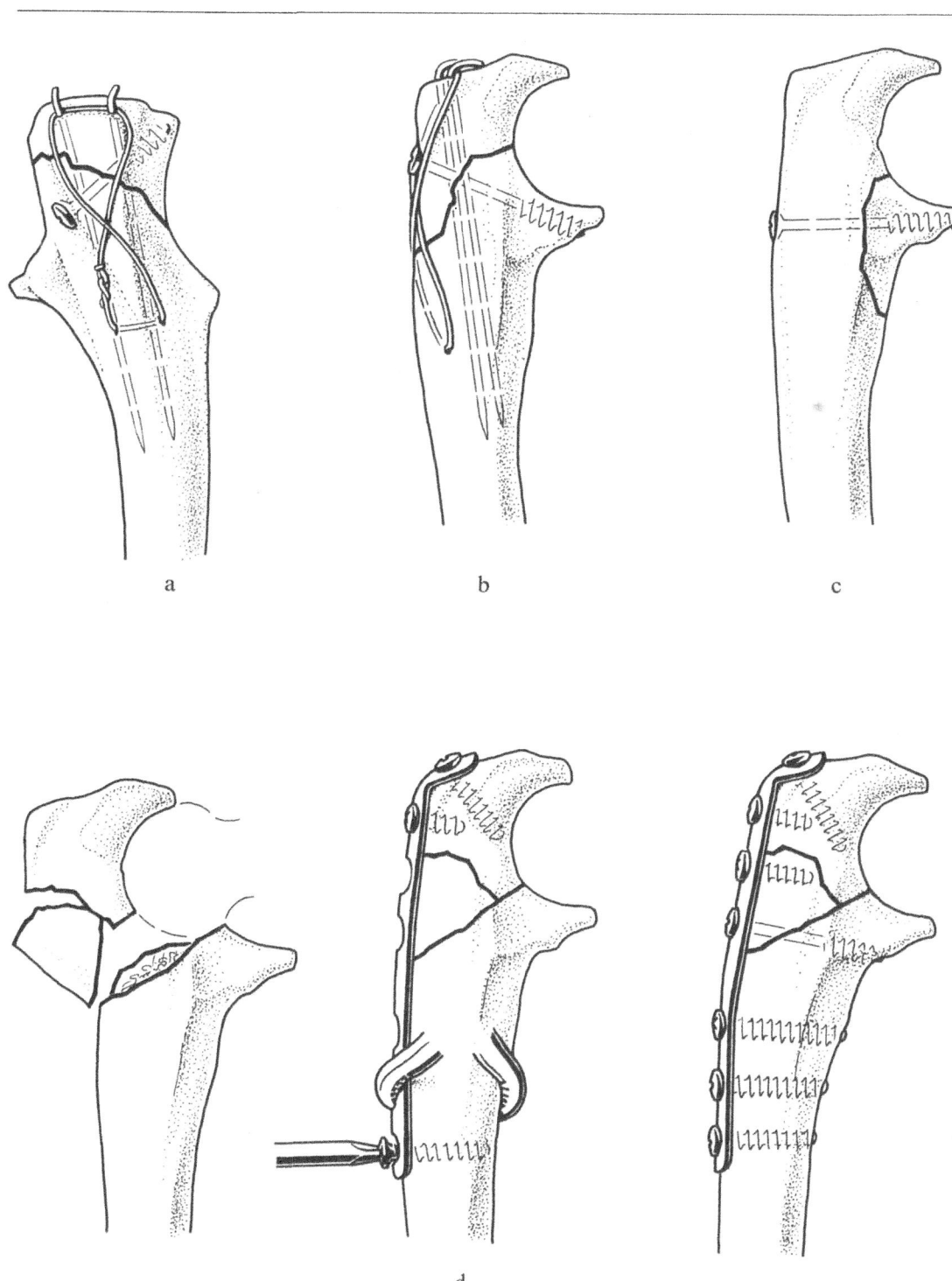

a

b

c

d

Fig. 42 Clinical example: Fracture of the radial condyle of the humerus
A housewife, aged 39. Fall on the outstretched hand

a   Fracture of the lateral condyle of the humerus

b   Internal fixation with small cancellous screw: A small step is still visible on the X-ray
No complications. Removal of the screw at 16 months

c   Final check after 18 months. No disability. Extension $-5°$, flexion $-10°$, pronation and supination
equal on both sides. Slight arthrosis. Patient was symptom-free

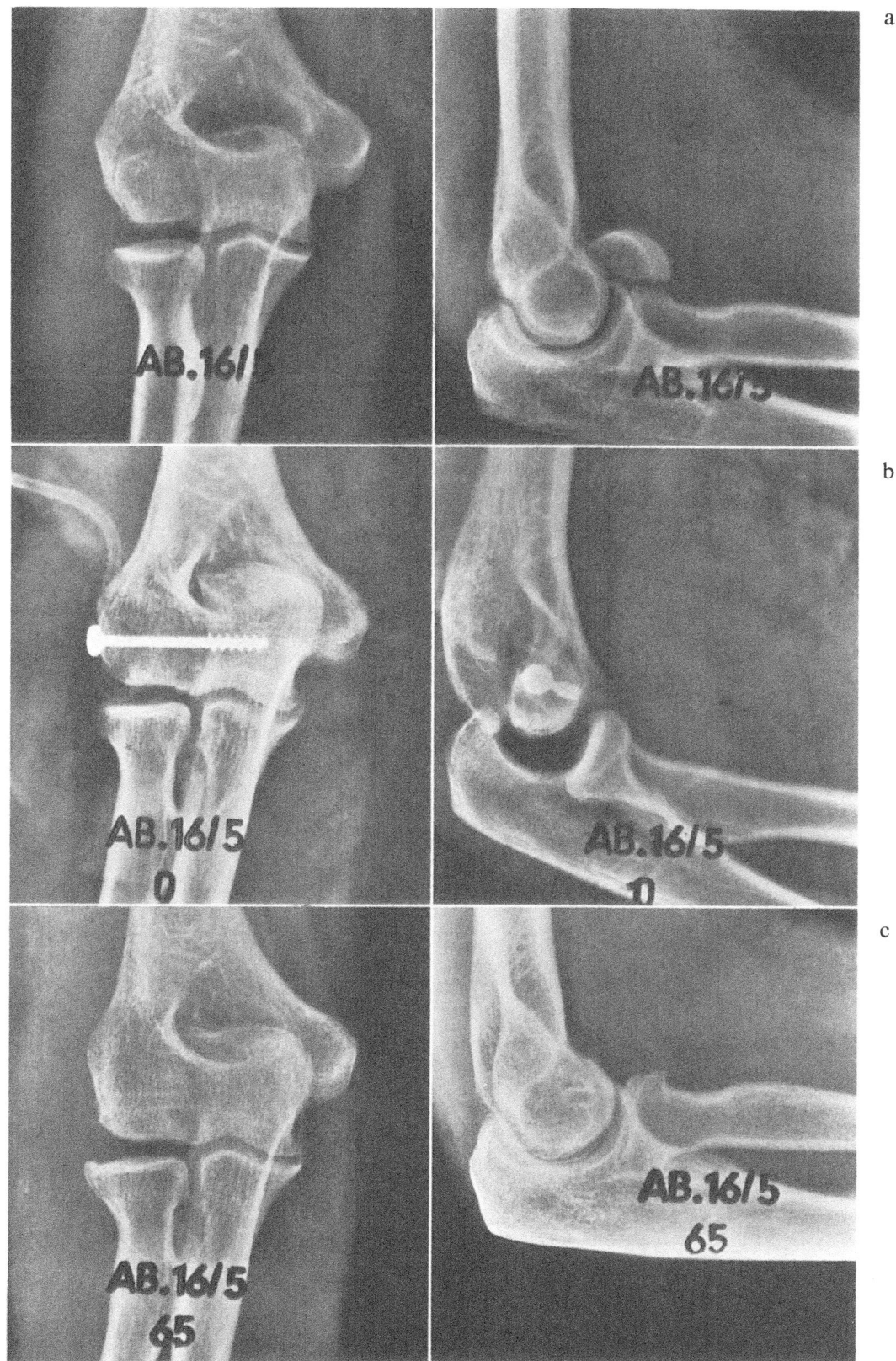

Fig. 43 Clinical example: simple fracture of lower humeral epiphysis
A female hotel keeper, aged 49. Fall at home

a   Partial intra-articular transcondylar fracture of the humerus

b   Emergency internal fixation with two small cancellous screws inserted from each side
No complications. Full working capacity after four months

c   Final check after two years: patient is symptom-free, extension −15°, flexion·and pronation equal
on both sides, supination −10°

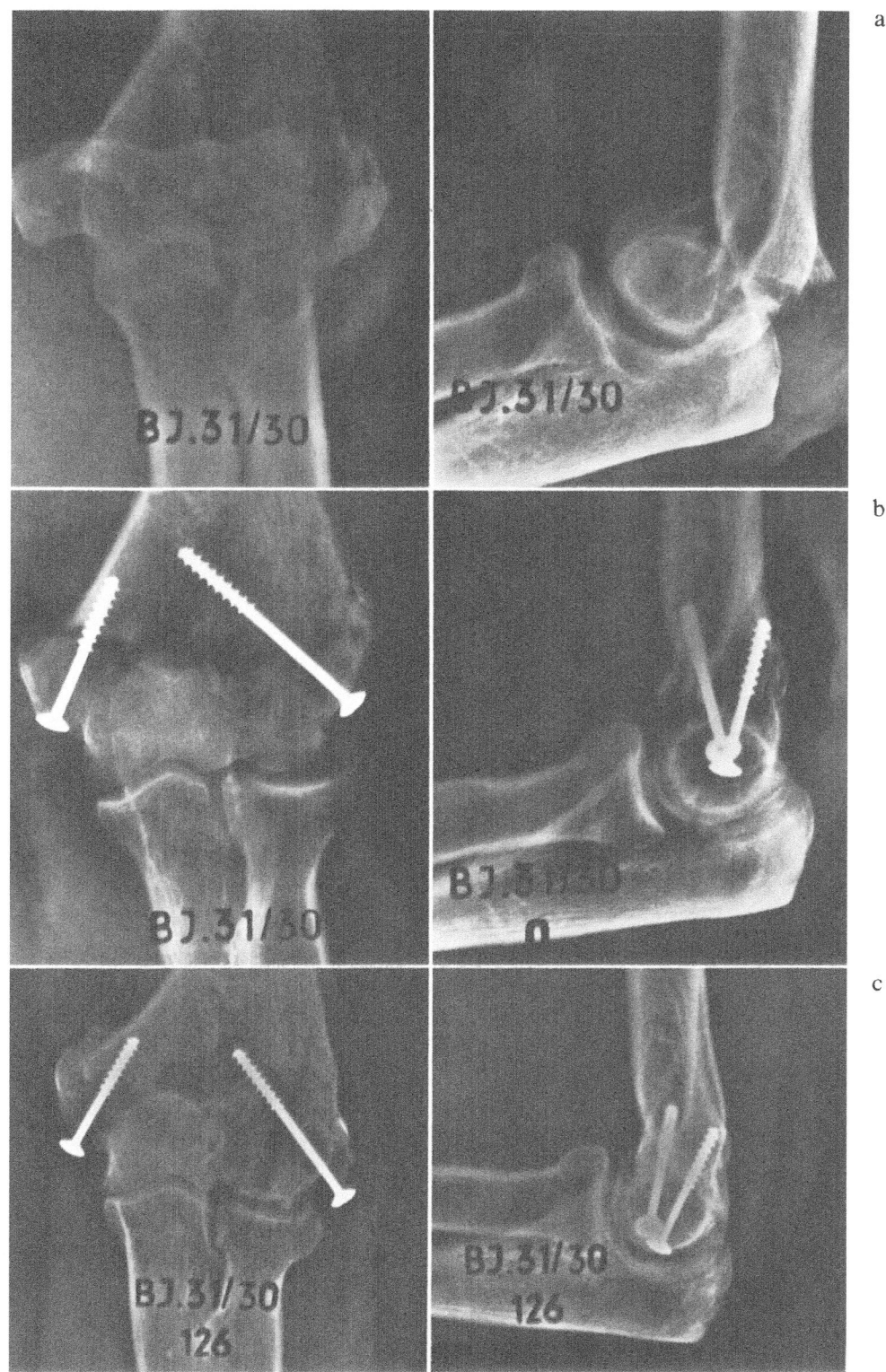

Fig. 44 Clinical example: Intra-articular comminuted fracture of the lower humerus
A 30 year-old manager of a health resort. Fall in the street

a   Intra-articular comminuted fracture of the lower humerus

b   Emergency internal fixation: osteotomy of the olecranon. Reduction of the trochlea with large cancellous screw, two small semi-tubular plates
No complications. A posterior plaster slab applied for six weeks. Removal of the plates and screws as well as anterior transposition of the ulnar nerve at nine months

c   A final review after 17 months: Occasional symptoms. Extension $-20°$, flexion $-15°$, pronation and supination equal on either side. No arthrosis

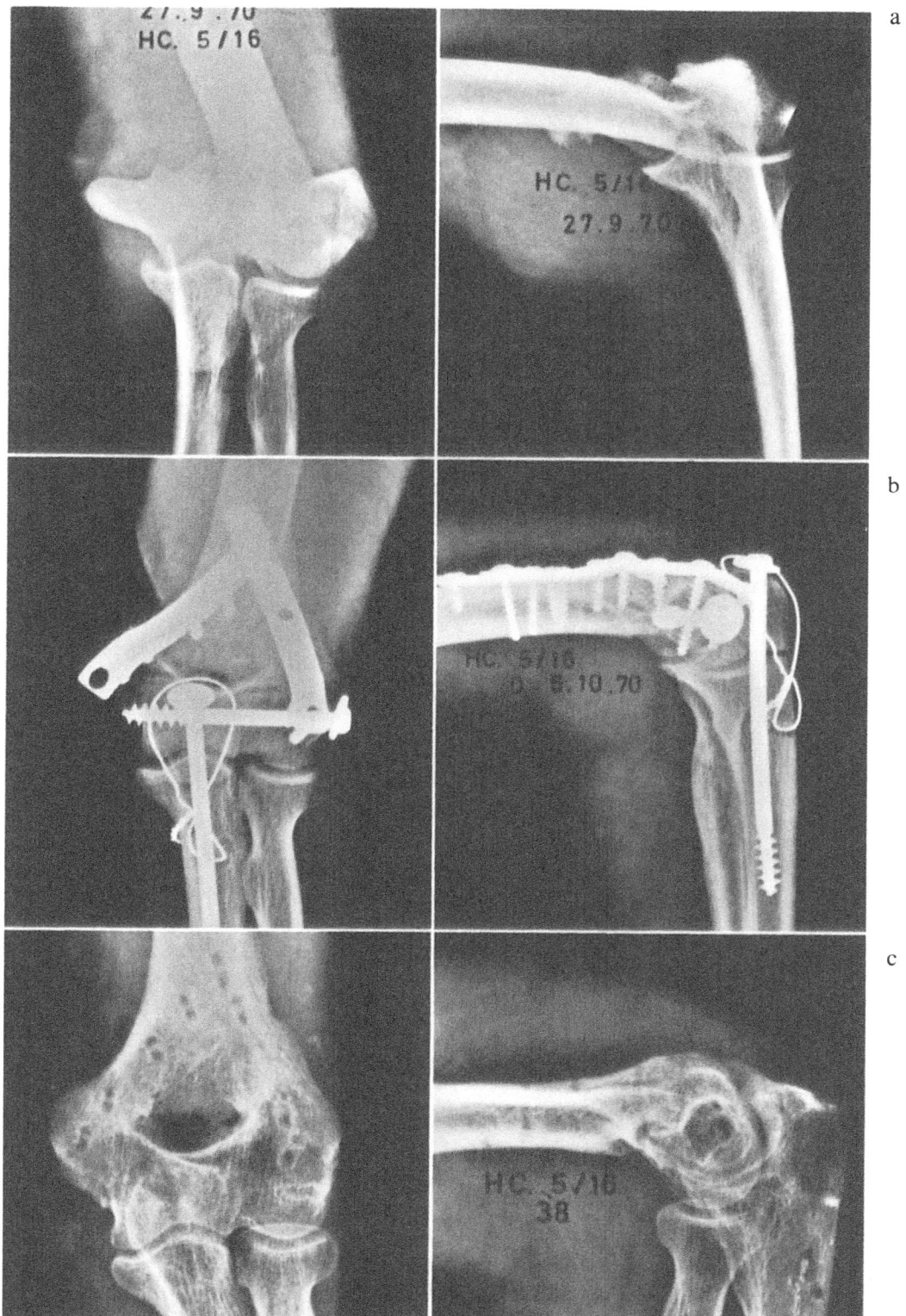

a

b

c

Fig. 45 **Clinical example: Impacted fracture of the radial head**
A housewife, aged 57. Fall on the outstretched hand

a   Cap-over-ear impacted fracture of the radial head with an additional fissure

b   Internal fixation with a single 2.7 mm cortex screw after four days. Complete reduction
No post-operative complications. Posterior plaster slab for three weeks. Removal of the screw at five months

c   A final review at $2^1/_2$ years: Symptom-free, joint function identical in either arm, no arthrosis

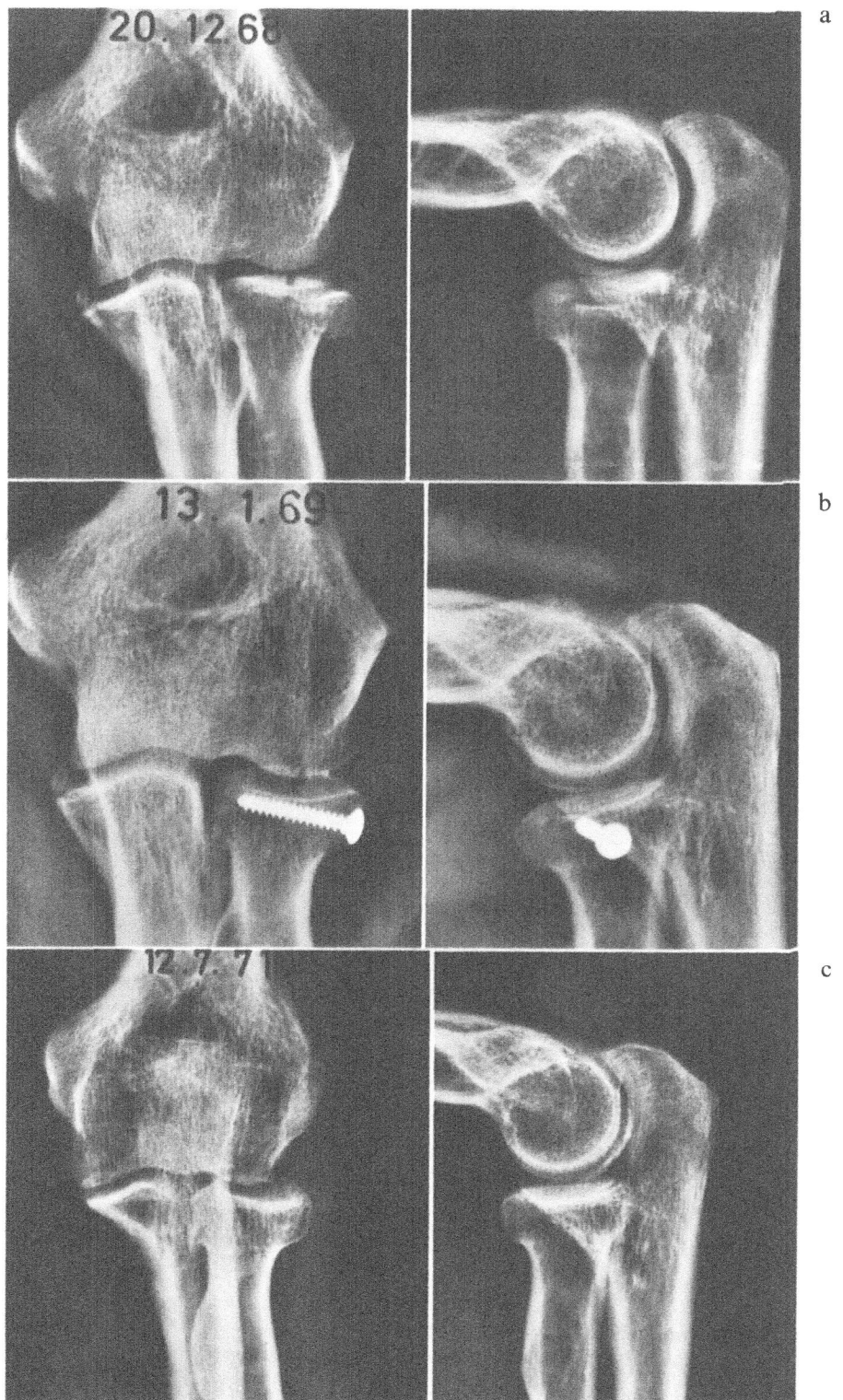

Fig. 46   **Clinical example: Oblique fracture of olecranon**
Patient was a manual printer who fell on his elbow

a   Oblique fracture of olecranon

b   Primary internal fixation with tension-band wire and an additional 3.5 mm cortex screw
Complications: Infection and fistula formation

c   Removal of metal after 28 weeks. Infection in the process of healing
Final check at 12 months: symptom-free, extension $-15°$, flexion equal on both sides, pronation and supination also equal

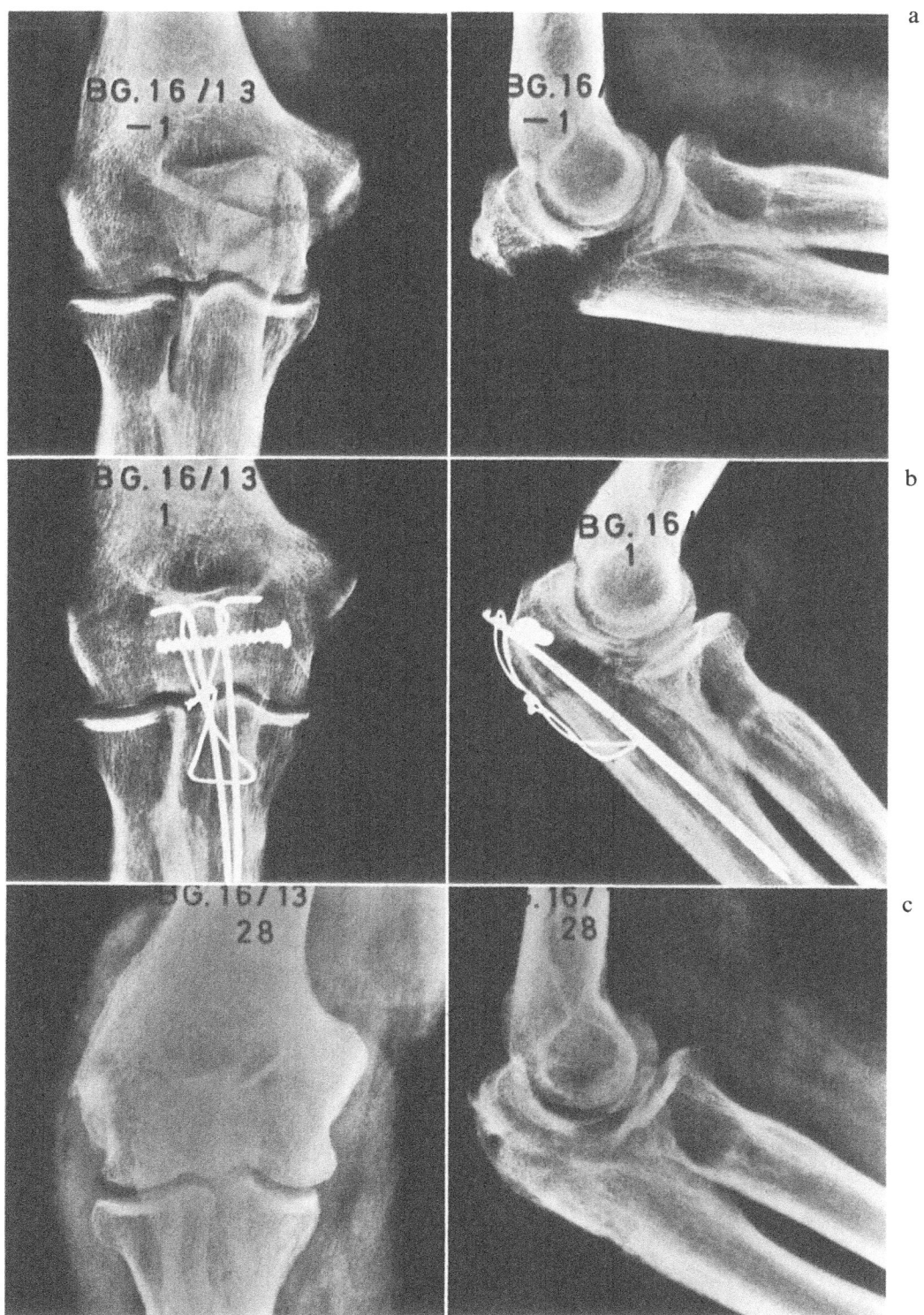

a

b

c

83

IX. The Wrist Joint

1. Lower End of Radius

The most frequent fracture in this region is the Colles fracture which is a compression fracture of the area of the lower radial epiphysis, the primary treatment of which is conservative. Where reduction is poor, this fracture has serious consequences. It is not justified to consider them as trivial cases simply because most of these patients are elderly so that disability does not affect their working life or their earnings. Certain cases need operative treatment, and reduction of a comminuted fracture can often be held by two Kirschner wires inserted percutaneously from the radial side. Larger defects may require an additional primary cancellous bone graft (Willenegger) (Fig. 47).

Internal fixation using the SFS is indicated in the following cases:

a) Isolated Fractures of the Radial Styloid Process

Most of these fractures can be fixed by screws alone, using small cancellous screws of 4.0 mm or small cortex screws of 3.5 mm (Fig. 48).

b) Fractures of Articular Fragments without any Depressed Areas

There is no satisfactory method of conservative reduction here, but these fractures can be securely fixed, either with screws or with the special T-plate. The type of fracture determines the right approach, either from the dorsal or the palmar aspect (see below).

c) Comminuted Articular Radial Fractures with Palmar Displacement of Fragments (Goyrand or Smith's Fracture)

These palmar fragments are suitable for open reduction as they compress flexor tendons together with the median nerve; there is moreover considerable shortening. This indicates the use of a buttress plate. We use the special T-plate for the distal radius and it is placed on the palmar side. As this plate does not fix the radial styloid process, comminuted fractures require additional Kirschner wires in order to increase stability here. Rare cases may require a cancellous bone graft (Fig. 49).

d) Approaches and Techniques of Internal Fixation

Experience has shown that surgeons are averse to operations on the wrist joint because of the complex anatomy. Particularly on the dorso-radial side the multiple layers of partly intersecting tendons and nerves impede an adequate approach to the bones if this is to be done without endangering the soft parts. Specially tested approaches for the above mentioned internal fixations will now be discussed in detail.

Approach to the Radial Styloid Process

Starting points for the incisions: *the tip of the styloid process and the radial edge of the radial fossa* respectively.

A sligthly curved incision on the radial side of the wrist joint. Identification of the superficial branches of the radial nerve followed by their retraction in an ulno-dorsal direction. Proceeding to the styloid process between the tendons of extensor pollicis brevis and extensor carpi radialis longus. Reflection of extensor pollicis brevis together with the parallel abductor pollicis longus in a radio-palmar direction. Thus we approach the periosteum, and a partial incision of the extensor retinaculum provides a good view of the styloid process and the immediately adjacent dorsal radial epiphysis.

Proximal extension of the incision however is rather restricted because of the intersection of the extensors carpi radialis (Fig. 50a and c).

Approach to the Back of the Distal Radius

The starting point of the incision is the *radial edge of the tendon of the extensor pollicus longus beneath the extensor retinaculum.*

The skin incision is similar to that for the radial styloid with an S-shaped elongation in a proximo-ulnar direction (Fig. 50a). The superficial branch of the radial nerve must be identified and retracted in a radio-palmar direction. The extensor retinaculum is incised longitudinally between the tendon of extensor pollicis longus and extensor carpi radialis brevis. The periosteum must be lifted from the cortex to which it closely adheres. Here we prefer the scalpel to the periosteal elevator. From here the radius can be exposed proximally to any desired extent, though a good exposure of the styloid process is not feasible (Fig. 50b, d, and e).

The distal part of the special T-plate must be contoured so as to fit the back of the radius. After internal fixation the extensor retinaculum is closed above the plate with several sutures (Fig. 50f). Thus the pulley of the extensor pollicis longus tendon in its osteocartilaginous channel is preserved.

Approach to the Lower Radius from the Palmar Surface

The incision begins at the *tendon of flexor carpi radialis.*

A long S-shaped incision on the distal forearm is continued to the thenar palmar crease (Fig. 51a). The incision is made close to the ulnar side of the prominent and strong tendon of flexor carpi radialis. The median nerve is identified. The flexor retinaculum is divided along its ulnar margin (Fig. 51b–d). The median nerve is retracted, together with the flexor tendons in the uninjured synovial sheath, in an ulnar direction (Fig. 52a). This provides access to the lower radius and the fracture. A limited reflection of pronator quadratus on the disto-radial surface is made with the help of a periosteal elevator. The wrist joint is opened followed by reduction of the articular surface (Fig. 52b). This procedure, however, does not provide any access to the radial styloid process.

Second Approach

Where the distal radio-ulnar joint must be exposed, the approach is made from the ulnar side, and the flexor tendon together with the median nerve are retracted laterally (Fig. 52c).

As the bend of the special T-plate fits the palmar surface of the radius, further bending is unnecessary. After insertion of the Redon suction drain, the wound is closed with simple skin sutures. In older clumsy patients, a posterior plaster slab is recommended.

Removal of metal entails reopening most of the incision which amounts to quite a major procedure. With dorsal incisions, protection of the superficial branch of the radial nerve may be difficult. Metal need not therefore be removed in older patients who are symptomfree.

e) Secondary Surgery

Pseudarthrosis of the distal radius rarely occurs. When treatment is required, fixation is obtained either with the special T-plate or a semi-tubular plate. The small semi-tubular plate seldom provides enough rigidity however. Cancellous bone grafting is often necessary, as most cases have bony defects.

Osteotomy is indicated in three different conditions:

In *malposition* after conservative treatment of a typical radial fracture. In this the articular surface is usually impacted and tilted dorsally. Functional disability and related symptoms may require some corrective procedure. Symptoms may sometimes be the result of compression of the median nerve in the carpal tunnel so that a careful electromyographic examination of the nerve is indicated before operation. Internal fixation of the fracture must then be combined with division of the flexor retinaculum to decompress the median nerve.

Fixation is achieved with a buttress plate which holds the lower radial epiphysis in the correct position. If there is a defect it is filled in with cancellous bone graft. In the presence of much osteoporosis however, a cortico-cancellous bone graft may be indicated (Fig. 58).

A *lengthening osteotomy* of the lower radius is seldom indicated, but when required is done by graft interposition. Fixation is then provided by one of the implants described above.

A *shortening osteotomy* of the lower radius is fixed with a semi-tubular plate applied radially.

2. Lower End of the Ulna

Since the distal ulna is an integral part of the forearm, its narrow lower end may sustain a transverse or short oblique fracture, both of which may be considered as "vassal" fractures. Stabilization of such a fracture is carried out with a small semi-tubular plate.

Secondary Operation

Secondary operations are quite often indicated on the lower ulna. Non-union of the lower end of the radius or arthrosis of the distal radio-ulnar joint are indications. As resection of the lower end of the ulnar does not detract from stabilitiy in the region of the wrist (Ricklin), we prefer this type of operation to a shortening osteotomy.

3. Scaphoid Bone

a) Indications

Undisplaced fractures of the scaphoid treated conservatively usually heal after 8–12 weeks with a suitable plaster cast, while fractures of the tubercle alone settle down after 3 to 4 weeks. From long experience it is clear that indications for primary internal fixation of the scaphoid are limited.

Internal fixation is justified in displaced fractures of the middle third which cannot be easily reduced by closed methods. This is especially true for the peri-lunate trans-scaphoid fracture-dislocation described by De Quervain, 50% of which end up with pseudarthrosis (Jahna). Internal fixation is also indicated for the rare vertical-oblique fracture which, like the fracture of the neck of the femur of Pauwels type III, is especially exposed to strong shearing forces so that the development of a Pseudarthrosis is six times as common as in all the other types of fracture (Trojan). The established method is screw fixation with the small cancellous screw (Willenegger, Pfeiffer, Koob).

b) Approach and Internal Fixation

A curved dorso-radial incision is made in the anatomical snuff-box. The superficial branches of the radial nerve and the tendon of extensor pollicis longus are retracted together posteriorly. The tendons of extensor pollicis brevis and abductor pollicis longus are retracted together with the radial artery, in a radial direction (Fig. 53a and b). The wrist joint is opened at the dorsal margin of the radial styloid. The hand should be kept in strong palmar and ulnar flexion. The fracture is exposed and reduced with the help of a fine elevator or hook. The articular cartilage must be carefully protected (Fig. 53c). Provisional transfixion with a fine Kirschner wire inserted from the tubercle is the next step. The position and length of the wire can be verified by X-ray.
Using the triple drill guide and 2.0 mm bit, an axial hole is drilled parallel to the wire. After tapping the thread, a small cancellous screw is inserted in this hole. In order to prevent rotation of the proximal fragment, the guiding wire should only be removed after the screw has been tightened up (Fig. 54). The primary partial excision of the radial styloid process to give improved exposure of the fracture is in dispute because it may disturb the blood supply.

c) Secondary Operation

Delayed consolidation of a fracture after conservative treatment provides an excellent indication for screw fixation. The bony fragments should be alive if success is to be achieved, and additional post-operative immobilization is indispensable.

A *real pseudarthrosis* with sclerosis and poor vascularity of the fracture surfaces resembles the atrophic pseudarthrosis in other bones. This type cannot be healed by a mere screw, but cancellous bone grafting, as described by Matti-Russe, is the most reliable method (Weber).

d) Statistics

Table 1. Scaphoid

	Number of fractures fixed with screws	Delayed union infection and pseudarthrosis	Final functional result			
			A	B	C	D
Primary internal fixation	22	3[a]	15	5	2	–
Secondary internal fixation	4	3[a]	2	2	–	–
Pseudarthrosis	12	3[a]	6	5	1	–

A: Full function, no symptoms.
B: Slightly impaired function, full working ability, occasional mild symptoms.
C: Considerable functional limitations, some handicap at work, permanent symptoms.
D: Functional result unknown, as patient not traceable.
[a] Cases where a subsequent Matti-Russe operation was required.

These figures include all the scaphoid fractures in which we used screw fixation, and which were followed up until the end of 1971.
The results confirm that the indications for screw fixation are limited: Disturbances in bone healing occurred in about a quarter of all cases. The number of poor final results amounted to about 8%.

minution in the wrist, early arthrodesis of the whole joint is recommended. This is performed with the help of an ASIF plate extending from the radius to the second metacarpal. The small semi-tubular plate does not often provide sufficient rigidity. An autogenous cancellous bone graft must always be used.
The same technique can be used when secondary arthrodesis is needed.

4. Other Parts of the Carpus

Fractures of other carpal bones are rare. Where they occur, internal fixation is indicated, provided that larger, easily approached fragments are present. This is sometimes true for displaced fractures. In the case of extensive com-

5. Clinical X-Ray Examples
Figs. 55–61, pages 103–113

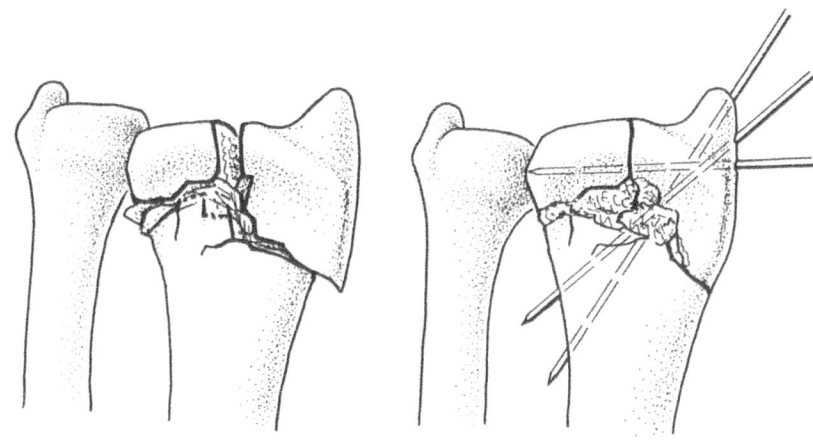

Fig. 47   Comminuted fracture of the lower radial epiphysis

with a defect in cancellous bone. Internal fixation with Kirschner wire and subsequent cancellous bone grafting (see also Müller *et al.*, Manual of Internal Fixation 1970, Fig. 132)

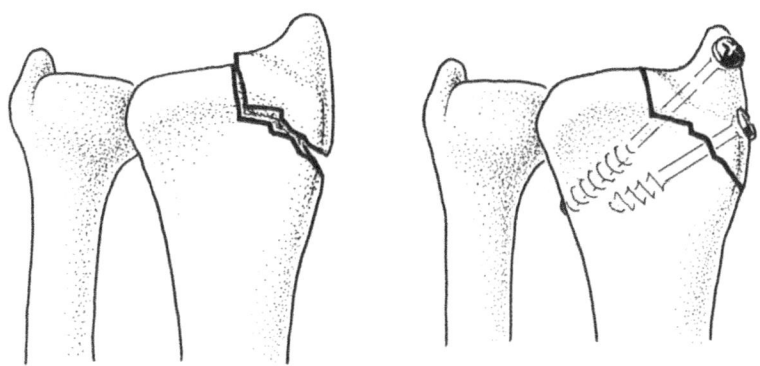

Fig. 48 **Isolated fracture of the radial styloid process**
Internal fixation with screws

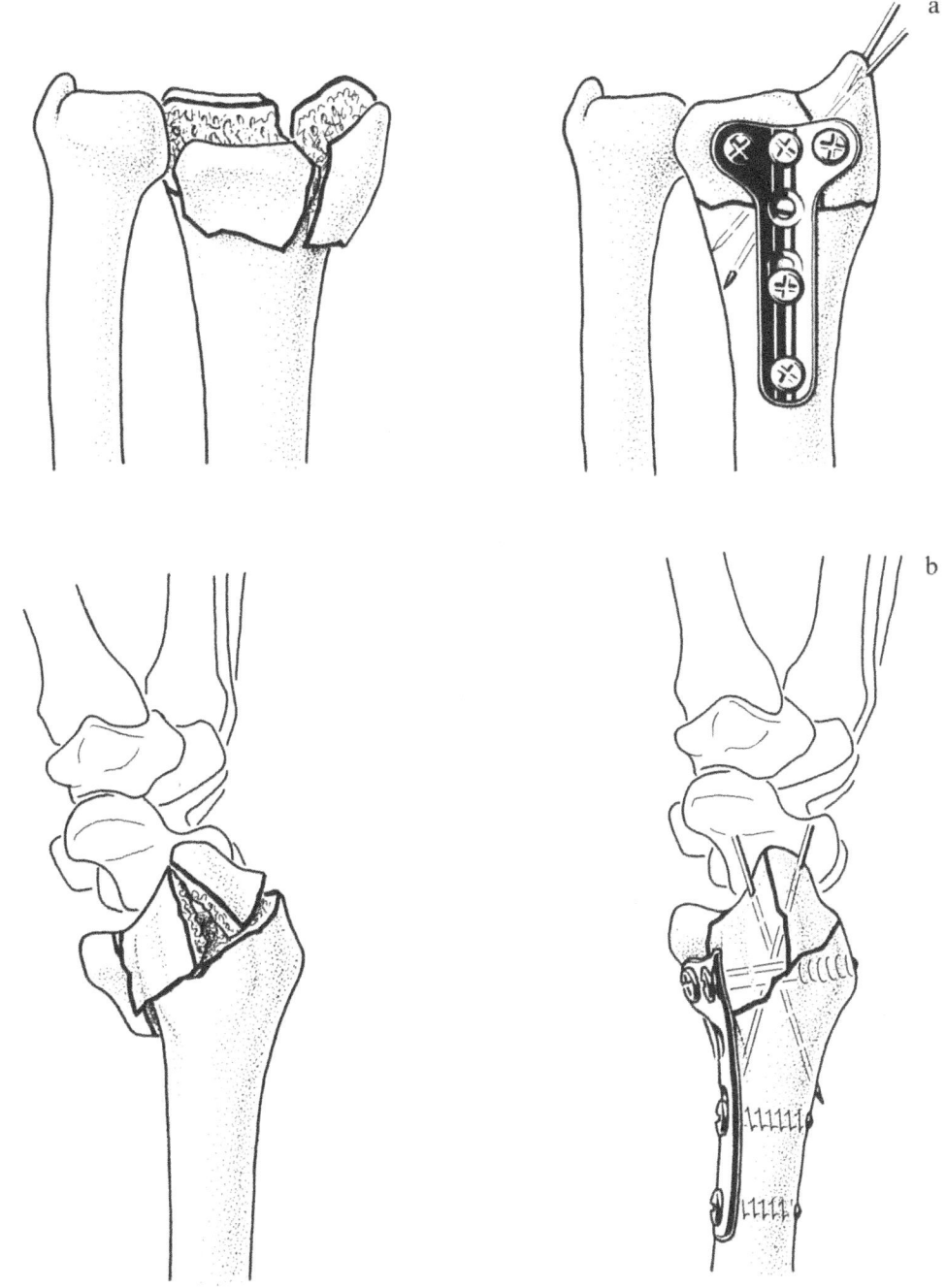

Fig. 49   Comminuted fracture of the radius with palmar fragments

Internal fixation using the special T-plate

a   Seen from the palmar aspect

b   Seen from the radial side

Fig. 50 Dorso-radial approach to the lower radius

a S-shaped incision:
1 Approach to the radial styloid process
2 Approach to the lower radial metaphysis

b Approaches shown in transverse section of lower forearm:
1 Between the tendons of extensor pollicis brevis and extensor carpi radialis longus
2 Between the tendons of extensor carpi radialis brevis and extensor pollicis longus

c Approach number 1: Leads directly to the radial styloid process. Partial division of the extensor retinaculum, retraction of the superficial branch of the radial nerve in a dorsal direction

d Approach number 2: Division of the extensor retinaculum close to the extensor pollicis longus and then extended proximally

e Approach number 2: After division of the extensor retinaculum it is elevated from its underlying bony attachment

f After completion of the internal fixation, the retinaculum is sutured back and the skin closed

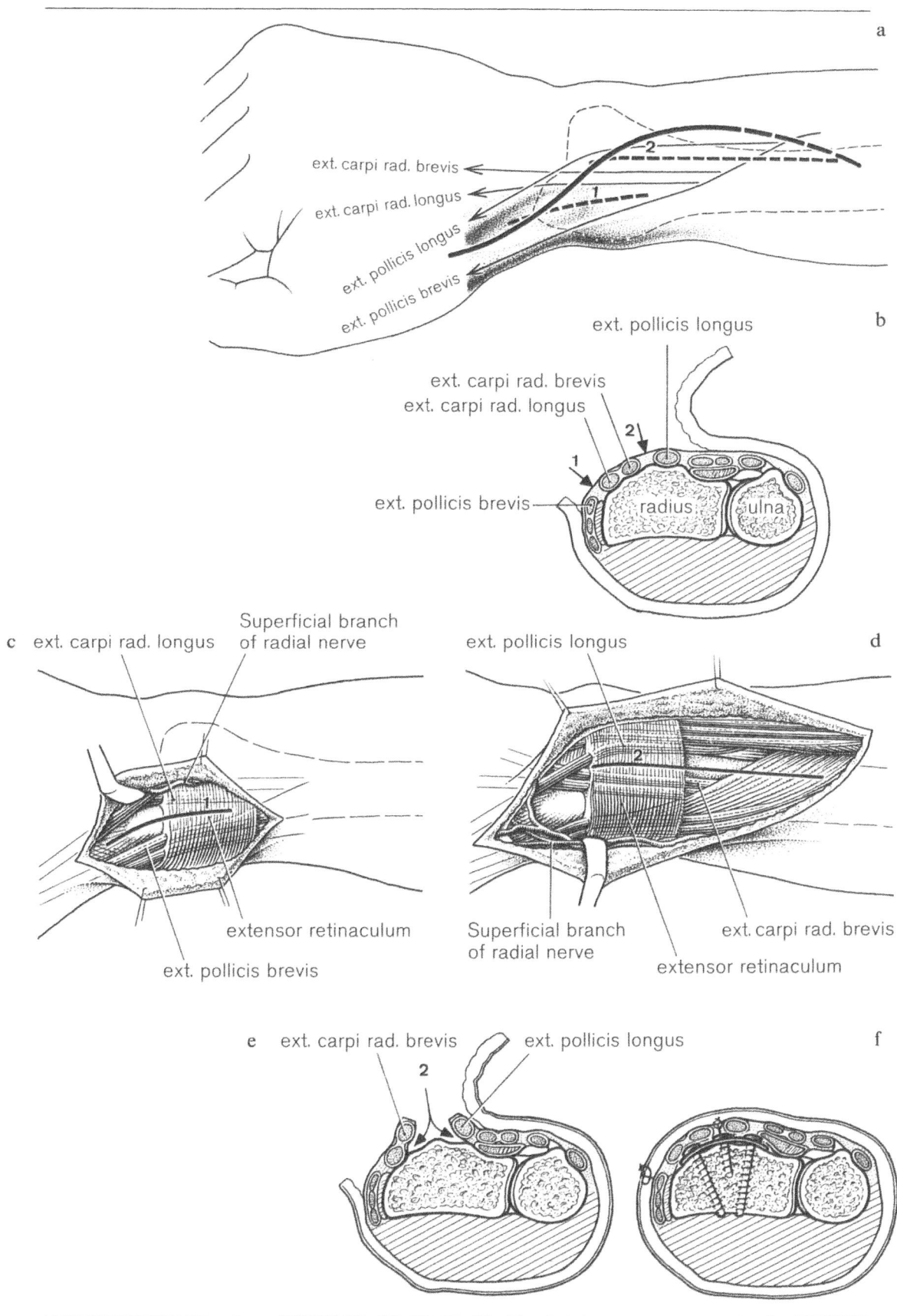

a

b
ext. carpi rad. brevis
ext. carpi rad. longus
ext. pollicis longus
ext. pollicis brevis

ext. pollicis longus
ext. carpi rad. brevis
ext. carpi rad. longus
2
1
ext. pollicis brevis
radius
ulna

c ext. carpi rad. longus
Superficial branch
of radial nerve
extensor retinaculum
ext. pollicis brevis

d ext. pollicis longus
2
Superficial branch
of radial nerve
extensor retinaculum
ext. carpi rad. brevis

e ext. carpi rad. brevis
2
ext. pollicis longus
f

93

Fig. 51 Palmar approach to the lower radius: Superficial layer

a Long S-shaped skin incision

b Approach by incising the flexor retinaculum and deepening the incision along the ulnar side of the tendons of flexor carpi radialis. A second approach is to enter on the ulnar side of the tendon of palmaris longus. This is shown as a dotted line

c Cross-section through the lower radius, level with the flexor retinaculum

d Cross-section at a more proximal level through the lower radius

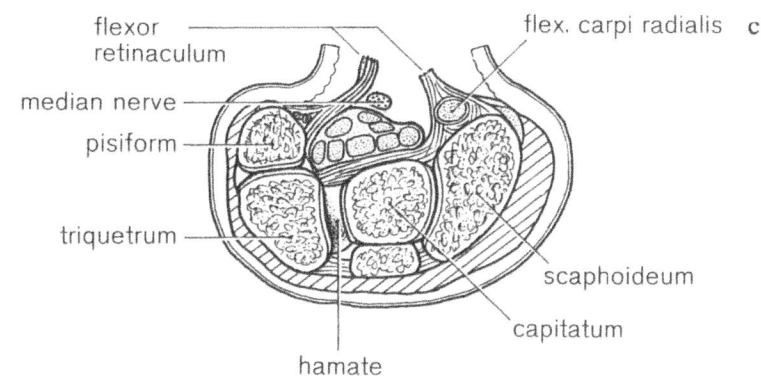

flexor
retinaculum

flex. carpi radialis   c

median nerve

pisiform

triquetrum

scaphoideum

capitatum

hamate

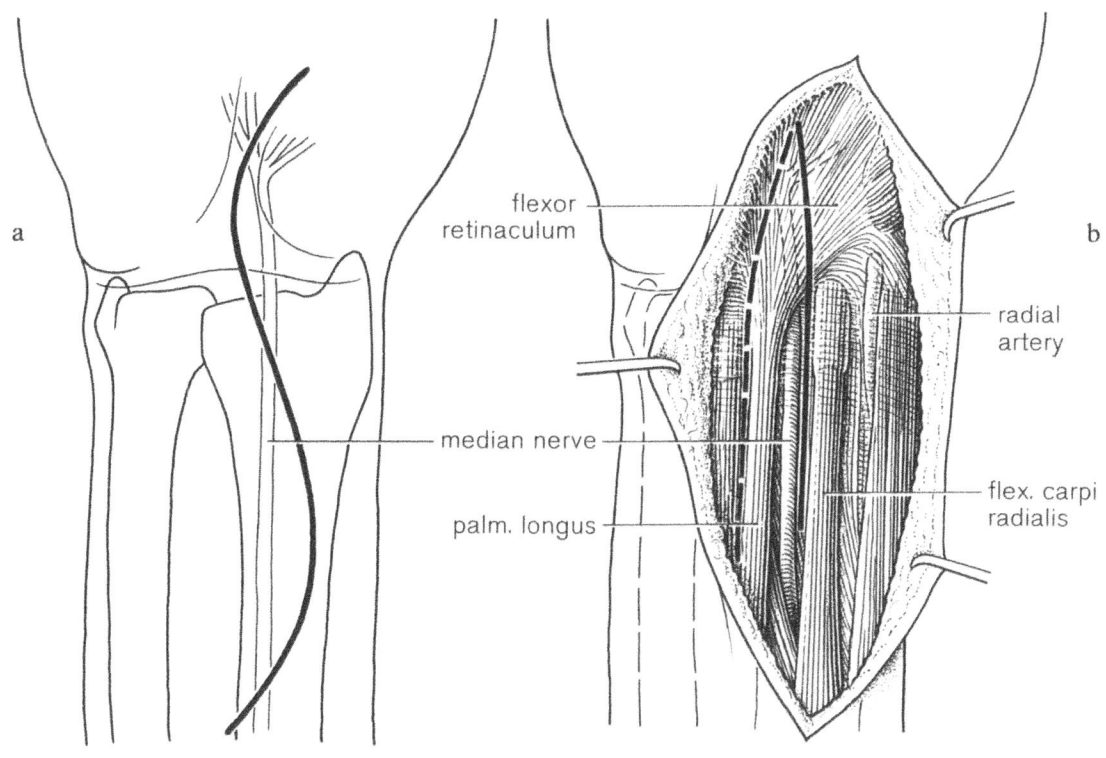

a

b

flexor
retinaculum

radial
artery

median nerve

flex. carpi
radialis

palm. longus

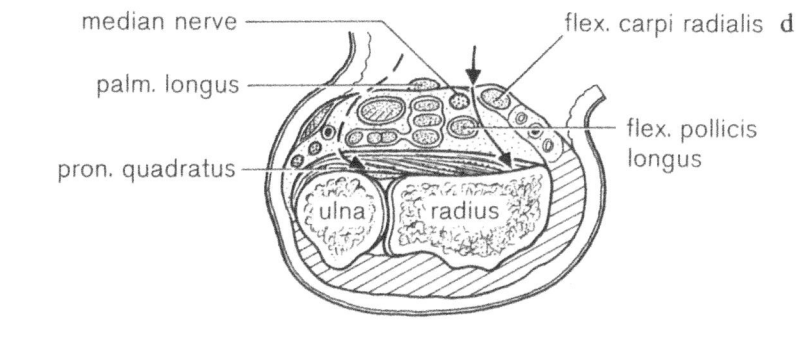

median nerve

flex. carpi radialis d

palm. longus

flex. pollicis
longus

pron. quadratus

ulna

radius

Fig. 52 Approaches to the lower radius from the palmar surface: deep layer

a Retraction of the median nerve and the flexors ulnarwards while the flexor carpi radialis is retracted towards the radial side. Exposure of the fracture and pronator quadratus

b Reflection of the pronator quadratus in an ulnar direction. Exposure of the wrist for the purpose of open reduction

c Second approach: retraction of the median nerve and the flexors radially. Exposure of the lower radio-ulnar joint

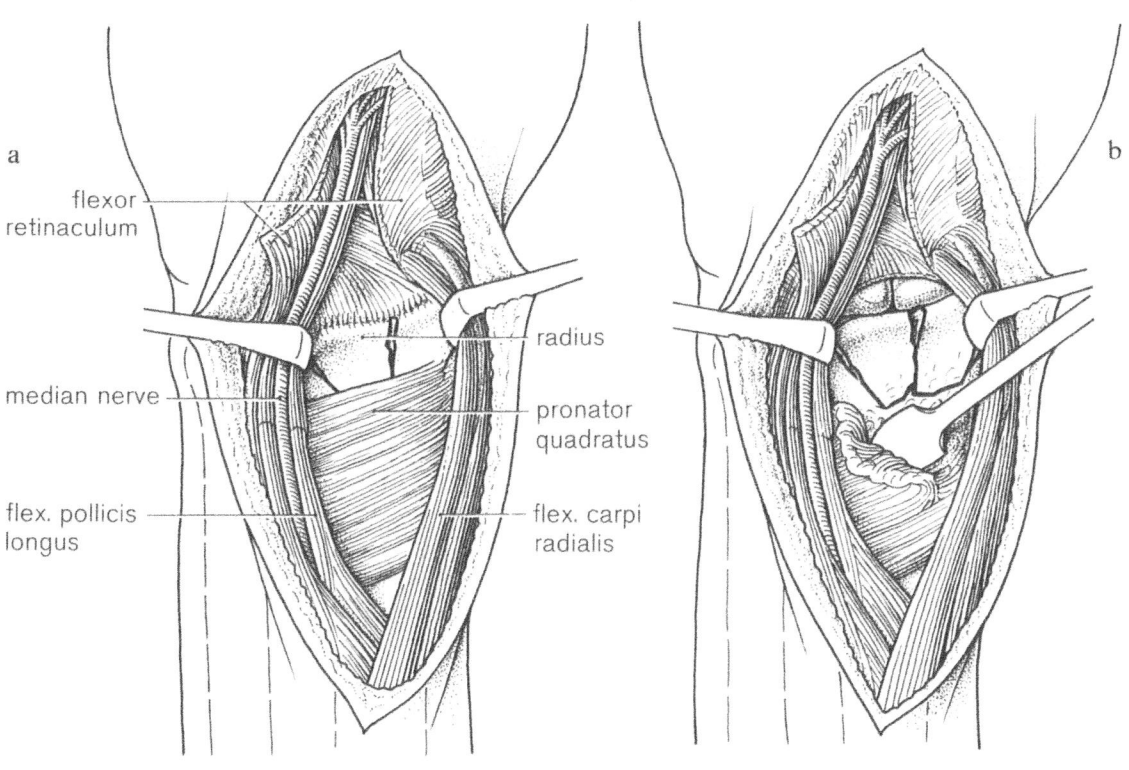

a

flexor
retinaculum

median nerve

flex. pollicis
longus

radius

pronator
quadratus

flex. carpi
radialis

b

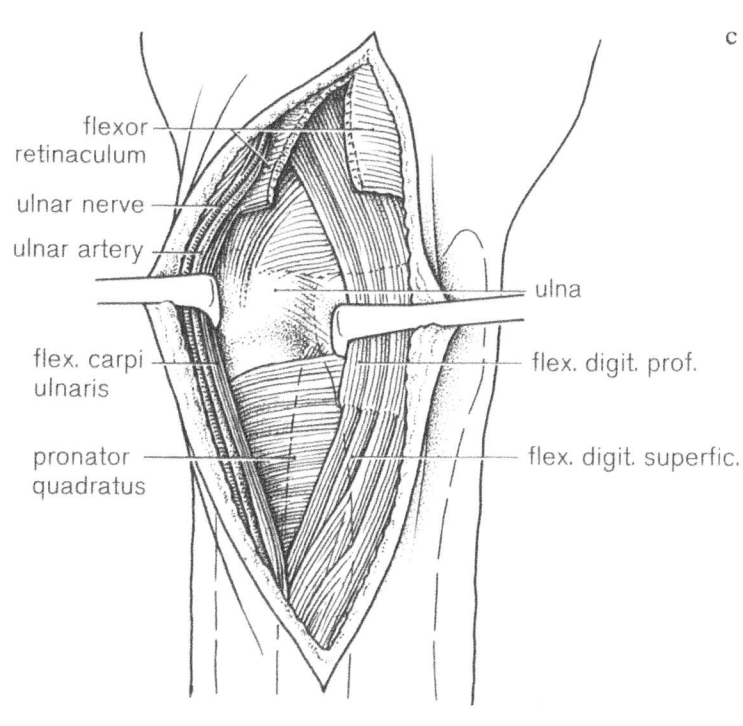

c

flexor
retinaculum

ulnar nerve

ulnar artery

flex. carpi
ulnaris

pronator
quadratus

ulna

flex. digit. prof.

flex. digit. superfic.

Fig. 53 **Fracture of the scaphoid: Incision and approach**

a Skin incision

b Topography: Tendons of extensor pollicis longus and extensor carpi radialis together with the superficial branches of the radial nerve are retracted dorsally, while the radial artery and another superficial branch of the radial nerve are retracted radially

c Exposure of the wrist joint at the dorsal margin of the radial styloid process. Reduction of the fracture by means of small hooks

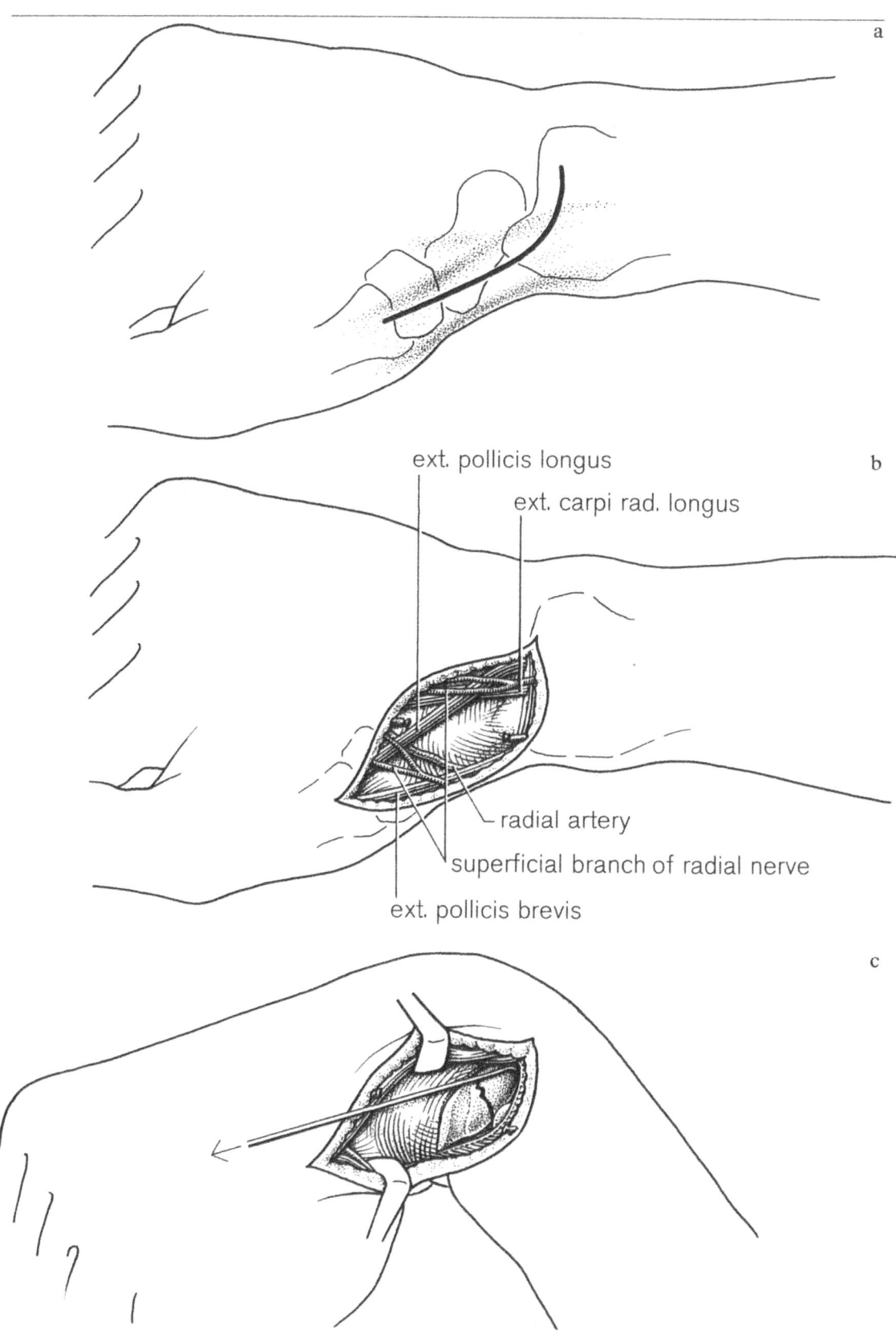

ext. pollicis longus

ext. carpi rad. longus

radial artery

superficial branch of radial nerve

ext. pollicis brevis

Fig. 54 **Fracture of the scaphoid: Internal fixation**

    a   Transfixion of the reduced fracture by a fine Kirschner wire. X-ray check

    b   Using the drill guide to place the drill hole parallel to the guide wire

    c   Tapping the thread

    d   Insertion of the screw and removal of the Kirschner wire

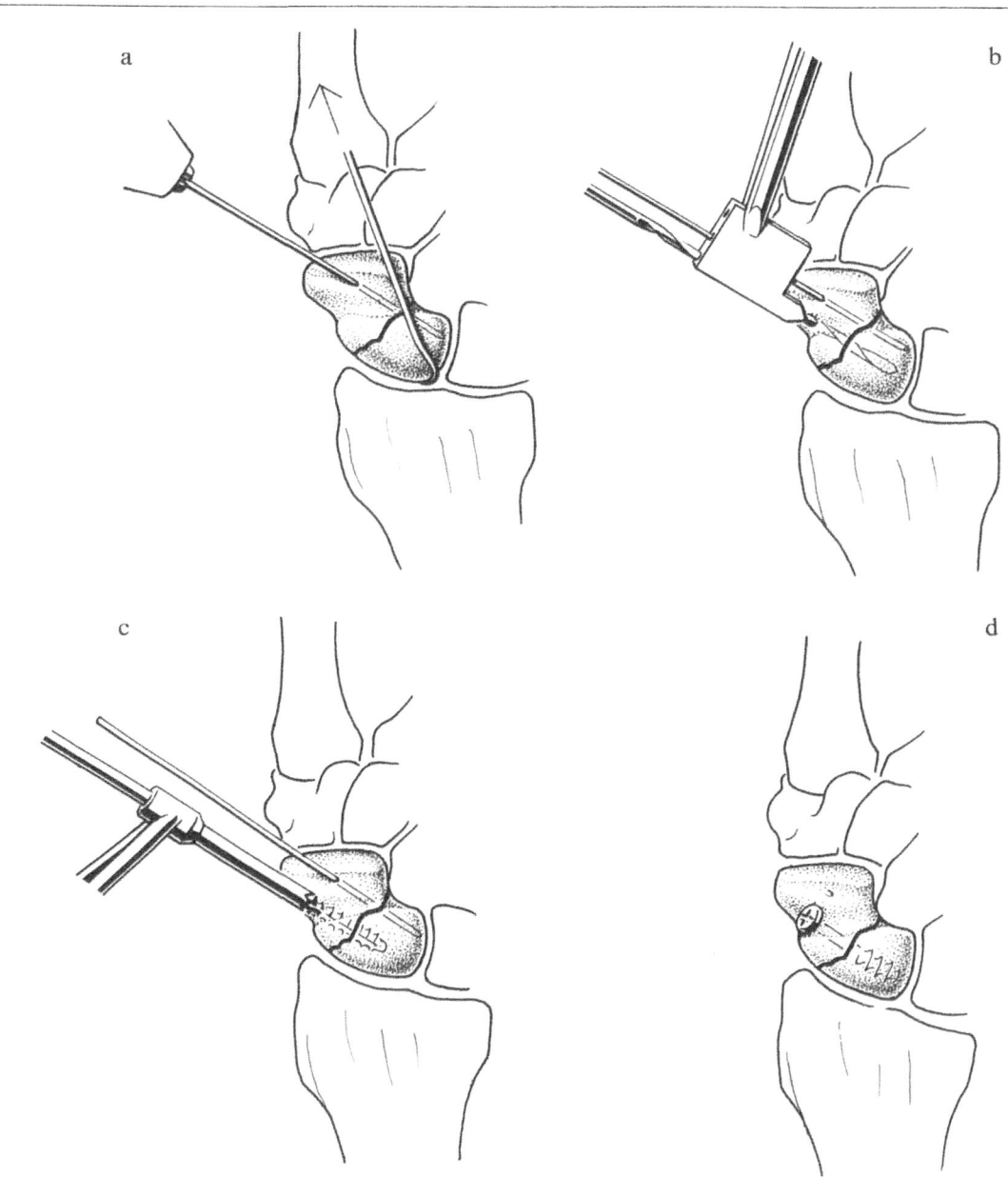

a

b

c

d

Fig. 55   **Typical example: Fracture of the radial styloid process**
The patient was a brewer, aged 42. Motor cycle accident

a   Irregular fracture of the radial styloid process

b   Primary internal fixation with small cancellous screws. Kirschner wire and fine figure-of-8 tension-wire
No complications

c   Removal of metal at twelve months
Final review at 14 months: Patient symptom free, slight restriction of movement in every direction

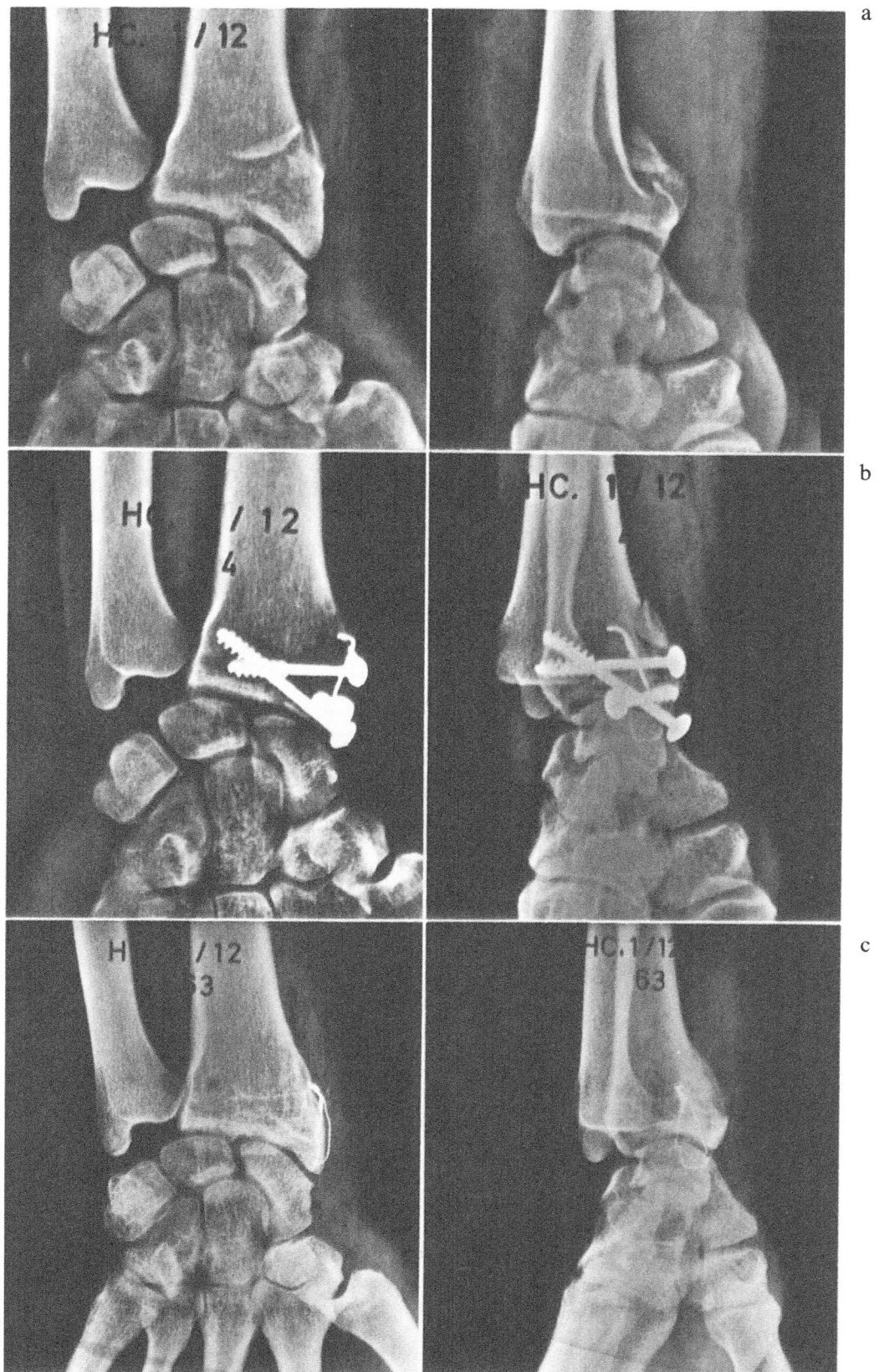

Fig. 56 **Clinical example: Comminuted fracture of the lower radius**
Patient was a carpenter, aged 29. He was injured in a traffic accident and had multiple injuries including cranial damage and eight fractures

a Unstable comminuted articular fracture of the left radius

b Secondary internal fixation with a posterior T-plate on the radius

c No complications. The fracture healed after six months
Clinical review after 12 months; patient symptom free, full working capacity, full function. He was booked for removal of the metal

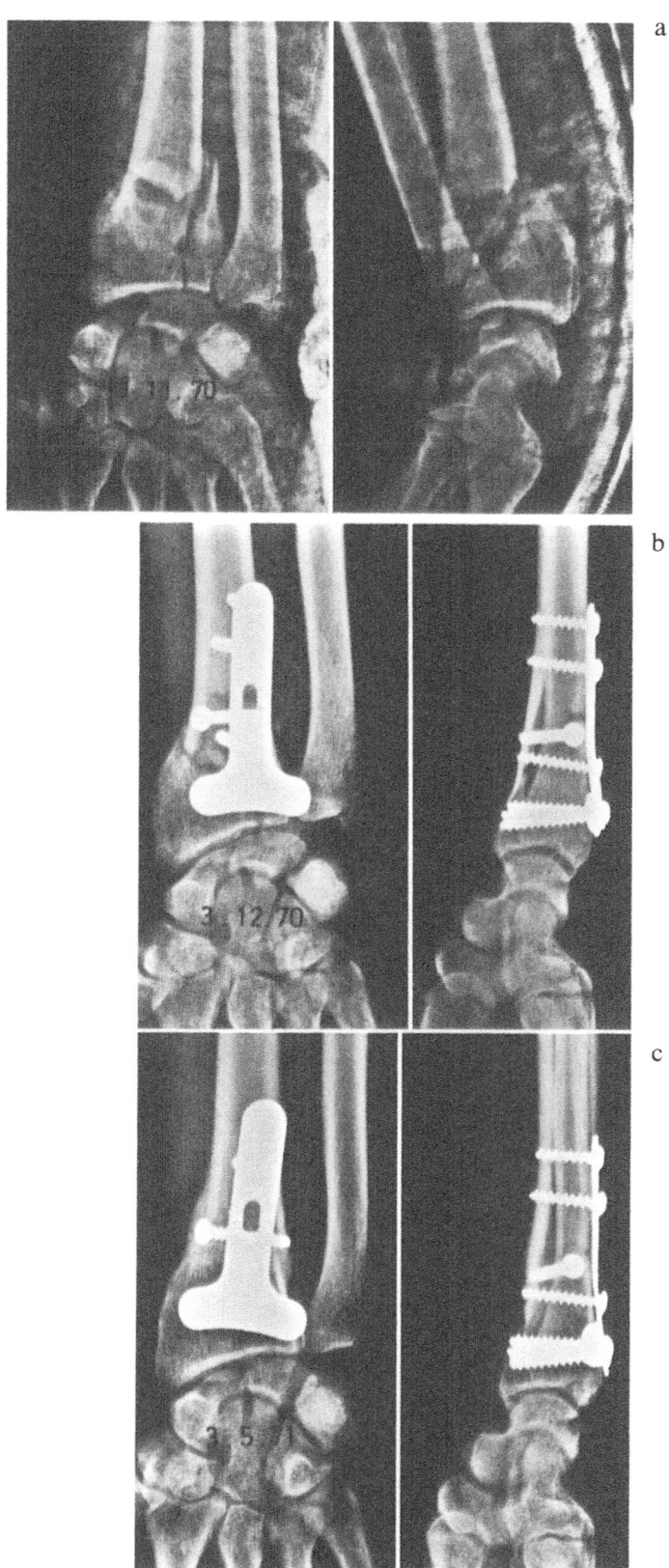

105

Fig. 57 **Clinical example: Comminuted fracture of the lower radial epiphysis with palmar displacement**
The patient was a housewife, aged 55, and had fallen on the outstretched hand

a   Comminuted fracture of the lower radius with palmar displacement

b   Primary internal fixation with a palmar T-plate and additional Kirschner wires to fix the radial styloid process. A plaster cast was applied for four weeks
No complications. Removal of the metal at five months

c   At final review after $1^1/_2$ years: symptom free, full strength, pronation $-10°$, ulnar adduction $-10°$, remaining movements full. Fracture healed

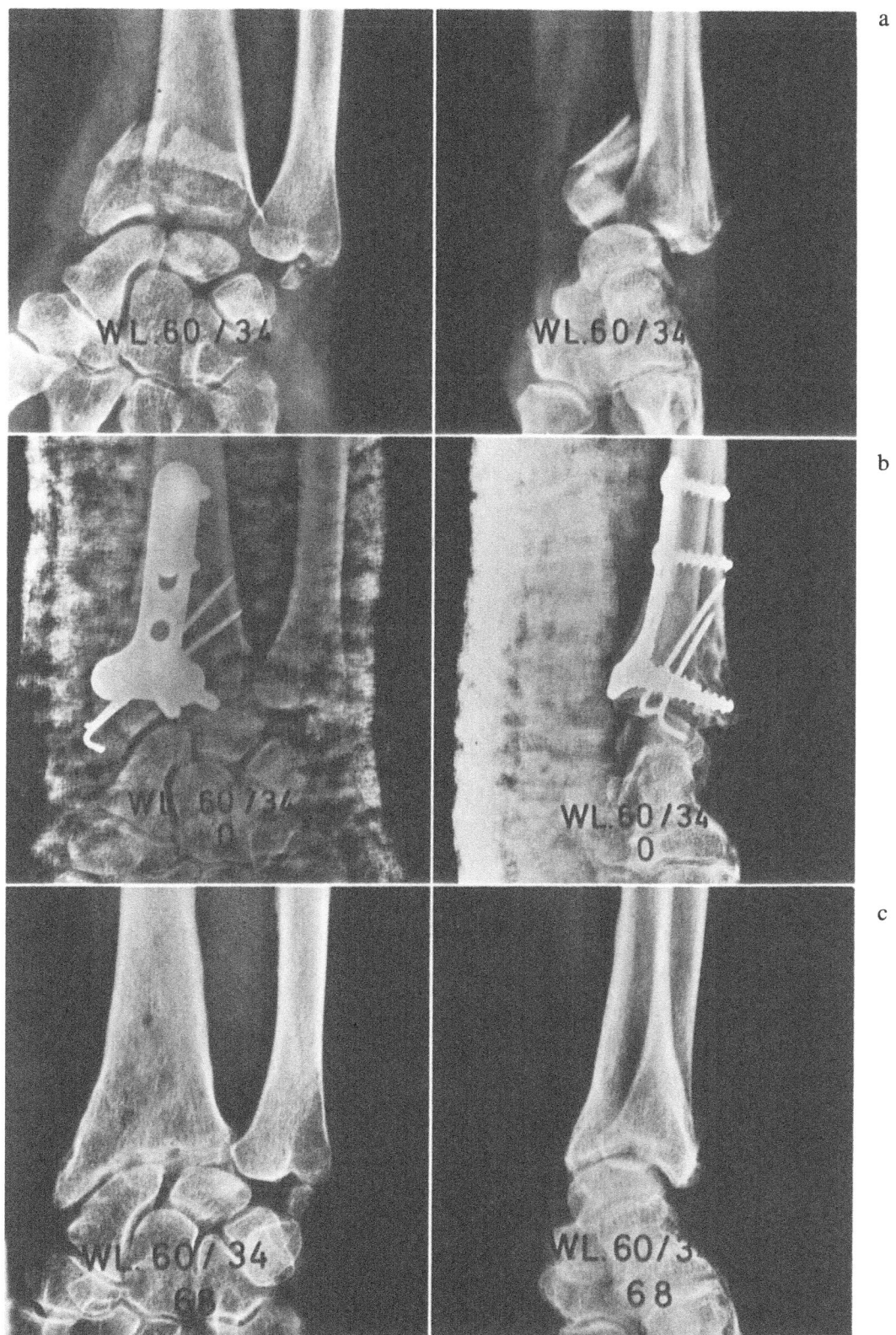

a

b

c

107

Fig. 58 **Clinical example: Malposition of lower radius**
A housewife, aged 41, who had fallen on her hand. Closed reduction and plaster cast, secondary displacement

a   Severe malalignment resulting in restricted movement which also affected the fingers; trophic disturbance and osteoporosis

b   Osteotomy together with cancellous bone grafting and a cortico-cancellous peg three months after the accident. Posterior T-plate

c   No complications. Physiotherapy. Metal removal at six months
Final review at seventeen months: moderate restriction of wrist movements. Full movements of fingers. Trophic changes had gone

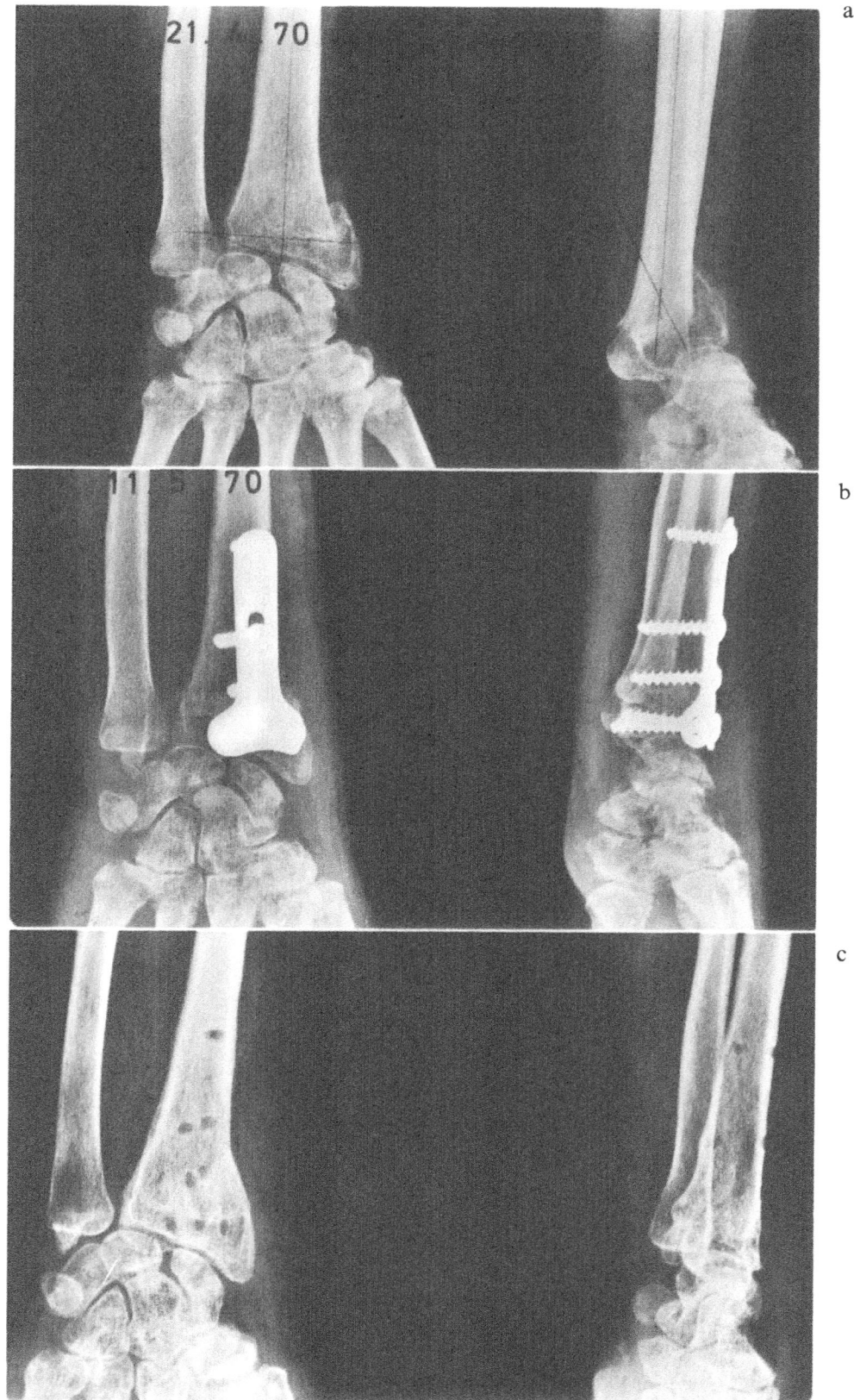

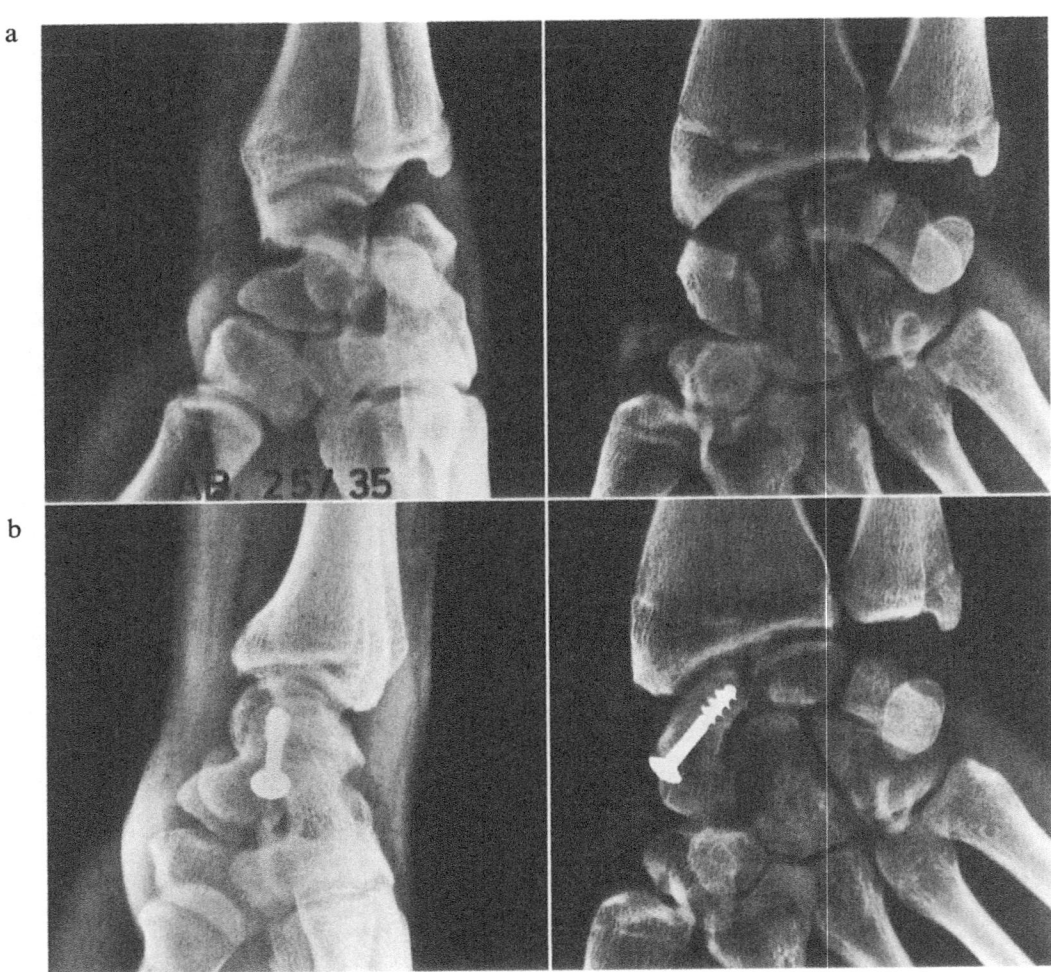

Fig. 59   Clinical example: Displaced fracture of the scaphoid with perilunar dislocation
A male student, aged 18. Fall from a small motor-cycle. A perilunar dislocation of De Quervain and displaced fracture of the scaphoid

a   Closed reduction of the dislocation, but the scaphoid fracture remained displaced

b   Screw fixation of the fracture one week after injury. Consolidation of the fracture at four months
Review at 10 months: Symptom free and full function. Booked for metal removal

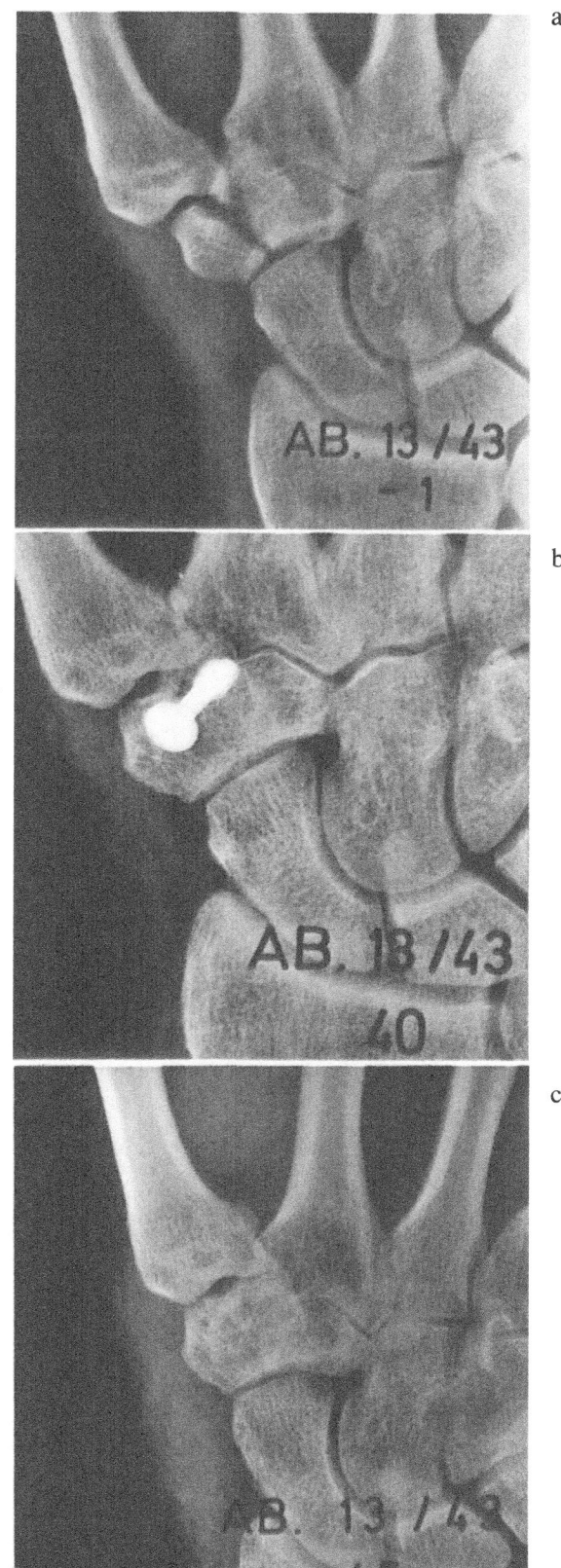

a

b

c

Fig. 60 **Clinical example: Fracture of trapezium**
Male elevator fitter, aged 30. Fall off a bicycle

a   Vertical fracture of trapezium. Internal fixation with small cancellous screw after one week

b   No complications. Consolidation of fracture and removal of metal at ten months

c   Final review at twelve months. Symptom free, thumb spread lacking 1 cm but remaining movements equal in both hands. No arthrosis

111

Fig. 61   Clinical example: Pseudarthrosis of scaphoid
The patient was a merchant, aged 41, who had fallen on his hand

a   Treated as a sprain for ten months. X-ray taken then showed a fracture of the scaphoid with
    live fragments and no displacement. A plaster cast was applied for three months, but union was
    not obtained

b   A screw fixation of the pseudarthrosis thirteen months after the accident. A plaster cast was
    applied after operation. The pseudarthrosis had consolidated at four months. The metal was removed
    eleven months after the operation

c   Final review at two years: Symptom free, full function, no arthrosis

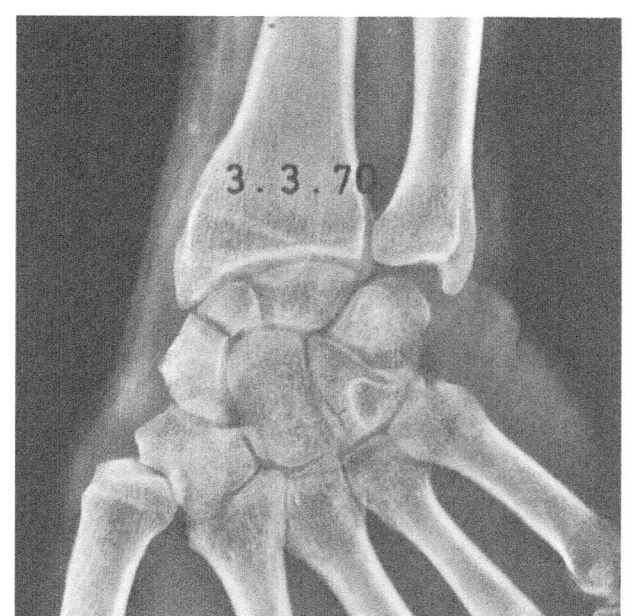

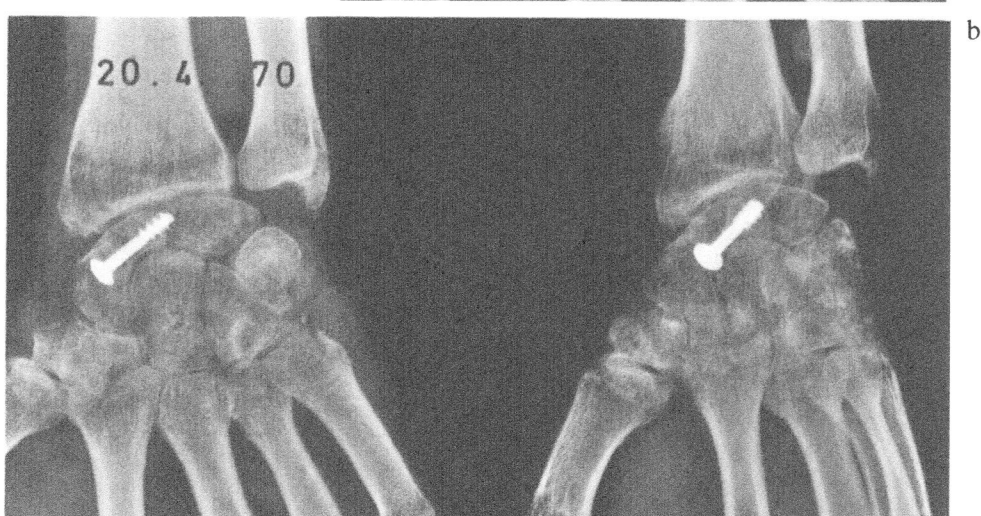

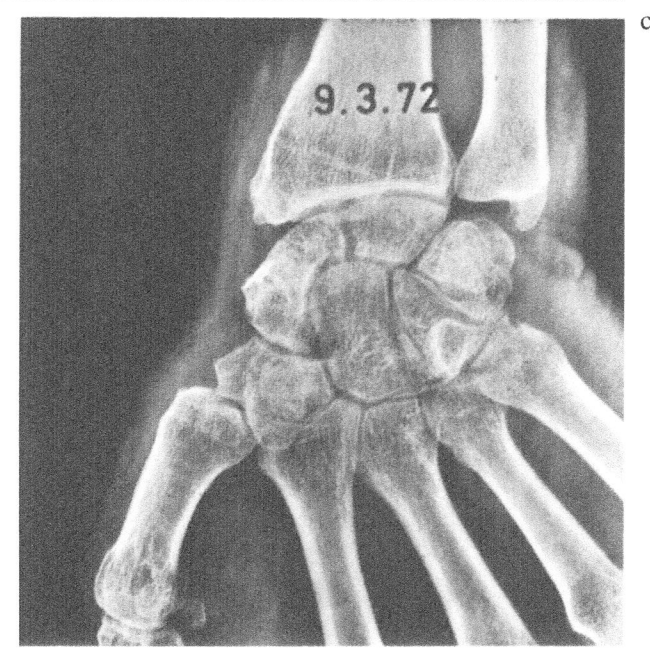

X. The Hand

A. Introduction

The technique of internal fixation in the peripheral bones of the hand is difficult and the surgeon assumes great responsibility. A thorough knowledge of the instrument set and familiarity with its contents, as well as a thorough knowledge of the functional anatomy of the hand, are indispensable prerequisites. Moreover, careful atraumatic treatment of the soft parts is very important for the preservation of full mobility. Unsuitable incisions and injury to the peritendinous layers and capsular structures of joints can result in permanent stiffness. Experience has, however, shown that rigid internal fixation enables us to achieve much better results than procedures known hitherto, provided that the described techniques are carefully adhered to.

This is particularly true for *open fractures of the bones of the hand* together with injuries to tendons and nerves. Rigid fixation of fragments facilitates post-operative treatment of the involved soft parts. Thus primary reconstruction of all the injured structures may be obtained in one step. Internal fixation of bony fragments also promotes wound healing, as the use of splints and plaster casts can be dispensed with.

Our team at the Basel University Department of Surgery has undertaken 25 internal fixations of open fractures of hand bones between 1967 and 1970, 11 cases involving multiple internal fixations, but no wound infection developed. There are, however, some limitations to the scope of comprehensive primary treatment, either because of circulatory impairment from crushing injuries, especially in the fingers, or because safe tourniquet time must not be exceeded. Where multiple open fractures and associated injuries of nerves, tendons or skin require time-consuming grafting procedures, the surgeon should consider whether simple Kirschner wiring, of oblique, axial or cross types, should be preferred to rigid internal fixation. Very small fragments are unsuitable for screw fixation. Instead we use the tension-band method either by a figure-of-eight system or by a trans-osseus wire inserted with the pull-out method as in Bunnell's tendon suture. Internal fixation is imperative where there are rotational deformities or articular steps which cannot be reduced.

B. Injuries to and Internal Fixation of the First Ray

There are three reasons why the first ray calls for special treatment; firstly basal fractures of the first metacarpal and associated conditions are important. Fractures in the region of the carpo-metacarpal and interphalangeal joints of the thumb are fairly common. Because of the considerable tensile strength of muscles and tendons, most shaft fractures are unstable so that conservative attempts at impaction are difficult. Internal fixation is then often indicated. Except for Bennett's fracture anatomical approaches to the thumb are relatively simple.

1. Fractures of the Base of the First Metacarpal

a) Bennett's Fracture

Bennett's fracture is a fracture-dislocation of the first carpo-metacarpal joint. The shaft fragment is displaced in a radio-dorsal direction in adduction. The small articular fragment remains fixed to the carpus. Unless the dislocation is completely reduced, it will certainly result in severe post-traumatic arthrosis, with pain and functional disability of the entire thumb. Full abduction of the thumb must be provided to give a broad grip between the thumb and index. Iselin's school has particularly emphasized this aspect. Although it is infrequent, Bennett's fracture features often in the surgical literature. Many surgeons have tried to find a desirable procedure for achieving and for holding the reduction of Bennett's fracture.

From our own experience, as well as that derived from ASIF publications, we are convinced that open reduction with screw fixation represents the best procedure, giving the best promise of a lasting good result. although there are some technical difficulties.

Approaches to the Carpo-Metacarpal Joint and Operative Techniques for Bennett's Fracture

Inadequate exposure of the small proximal joint fragment is the chief impediment to complete reduction and operative fixation of this fracture.

Radio-Palmar Approach Described by Gedda and Moberg

This approach gives the optimal exposure. A radio-palmar sickle-shaped incision at the level of the first carpo-metacarpal joint is extended in a dorsal direction. The tendon of abductor pollicis longus must be carefully protected (Fig. 62). The joint is opened from the palmar surface and, if necessary, from the dorsum. Open reduction of the fracture and temporary fixation with a fine Kirschner wire inserted from the palmar side is carried out (Fig. 64).

Radio-Dorsal Approach (Second Approach)

A slightly curved skin incision is made along the radial border of the metacarpal, extending proximally towards the radial styloid process, with partial reflection of the thenar muscles. (Fig. 63). The carpometacarpal joint is now opened anterolaterally. The fracture is reduced and provisionally fixed with a Kirschner wire inserted from the dorsal side. Though the exposure of the joint and the articular fragment is limited in this procedure, there is better protection of the soft parts and especially of the joint capsule.

In both approaches, *screw fixation* is carried out *from the dorsal aspect* (Fig. 64): A hole is drilled with the 2.0 mm bit, and a thread is then tapped. A small cancellous screw of the right length fixes a larger fragment, while a smaller fragment may need to be held with a small lag screw of 3.5 mm or sometimes 2.7 mm. The strength of interfragmentary compression is still somewhat inadequate, as the channel in the larger shaft fragment must be very accurately converted into a gliding hole. Though this detail must not be overlooked, a review of our cases has shown that post-traumatic arthrosis does not appear, even if the reduced position is not quite perfect. The main aim is the permanent correction of the dislocation.

The guide wire should be removed only after the screw has been tightened so that it can prevent any secondary rotation of the small fragment.

Where screw fixation fails for some technical reason as when fragments are small or too many, we can insert multiple Kirschner wires in different directions to secure the fragment.

b) Rolando's Fracture

This is an intra-articular Y-fracture of the base of the thumb, and is in most cases complicated and comminuted. Internal fixation is technically difficult and operation is indicated when there is an articular step, adduction of the distal fragment, or shortening due to muscle pull. The last can lead to secondary effects.

Approach and Internal Fixation

The best exposure of this comminuted fracture is obtained by the *incision described by Gedda-Moberg*. A sickle-shaped incision is extended distally to the ulnar edge of the first metacarpal

(Fig. 62). The first carpometacarpal joint is opened widely.

Second approach: in simpler articular fractures, sufficient exposure is obtained by the *dorso-radial incision* described for Bennett's fracture. In this case too, the incision is helpful in protecting soft parts (Fig. 63).

The first step is to reduce the joint surface accurately. This reduction is held by Kirschner wires which in suitable cases can be replaced by a screw (Fig. 65 b). The articular part is then held to the shaft fragment with the help of a buttress plate in the form of a reversed finger T-plate (Fig. 65 c). If absolute rigidity is not thus obtained, a palmar plaster splint is applied with the thumb in abduction and opposition for 4 to 6 weeks.

c) Extra-Articular Fracture of the Base of the Thumb Metacarpal

This fracture is much more common than Bennett's or Rolando's fracture. Here there is always an adduction crack in the shaft fragment and a narrowed web between the thumb and the index. Since reduction and its maintenance by plaster cast is difficult, internal fixation is often indicated. The rigidity thus obtained is complete, so that early mobilization and rapid resumption of work is usually possible.

Approach and Internal Fixation

We use the dorso-radial longitudinal incision, the second approach described in the paragraph on Bennett's fracture (Fig. 63). In most cases, it is unnecessary to open the carpo-metacarpal joint and stabilization of oblique fractures can be obtained by simple screw fixation, while transverse fractures need to be held with a reversed finger T-plate fixed as a tension-band system. The plate should be slightly bent to guarantee sufficient abduction of the thumb. It is first screwed to the proximal fragment, and then the distal shaft fragment can be lifted-up towards it with the help of forceps. It is then in a reduced position (Figs. 66 and 67).

2. Peripheral Fractures of the First Ray

a) Articular Fractures

Fractures of the carpo-metacarpal and interphalangeal joint of the thumb are quite common. They often consist of small fragments which can be completely stabilized with a single screw. The gauge of the screw is determined by the individual size of the fragment (Fig. 68 c).

b) Fractures of the Shaft of the First Metacarpal and the Proximal Phalanx of the Thumb

Internal fixation has become the approved method here, particularly when there are associated injuries. It facilitates early mobilization which is very important in the first ray, and it makes external fixation unnecessary. To get enough rigidity, internal fixation with plates is to be preferred.

Approach: a dorso-lateral incision is made. The fracture is exposed while the extensor tendon is protected (Fig. 67a and b).

3. Secondary Operation on the First Ray

a) Carpo-Metacarpal Joint

Here post-traumatic arthrosis is important. In most cases it either follows an inadequately reduced Bennett fracture or instabilitiy of the joint due to a ligamentous injury. It is painful and involves a long period of incapacity. Four surgical approaches are available:

Excision of the trapezium which is often carried out in rheumatoid arthritis in the female hand. The resulting defect can easily be filled in by part of the longitudinally split tendon of the flexor carpi radialis (Buck-Gramcko). Functional restriction of the thumb chiefly involves some loss of strength.

A new method of treatment for the excised trapezium is to replace it with a *silastic prosthesis* but this method has not been sufficiently tested yet, though it seems to be promising for elderly patients (Swanson).

In younger patients where a powerful grip must be maintained, *arthrodesis* is the treatment of choice. Some workers rate the functional limitations highly (Leach and Bolton). In our experience however, they are less than one would expect, probably because of the plaster-free post-operative treatment and the mobilization of neibouring joints. The most important advantage for the patient is the relief of symptoms which allows an early return to his occupation.

Operative Technique

The approach is similar to that for Rolando's fracture and involves an accurate exposure of the carpo-metacarpal joint and trapezium. Excision of the joint is obligatory and the resulting defect must be filled in with cancellous bone graft. Special attention must be paid to the accurate opposing position of the thumb. The operation is carried out following the technique which uses a compressed bridging graft. Here the bed for the graft is made in the trapezium and in the base of the thumb metacarpal. We use a reversed finger T-plate fixation. Both the proximal cortex screws of 3.5 mm have to fit accurately in the trapezium (Fig. 68). Complete rigidity is thus achieved but as consolidation may require several months, the metal should not be removed before one year has elapsed.

Opposition Block Procedure: In post-traumatic adduction contracture of the thumb, opposition can be passively restored by a graft interposed between the first and second metacarpal. Fixation of the graft is obtained either with a transfixation screw or with a straight plate (Fig. 69).

b) Metacarpo-Phalangeal Joint of the Thumb

This joint of rather simple structure has the least physiological range of motion in the first ray. Arthrodesis in a position of less than 10 degrees of flexion results in insignificant functional limitation.

The following operations can be considered. The first is excision of the joint with subsequent application of a tension-band plate, and the second adds the compressed bridging graft to the plate (Figs. 28 and 30).

c) Interphalangeal Joint in the Thumb

Comminuted fractures of this type may indicate either a primary or secondary arthrodesis. The appropriate technique is to use a bone-peg fixed with a screw, or excision of the joint with screw fixation alone (Figs. 29 and 30). The best position is either in full extension or very slight flexion. In patients whose profession especially requires a tip-to-tip pinch, flexion may be allowed up to 15°. When the metacarpo-phalangeal and carpo-metacarpal joints are uninjured, functional limitations are insignificant.

d) Malposition of the First Ray

A considerable adduction malposition may require osteotomy of the first metacarpal bone whereas this is rarely indicated for the proximal phalanx. Osteotomy is carried out using a compressed bridging graft fixed with a tension-band plate (Figs. 28 and 30). The resulting rigidity is enough to allow early mobilization.

e) Pollicisation

In transposing a finger ray to the remains of the thumb, the use of a small plate for fixation has become an accepted method (Simonetta, Pannike). Post-operative treatment can thus be concentrated on the soft parts.

118

4. Statistics Referring to the First Ray

Table 2. Thumb ray

	Number of fractures	Screw fixation	Plate fixation	Disturbed bone healing (infection or pseud-arthrosis)	Final functional result			
					A	B	C	D
Internal fixation								
Bennett's fracture	13	13	—	2	6	5	1	1
Rolando's fracture	8	1	7	—	7	1	—	—
Extra-articular fracture of the base of the metacarpal	15	7	8	1	9	6	—	—
Fracture of the shaft and head of the first metacarpal	15	6	9	2	6	7	1	1
Fracture of the proximal phalanx of the thumb	9	8	1	—	5	3	1	—
Arthrodesis								
Carpometacarpal joint	6	1	5	3	3	1	1	1
Metacarpo-phalangeal joint	12	1	11	1	11	—	1	—
Interphalangeal joint	12	12	—	—	10	2	—	—

A: Full function, no symptoms.
B: Slightly impaired function, no working handicap, occasional mild symptoms.
C: Considerable functional limitation, some handicap at work, permanent symptoms.
D: Functional result unknown because the patient could not be traced.

Summary of Table 2

The statistics comprise all the patients treated by us until the end of 1971. The figures confirm that primary internal fixation of fractures of the thumb gives a favourable prognosis. They also show that arthrodesis in the thumb gives good functional results. Delays in bone healing were infrequent.

5. Clinical X-Ray Examples
Figs. 70–79, pages 128–143

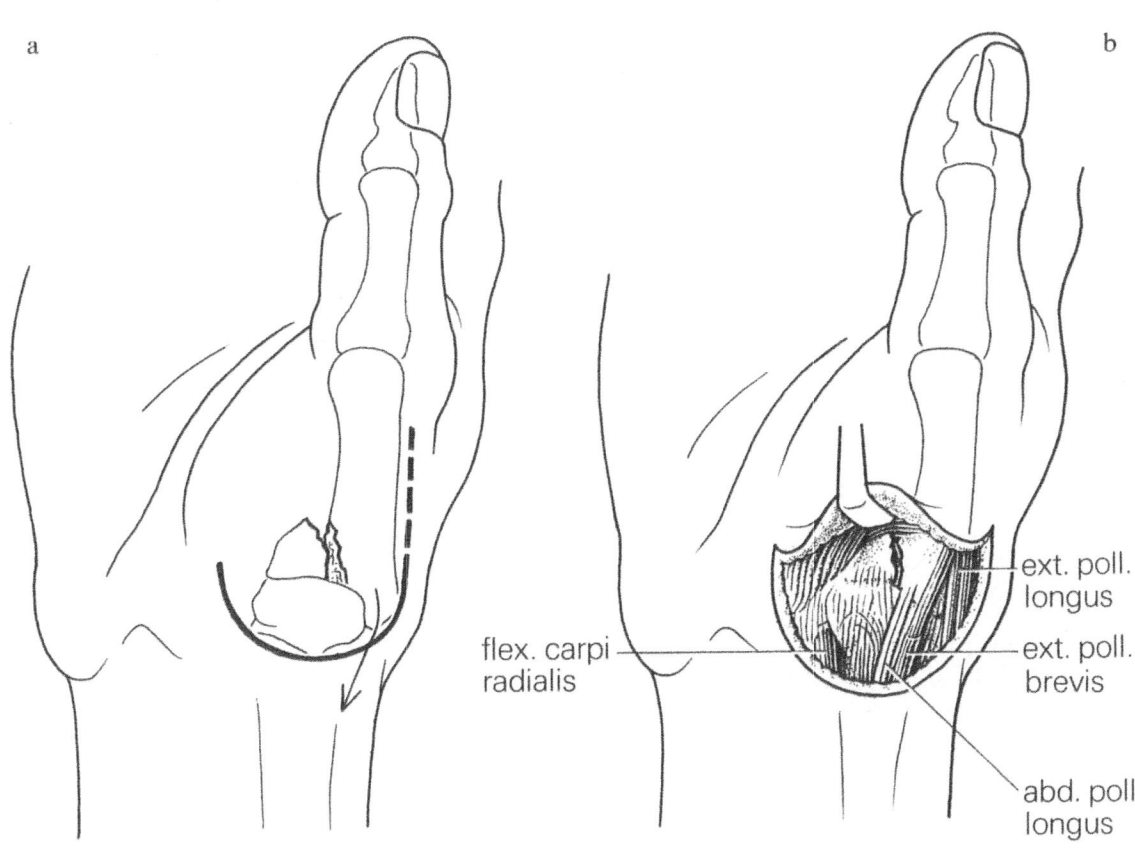

a

b

flex. carpi
radialis

ext. poll.
longus

ext. poll.
brevis

abd. poll.
longus

Fig. 62   **Bennett's fracture, the Gedda-Moberg radio-palmar approach**

    a   Incision (Distal extension for internal fixation of Rolando's fracture)

    b   Topography: Exposure of joint fragment and tendons

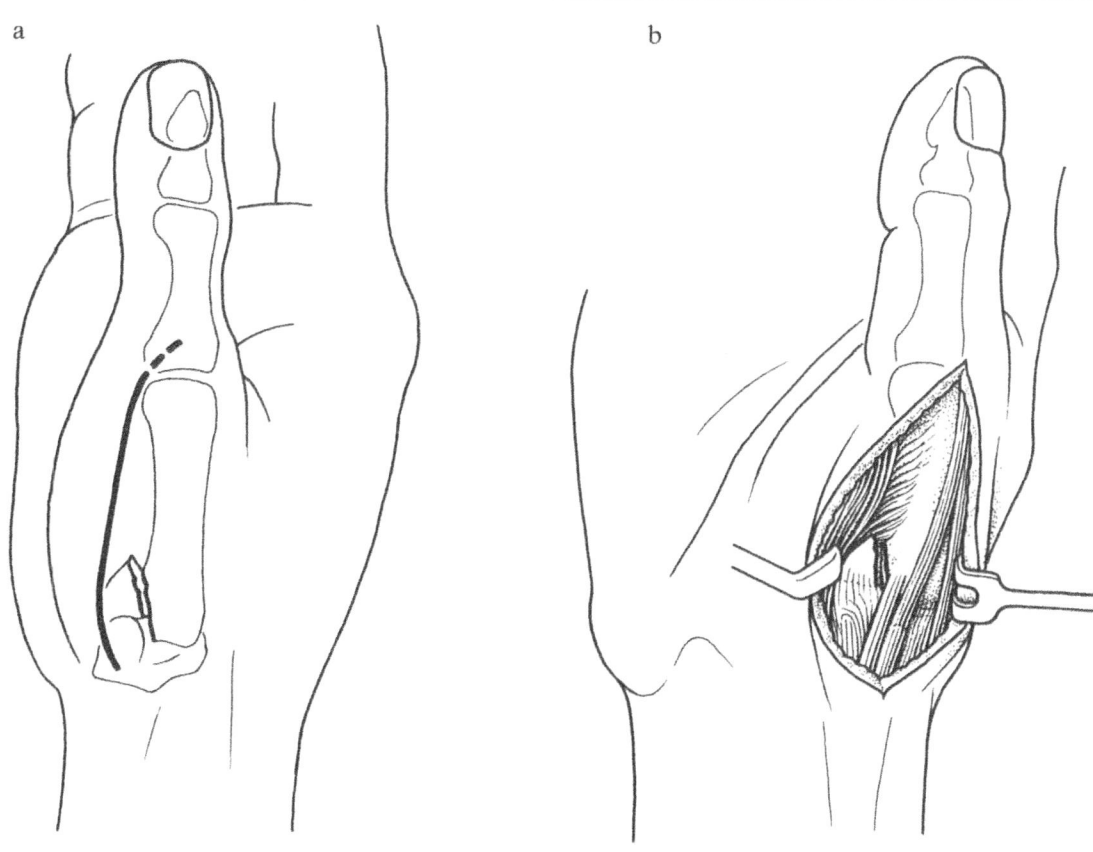

Fig. 63   Bennett's fracture, radio-dorsal approach

    a   Incision

    b   Topography: Exposure of joint fragment and tendons

Fig. 64 Bennett's fracture: Steps of the internal fixation

    a   Initial situation

    b–d   Internal fixation by Gedda-Moberg's approach. Reduction with forceps, temporary fixation with Kirschner wire from the palmar aspect and screw fixation from the back

    e–g   Internal fixation using the radio-dorsal approach: Reduction with a small hook, temporary fixation with Kirschner wire from the dorsal surface and screw fixation also from this aspect

    h, i   Completed internal fixation: Large fragments require small cancellous screws, small fragments small cortex screws but in this case the gliding hole must be made in the shaft fragment

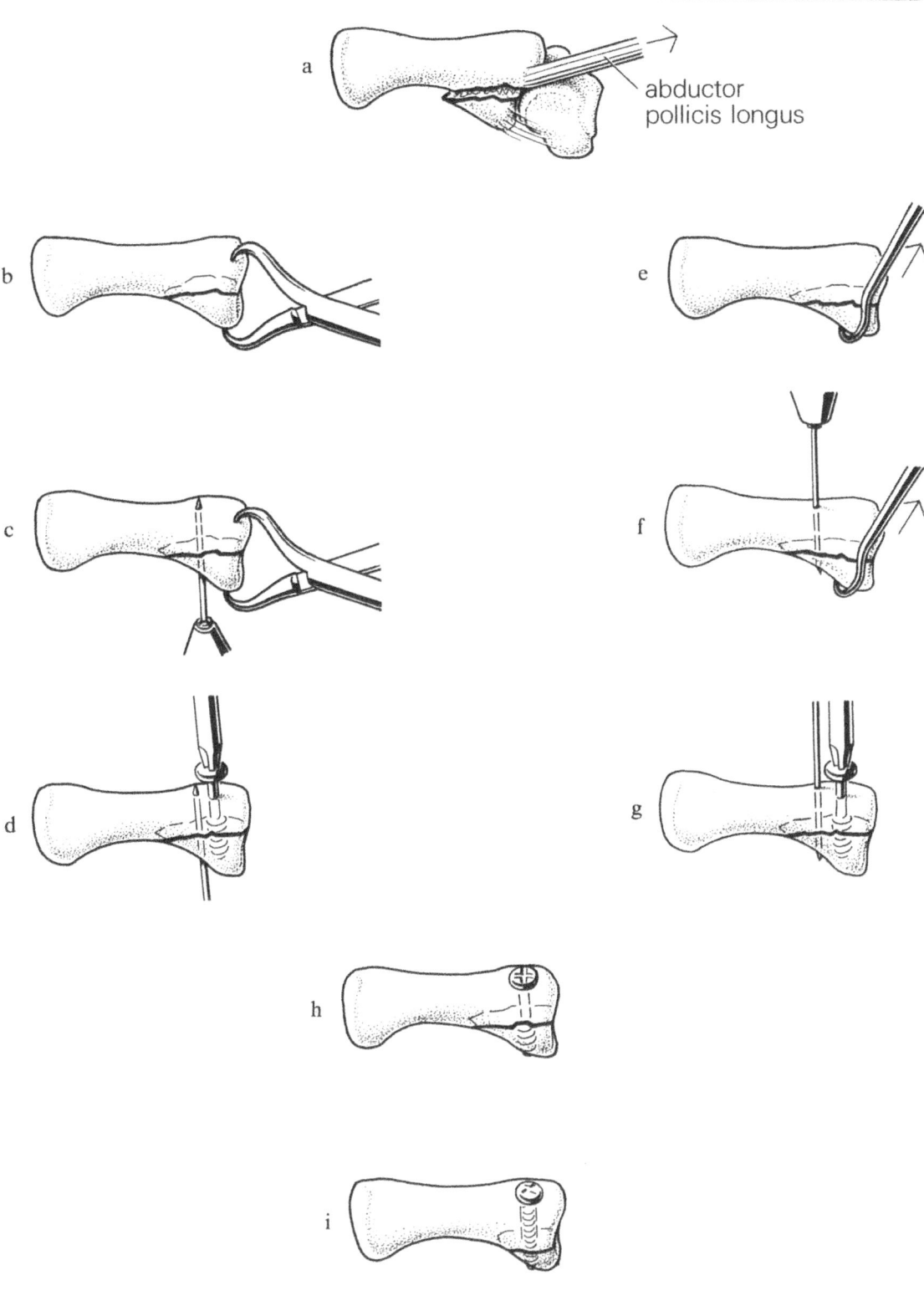

abductor
pollicis longus

123

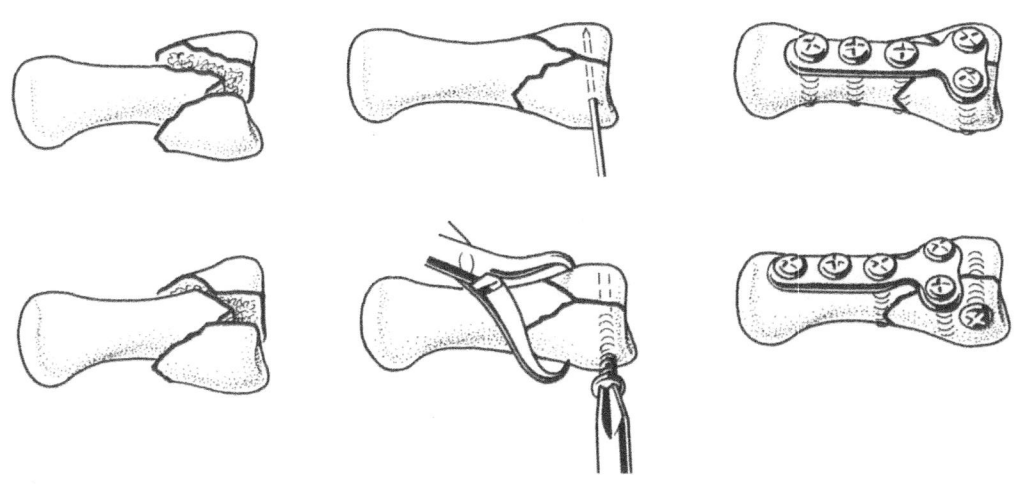

Fig. 65 Rolando's fracture: Method of internal fixation

Depending on the type of fracture, either using a reversed finger T-plate alone or combined with preliminary screw fixation of the joint fragments

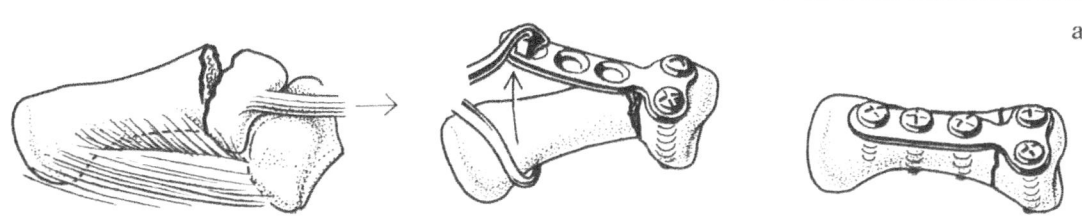

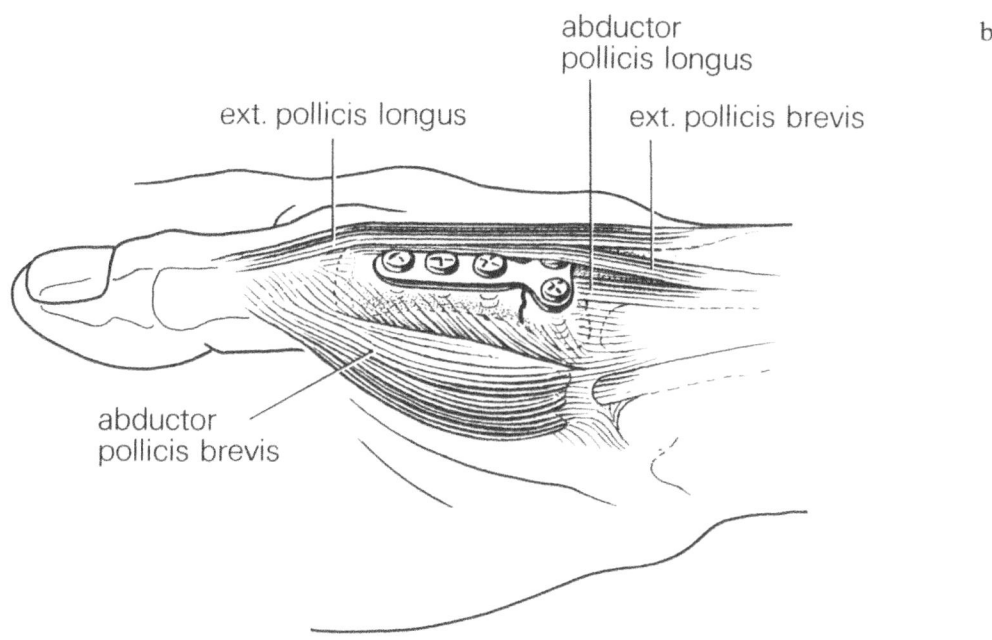

abductor
pollicis longus

ext. pollicis longus

ext. pollicis brevis

abductor
pollicis brevis

Fig. 66 **Extra-articular fracture of the base of the thumb metacarpal: internal fixation**

a The reversed finger T-plate is first fixed to the proximal fragment and then used as a lever to achieve reduction

b Topography of the internal fixation using a plate on the base of the first metacarpal

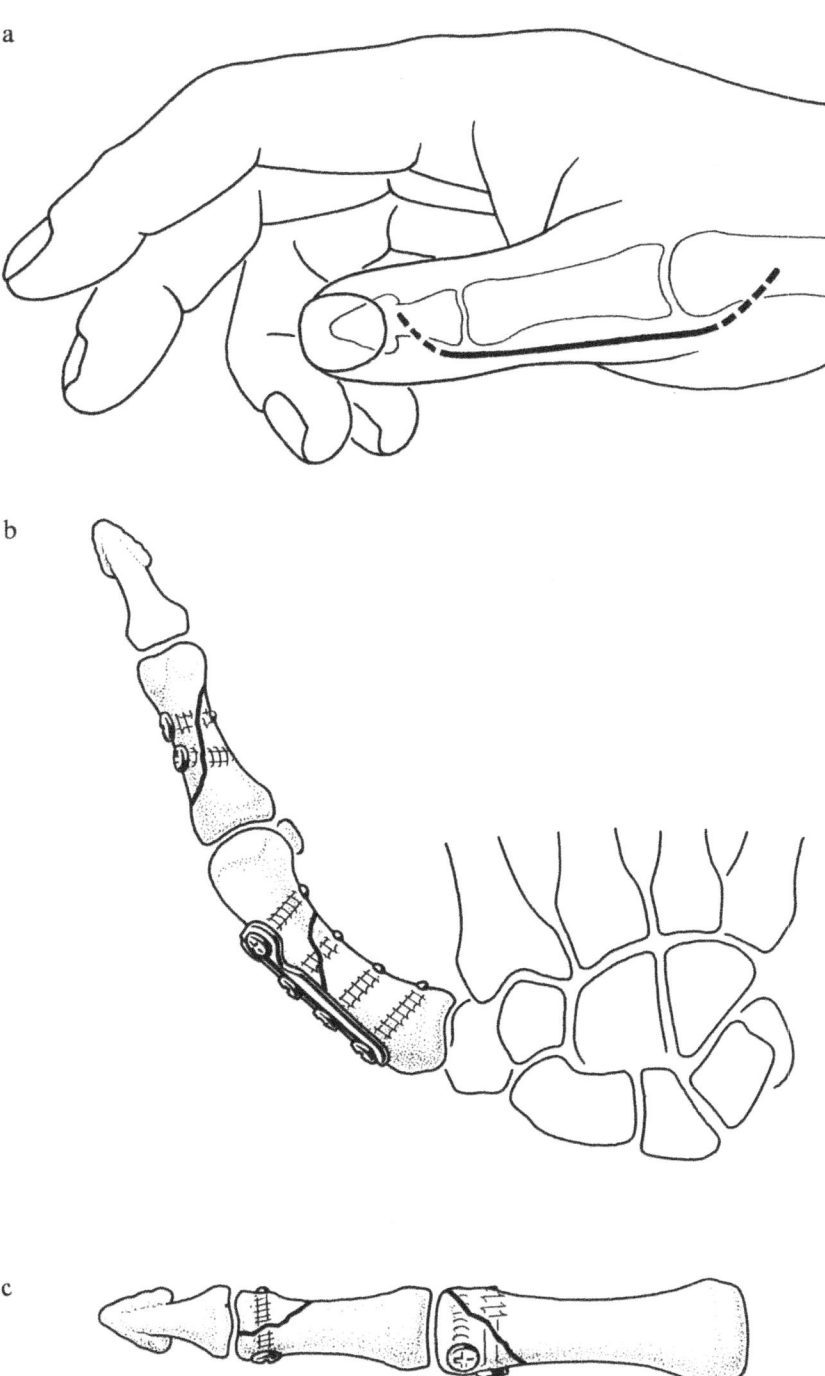

Fig. 67   Internal fixation of the bones of the thumb

    a   Incision

    b   Internal fixation of fractures of the shaft

    c   Internal fixation of articular fractures

Fig. 68 **Arthrodesis of the carpo-metacarpal joint**

Excision of joint, compressed bridging graft using a tension-band plate

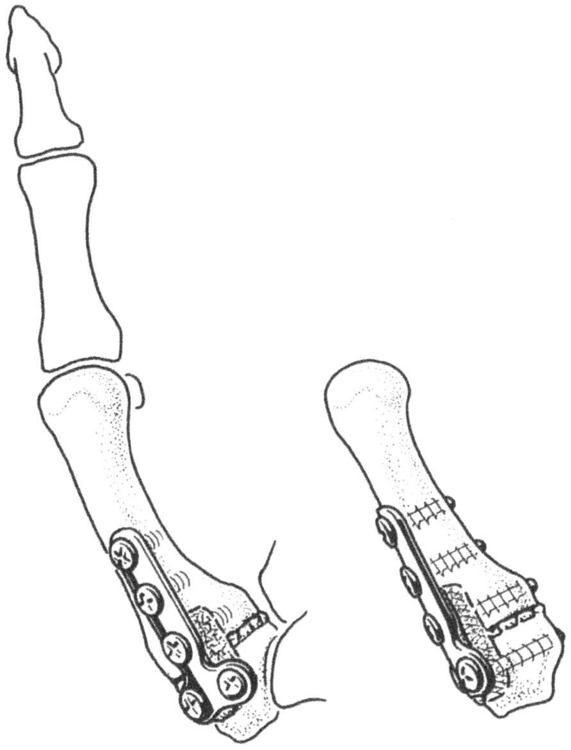

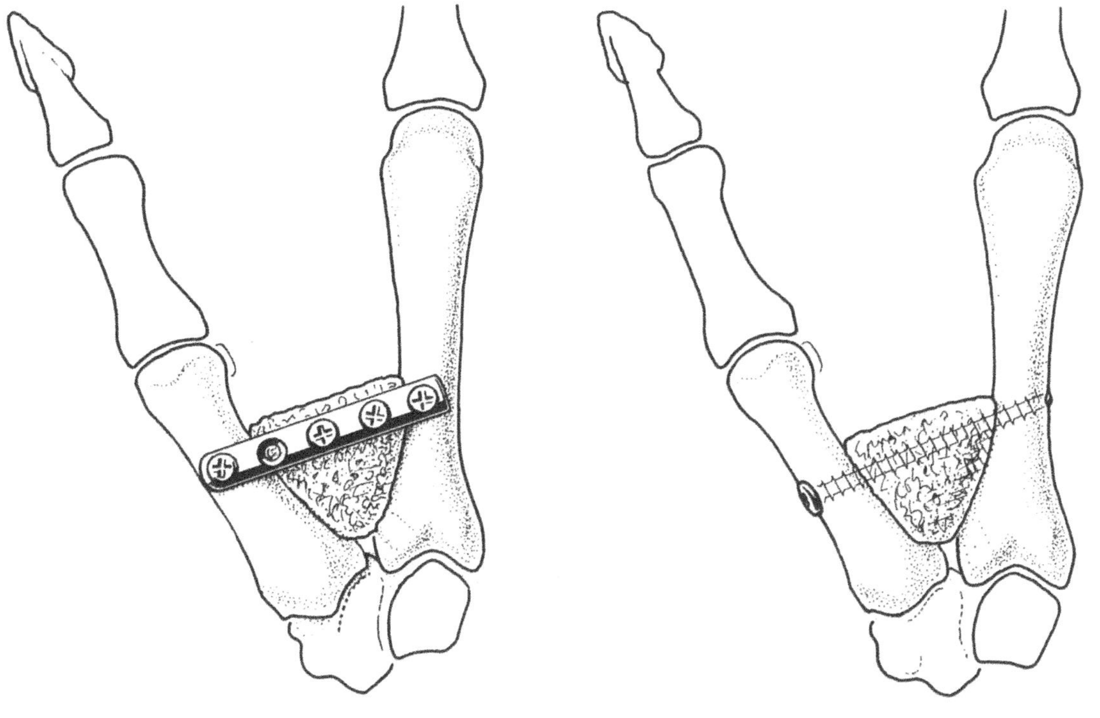

Fig. 69   Opposition block procedure in contracture of the first web space

Graft interposed between the first and second metacarpal, fixed either with a small semitubular plate or with a small cortex screw

a

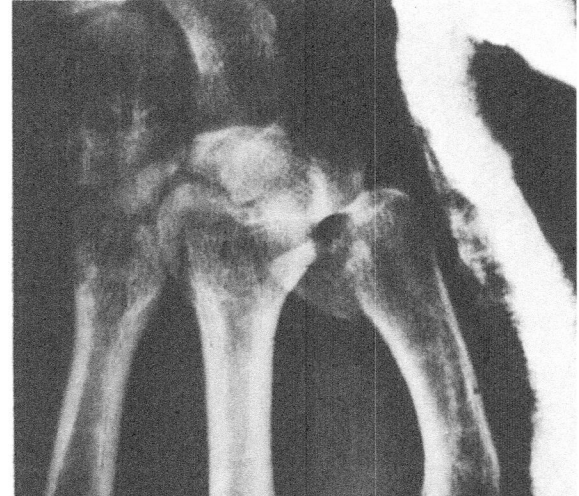

b

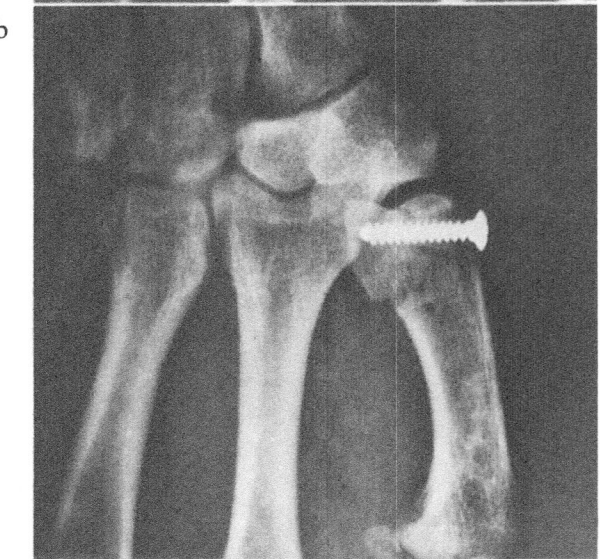

c

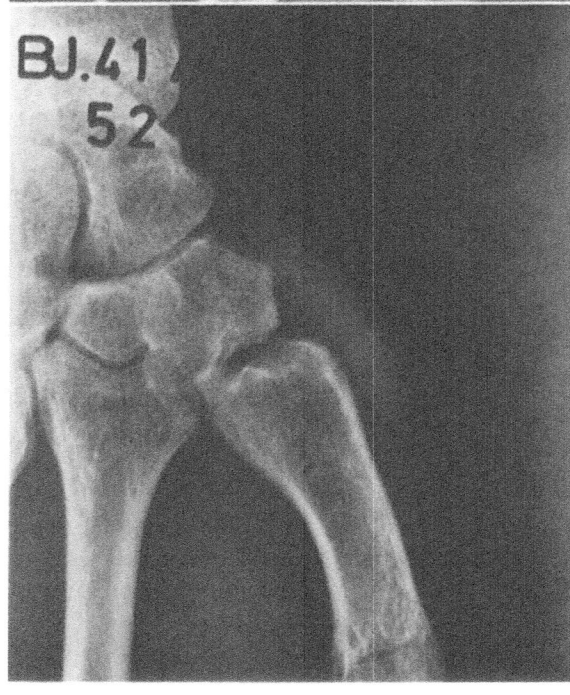

Fig. 70 **Clinical example:**
Bennett's fracture
Patient was a male electrical engineer, aged 29. Traffic accident

a Bennett's fracture with a rather small articular fragment

b Primary internal fixation with a small cortex screw
A small scar neuroma of a superficial branch of the radial nerve. Screw removed at twelve months

c Final review: Symptom-free, full function, no arthrosis

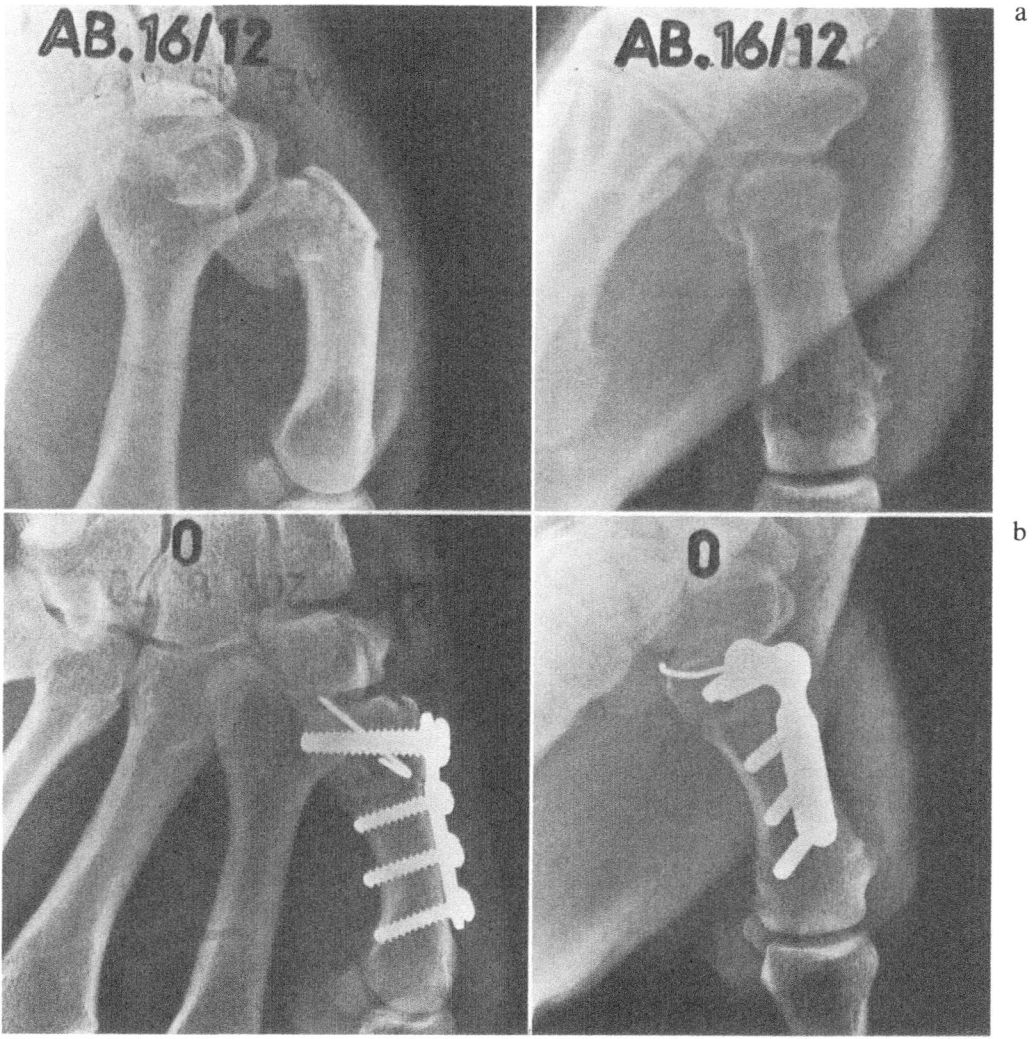

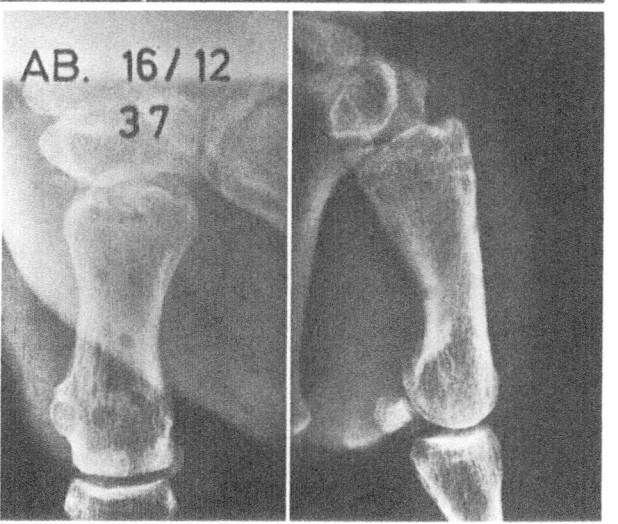

Fig. 71 Clinical example:
Rolando's fracture
Patient was a male workman in the chemical industry, aged 38. Traffic accident

a Rolando's fracture

b Internal fixation five days after the injury: a reversed L-plate and Kirschner wire
No complications

c Removal of metal after eight months
Final review after eleven months, symptom-free, full working ability, identical function in both hands

Fig. 72 **Clinical example: Extra-articular fracture of the base of the thumb metacarpal**
Patient was a nightclub pianist, aged 30. Skiing accident

a Extra-articular fracture of the first metacarpal with malposition in adduction

b Primary internal fixation with a reversed T-plate
No complications. Resumption of work as night-club pianist after one week

c Removal of metal and final check after eight months: Symptom-free, full function, no arthrosis

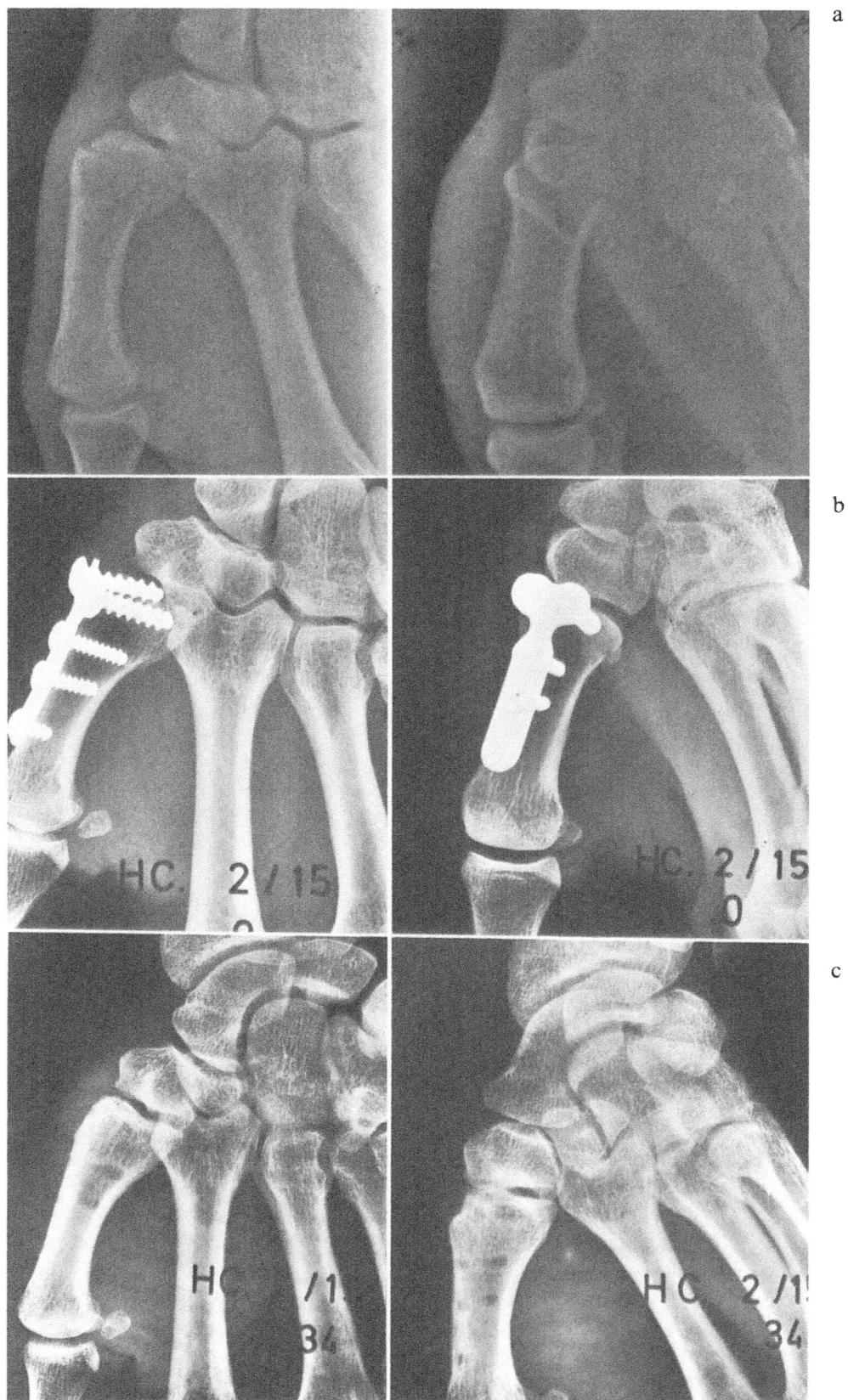

Fig. 73 **Clinical example: Multiple fractures of metacarpals**
Patient was a building worker, aged 29, his hand was caught in the gears of a crane

a   Open fractures of all metacarpals together with laceration of the first web space, avulsion of adductor pollicis and of dorsal interosseus from their origin

b   Primary internal fixation: Reversed T-plate applied to thumb metacarpal, and fixation of all the other metacarpals by double Kirschner wires following the "Eiffel Tower" method

c, d   No complications in fracture healing. Trophic disturbances. Z-plasty undertaken at a later date because of contracture of the first web space. Removal of Kirschner wires at two months (c) Removal of plate at one year (d)
Final review at fourteen months: Symptom-free, Limitation of power and moderate restriction of movement in several finger joints

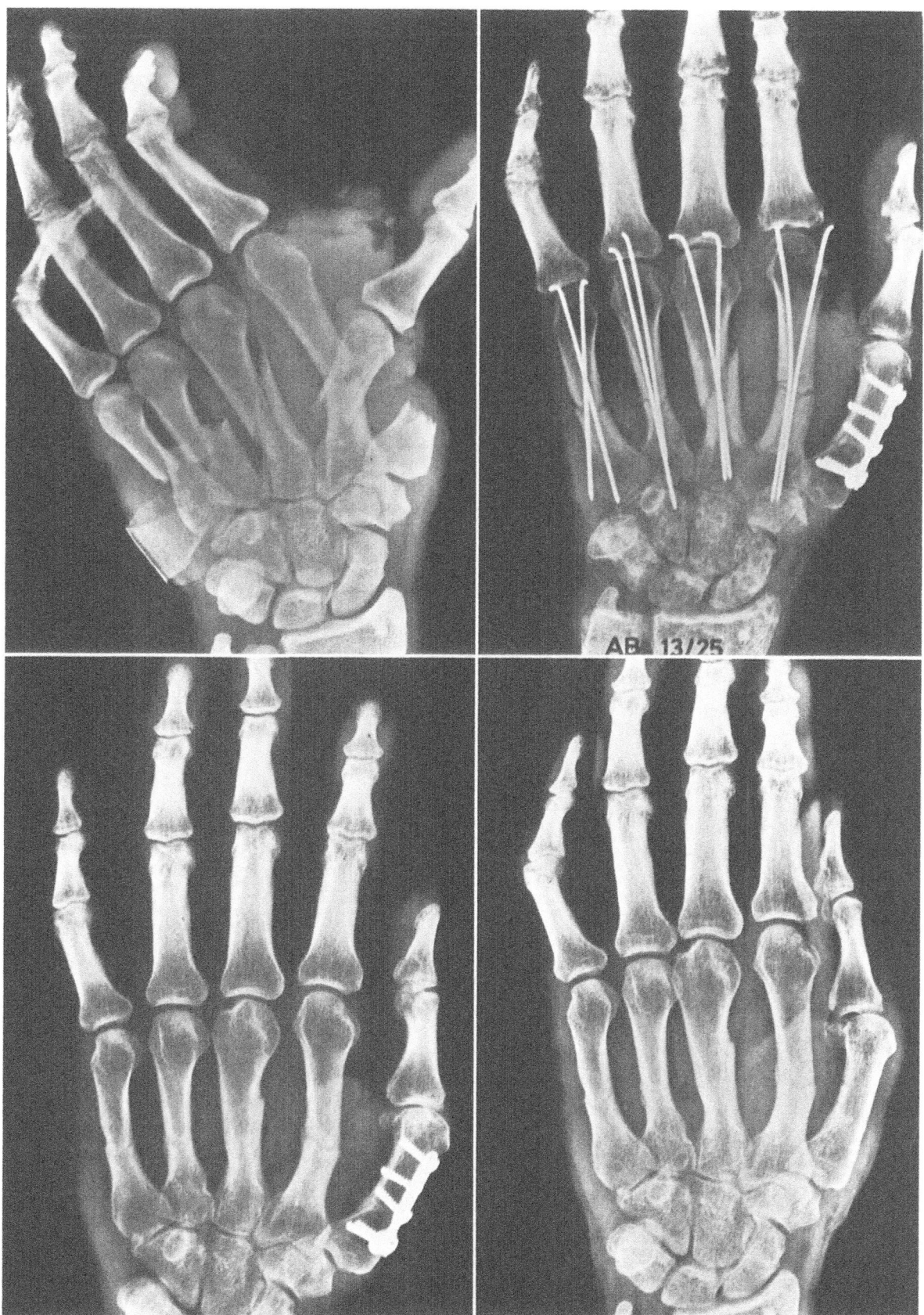

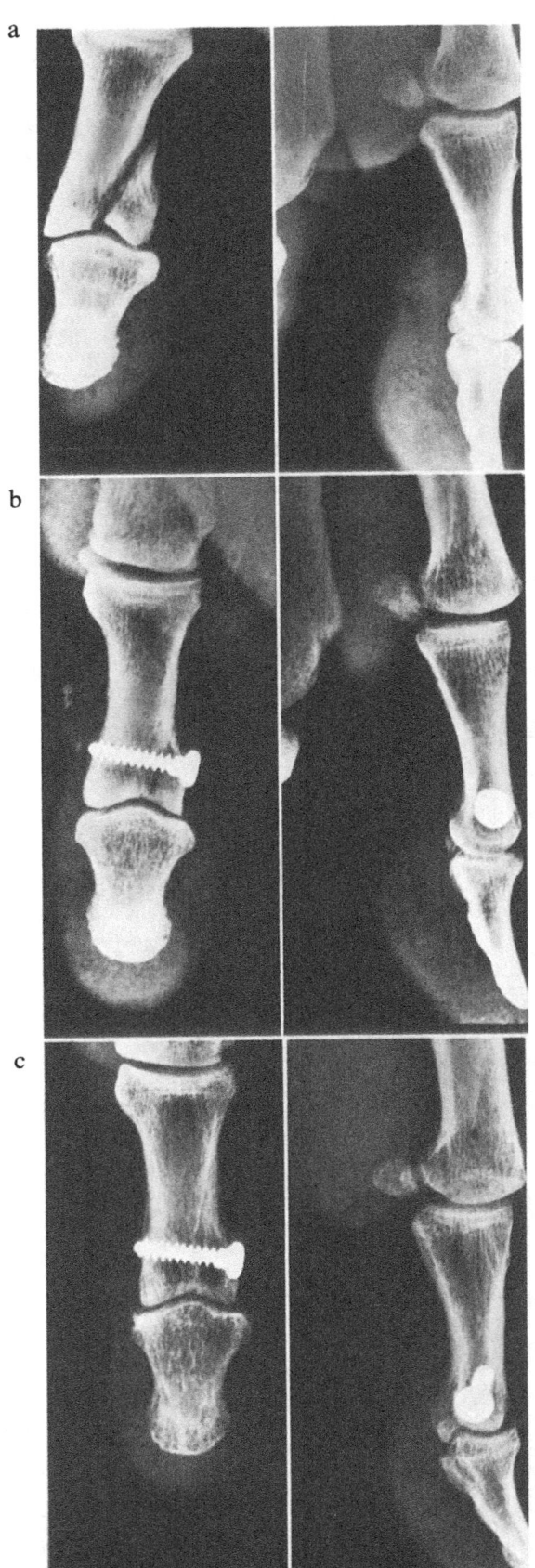

Fig. 74 Clinical example: Articular fracture of the head of the proximal phalanx of the thumb
The patient was a merchant, aged 34, who had fallen on his hand

a Open fracture of the head of the proximal phalanx of the thumb

b Primary treatment of the wound. Internal fixation with a screw three weeks after the accident
No complications

c Final review at sixteen months: Symptom-free. Flexion of I.P. joint −20°, otherwise movement identical on both sides. Moderate arthrosis. Screw left in situ

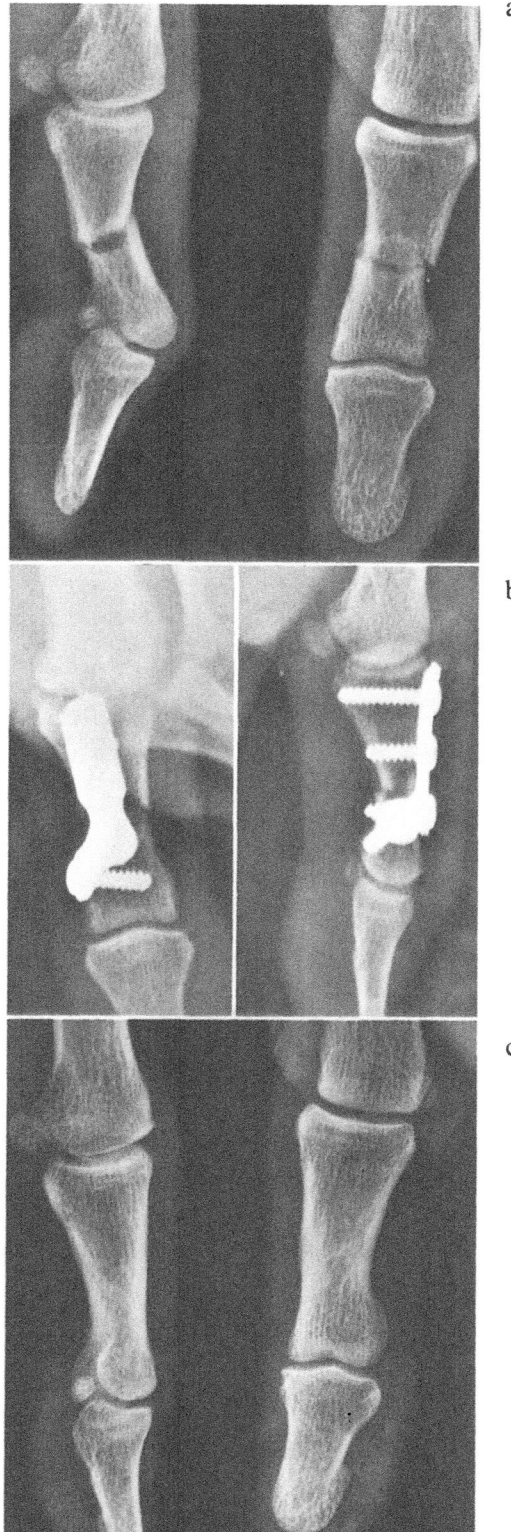

Fig. 75 **Clinical example: Transverse fracture of shaft of proximal phalanx of thumb**

Patient was an apprentice, aged 17. He had been hit on the thumb while playing ice-hockey

a   Transverse fracture of proximal phalanx of the thumb. The fracture was reduced and a plaster cast applied. Reduction could not be maintained and there was also a flexed position of the interphalangeal joint

b   Internal fixation undertaken with an oblique finger L-plate after two days
No complications. Early mobilization without any external support. Removal of metal after six months

c   Final review at $2^1/_2$ years: Symptom-free, identical function in both hands

135

Fig. 76 **Clinical example: Fracture of the shaft of the proximal phalanx of the thumb involving both joints**
Patient was a foreman bricklayer, aged 35. Injury was caused by a milling tool

a Open articular fracture of the proximal phalanx of the thumb with injury to the skin and laceration of the extensor tendon

b Primary internal fixation with a small cortex screw and Kirschner wire, suture of the extensor tendon and a skin graft
No complications

c Removal of the Kirschner wire after one month, removal of the screw after $3^1/_2$ months
Final review after seven months: Patient was symptom-free, and was working fully. Flexion of the metacarpophalangeal joint $-20°$, extension $-5°$

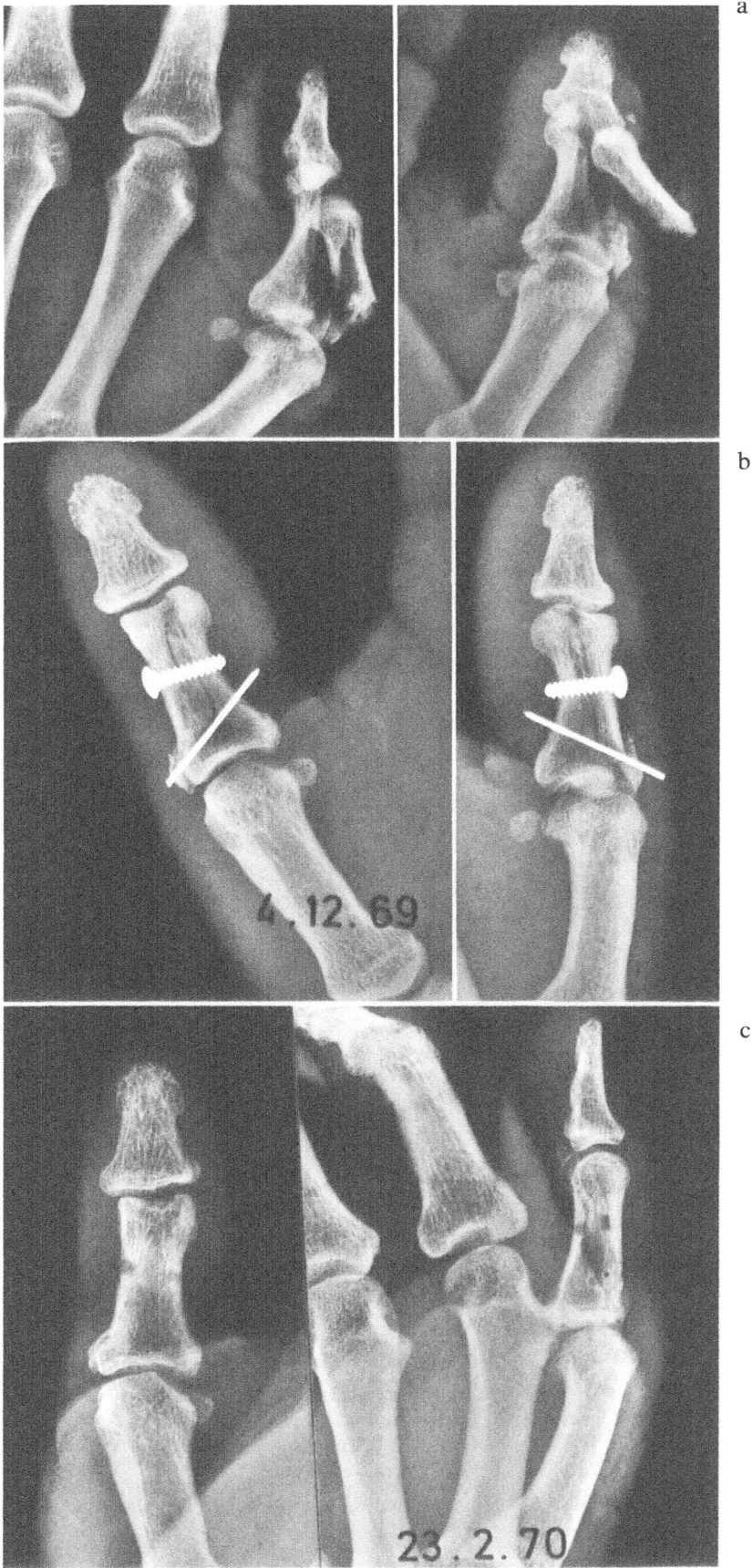

a

b

4. 12. 69

c

23 . 2. 70

Fig. 77   Clinical example: Arthrodesis of carpo-metacarpal joint
Patient was an ironer, aged 39. She had fallen on her hand and sustained a Bennett's fracture. She had been treated conservatively in plaster

a   After $1^1/_2$ years the patient was transferred because of a painful pseudarthrosis

b   Arthrodesis of the carpo-metacarpal joint. The joint was excised and a compressed bridging graft applied, fixed by a reversed finger T-plate
No complications. No external splinting required. Bony consolidation and restoration of full working capacity was obtained after three months

c   Removal of metal and final review after eight months. Mild symptoms. Complete bony union. Full function of peripheral joints

138

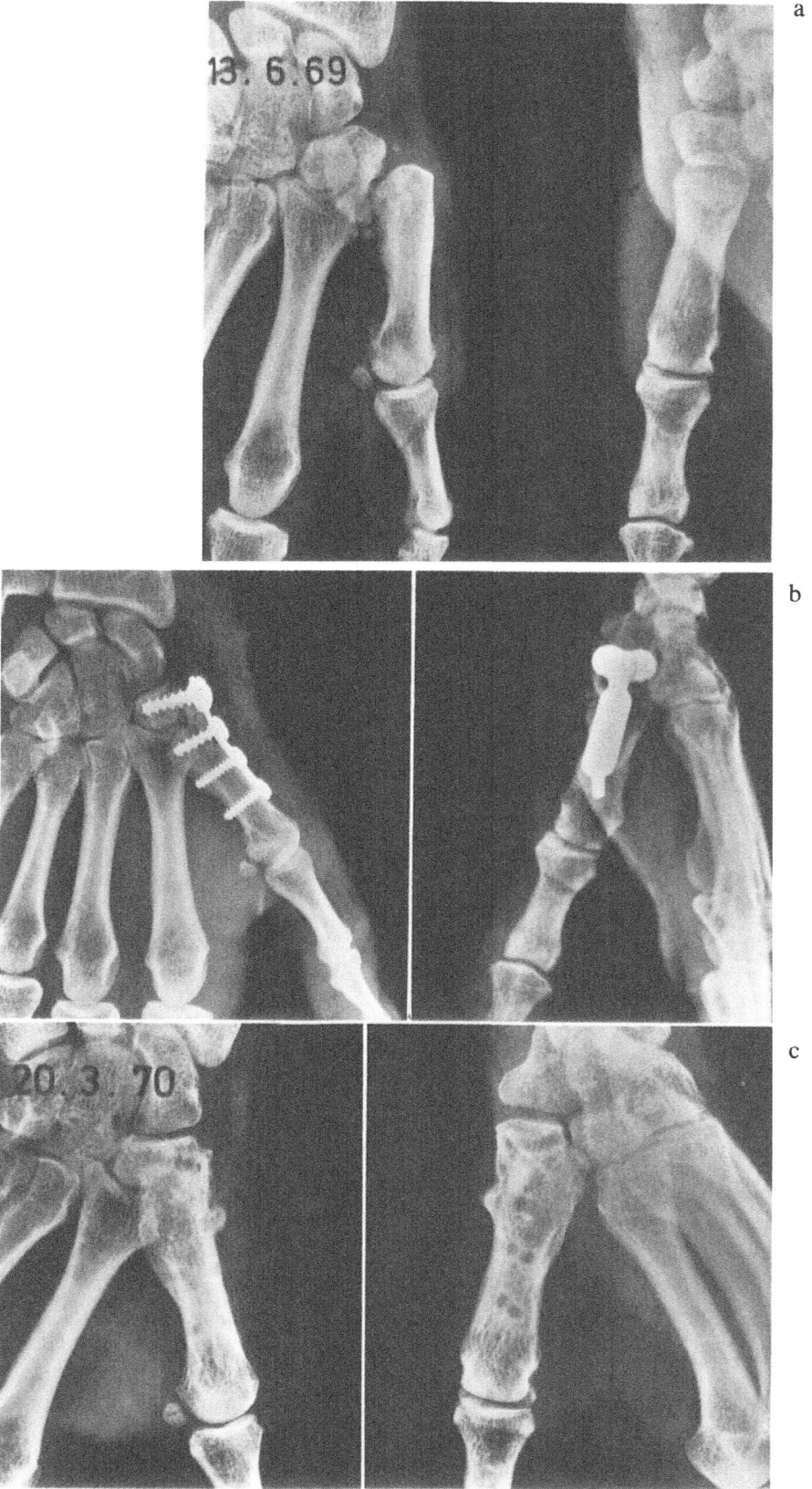

Fig. 78   Clinical example: Arthrodesis of M.P. joint of the thumb with a plate
The patient was a female warehouse worker, aged 47. She had fallen on her hand and ruptured
the ligaments of the M.P. joint of the thumb with subsequent dislocation and painful arthrosis

a   Arthrodesis of the M.P. joint by joint excision and tension-band plate
No complications

b   Removal of the metal at thirteen months
Final review at twenty months: Patient was pain-free and had a normal tip-to-tip pinch of all
the fingers. Flexion in the I.P. joint $-20°$

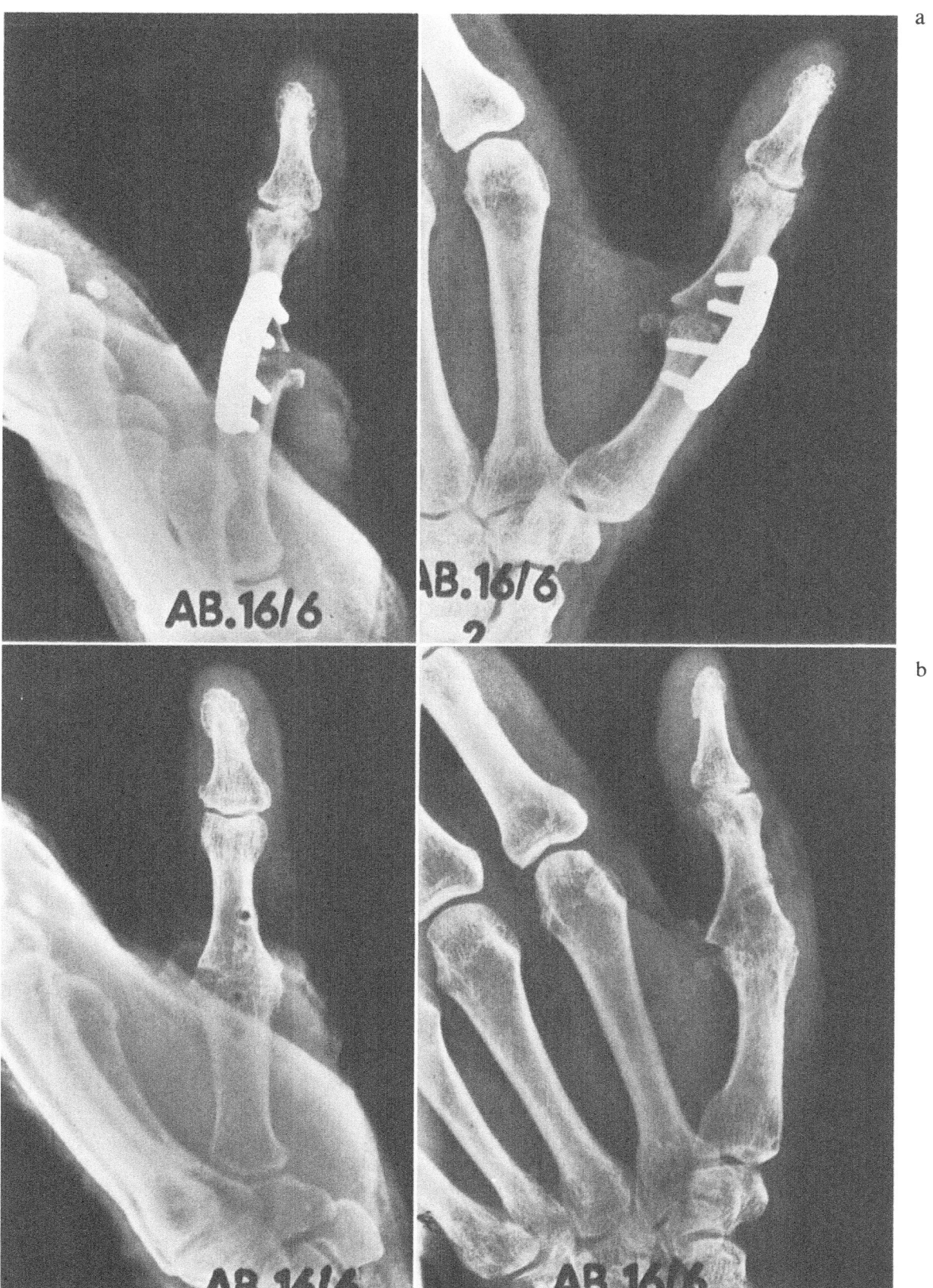

a

b

141

Fig. 79 **Clinical example: Screw arthrodesis of interphalangeal joint**
The patient was a bricklayer, aged 21. Injury to right thumb and index finger when these were caught in a milling tool. There was additional damage to the extensor aponeurosis. Flexion contracture of the thumb and index finger developed at the interphalangeal joints

a Screw arthrodesis of the I.P. joint of the thumb and the terminal interphalangeal joint of the index after five months
No complications

b Removal of the metal and final review after ten months

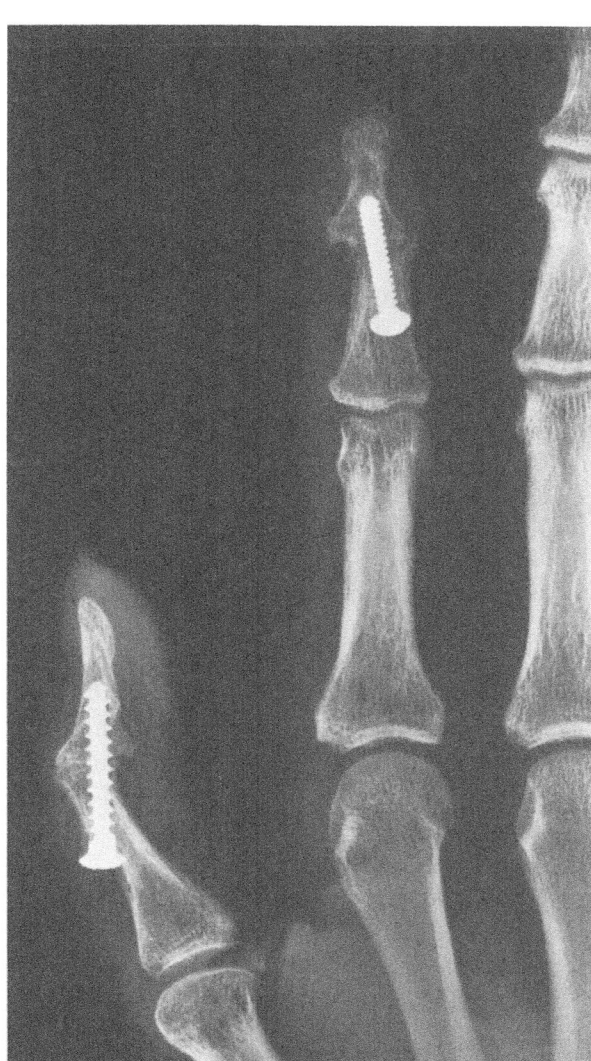

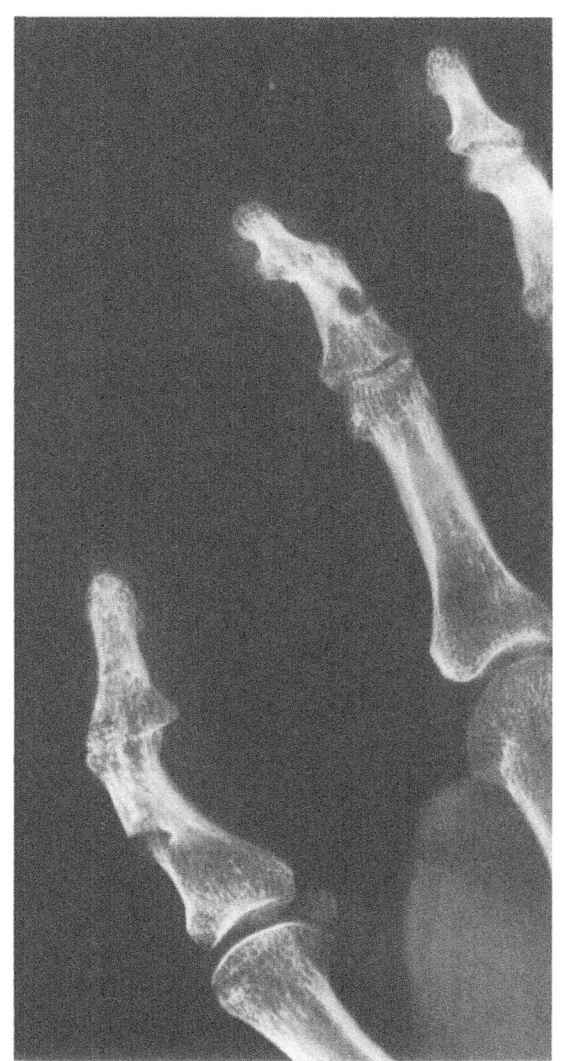

143

C. Injuries to, and Internal Fixation of the II–V Rays

These rays which are also called the palmar rays as they form the palm proximally and emerge from it distally, form a distinct functional unit. This chapter, therefore, deals with them collectively. Detailed advice is provided for the II ray and more expecially for the V ray.

The SFS has acquired an important place in the management of metacarpal fractures in which access is quite convenient and where the technical aspects of the operation usually present no great difficulty. Excellent final results can be obtained by functional treatment after operation.

The indications for internal fixation of the fractures of the phalanges, however, are subject to more discussion. In most cases, the approach inflicts additional trauma to tendons, and the extensor tendons particularly show a considerable tendency towards adhesion to underlying bone. Final results of postoperative treatment can be unsatisfactory and the operation itself can be very difficult. A careful selection of indications, therefore, and a large measure of self-criticism are the chief requirements.

1. Approaches

As the approaches are little known, they are here described in detail.

a) Approach to the II and V Metacarpal

A postero-lateral longitudinal incision with a curve at the distal or proximal end. Fine nerve fibres, especially over the V metacarpal are carefully retracted and the extensors must be elevated. The underlying bone is thus easily approached (Fig. 80).

b) Approaches to the III and IV Metacarpals

For operation on these metacarpals, either separately or together, as well as in combination with the II and III, and the IV and V, S shaped incisions have proved to be the best with regard to exposure and cosmetic result. Distal extension of these incisions to a finger is practicable. In multiple fractures of metacarpals it is sometimes unavoidable to use an approach which is less suitable cosmetically, i.e. a transverse incision with T- or L-shaped extensions at each side of the metacarpus (Fig. 80).

It is of utmost importance to protect the fine nerves at the back of the hand and above all the veins, since the latter carry the main return of blood from the peripheral hand. To protect the paratenon the exposed extensor tendons must be retracted with fine Hohmann retractors. In rare cases, the peripheral attachment of an intertendinous connection must be divided (Fig. 81).

c) Approach to the Metacarpal Head

Articular and neck fractures of metacarpals require special approaches:

— For the second and fifth metacarpals, incision has to extend beyond the joint at its end, so that it is curved at this point (Fig. 80).

— For the treatment of multiple fractures, a transverse incision over the metacarpal heads is used as in rheumatoid surgery and this has proved to be the best, even from the cosmetic view point (Fig. 80).

— Under certain circumstances, a Y-shaped inter-digital incision may give appropriate access where, however, the web space must be preserved.

The extensor hood must be sufficiently exposed. It is lifted up gently from the underlying bone or incised longitudinally if necessary. Thus the metacarpo-phalangeal joint can be exposed without any detriment and this facilitates open reduction. The collateral Ligaments must be preserved.

d) Approaches to the Proximal and Middle Phalanges

In most operations on fingers, we use dorso-lateral incisions with curved ends (Fig. 82a and b). Double S-shaped incisions which avoid joint creases and can be extended to the back of the hand may occasionally be of advantage (Fig. 82c). To reduce skin damage, the incisions must extend beyond the relative joint. Wherever possible, the dorsal subcutaneous venous network must be preserved. Protection of the palmar neurovascular bundle is obtained by keeping it continuously connected to the skin. This standard incision give us four different approaches to the bone. The choice of one of these depends upon the type and site of the fracture.

— Dorsal longitudinal incision through the extensor aponeurosis to expose the proximal part of the proximal phalanx (Fig. 83a).
— Lateral approach with partial incision of the lateral band of the interosseus tendon, exposing the middle of the shaft. The divided portion of the tendon has eventually to be closed with fine atraumatic sutures (Fig. 83b).
— Lateral approach to the distal part of the proximal phalanx with elevation of the lateral band without dividing it (Fig. 83c).
— Palmar approach. Exposure of the flexor sheath and retraction of the flexor tendons with a blunt hook. This approach gives a good access to articular fragments in the proximal interphalangeal joint. Tendon sheaths must not be sutured. Early postoperative movements prevents subsequent adhesion of tendons (Fig. 83d).

e) Exposure of the P.I.P. Joint

can be obtained by two different approaches, neither of which presents any difficulty.

— Either between the middle and lateral band of the extensor communis tendon, or between the lateral band and the collateral ligament.
— Under certain circumstances, division of the lateral ligament may be required to complete the exposure of the P.I.P. joint. This calls for the final suture of the ligament (Fig. 83e).

2. Fractures of the Second to Fifth Metacarpals

a) Basal Fractures

These uncommon injuries are mostly compression fractures which are not amenable to internal fixation. Avulsion fractures at the base of the second metacarpal, where the extensor carpi radialis longus is inserted, as well as transverse and oblique fractures of the fifth metacarpal analogous to Bennett's fracture occasionally occur. Because of the special position of the fifth ray, internal fixation with accurate reduction should be carried out wherever possible. Either screw fixation or the application of a reversed finger T-plate can be considered (Fig. 84a).

Where small fragments or comminuted fractures have to be reduced, an extension of the plate fixation up to the wrist may be required.

b) Shaft Fractures

We often have to deal with spiral fractures of the middle metacarpals. A 2.7 mm screw or on occasions a 2 mm screw are the best means of providing fixation, as rotational deformities can then be prevented. The second and fifth metacarpals are more exposed to external forces and these should, therefore, be fixed with plates. Either a tension-band or neutralization plate combined with screw fixation are used, while a transverse fracture is fixed with a straight or T-plate (Fig. 84). Small semi-tubular plates may occasionally be used in the very broad metacarpals of manual labourers whose hands are continually exposed to stress.

c) Fracture of the Metacarpal Neck

This fracture often occurs in the fifth metacarpal. As there is always a palmar crack of the head, reduction can be difficult and internal fixation is a matter of dispute. Some surgeons maintain that deformities of up to 30° are acceptable, while others advise percutaneous transverse fixation of the reduced metacarpal head to the neighbouring fourth metacarpal head with a Kirschner wire. We prefer internal fixation with a tension-band in the form of a finger L- or T-plate (Fig. 84), as this gives reliable reduction of the head as well as early postoperative movement. The extensor tendon must be lifted from the underlying bone and the metacarpo-phalangeal joint must be opened to obtain a satisfactory exposure. The surgical techniques are shown in the general section (Fig. 19).

When early movement is not imperative, open reduction and transfixation with one or two medullary wires inserted from the tubercles is still a successful procedure in fractures of the necks of the third and fourth metacarpals; the medullary wires must be removed after four weeks. In young patients this is the correct method of managing displaced fractures of metacarpal necks (Durband, Heim, Iselin).

3. Articular Fractures

a) Fractures of the Metacarpo-Phalangeal and Proximal Interphalangeal Joints of the Second to Fifth Metacarpals

Internal fixation is imperative in articular fractures of the metacarpal heads as well as in depressed fractures of the bases of the proximal phalanges. Here the main aim is a precise reconstruction of the joint surface which may, however, be very difficult to obtain. This is also true for displaced fractures of the proximal interphalangeal joint, the approach to which is especially intricate. Screw fixation will be best, but sometimes it is only possible to employ Kirschner wires or fine cerclage wiring. Further experience with the small 2.0 mm cortex screw may open up new possibilities here.

b) Comminuted Articular Fractures

When such fractures occur in the M.P. and I.P. joints, primary arthrodesis is sometimes the best method. In the P.I.P. joint it is carried out by means of a small tension-band plate or a single axial screw. Because of the nail matrix, screw fixation in the terminal interphalangeal joint is difficult. In such cases Kirschner wire fixation is still the best procedure.

4. Shaft Fractures of the Proximal and Middle Phalanges

Since reduction of oblique and spiral fractures is difficult, and as such fractures often produce secondary shortening and rotational deformity, operation is indicated. In most cases, screw fixation is the best procedure, while the use of plates is limited for anatomical reasons (Fig. 84). There is also disagreement about the indications for the infrequent transverse fractures. Conservative treatment is to be preferred in those cases where early mobilization is unnecessary. Oblique or crossed Kirschner wires are quite suitable in open reduction of displaced fragments. Transfixion of the terminal interphalangeal joint is usually contraindicated (Doliveux).

5. Secondary Operations of the Second to Fifth Rays

a) Pseudarthrosis

Pseudarthroses in the second and fifth metacarpals are commoner than those in the third and fourth. There is always a palmar crack of the distal fragment which gives pain in the palm as well as rotational deformity. After correction of the latter, fixation can be obtained by bone-pegging together with a tension-band plate, or with a compressed bridging graft (Figs. 26 and 28). Early movement guarantees a rapid return of function.

The infrequent pseudarthrosis in a finger is treated according to the principles for the metacarpal, though smaller implants should be used.

b) Osteotomy

When conservative fracture treatment has resulted in a rotational deformity or when there is a palmar crack and relative shortening, osteotomy in metacarpals and phalanges is indicated. The technique is similar to that used for pseudarthrosis. In the case of metacarpals, functional results are excellent but they are often disappointing in phalanges.

c) Secondary Arthrodesis

Wherever possible arthrodesis of a metacarpophalangeal joint should be avoided as it results in stiffness of the finger. Arthroplasty is sometimes of use. Swanson's joint prosthesis which has proved to be useful in rheumatoid surgery is seldom used in post-traumatic arthrosis, as the traumatic periarticular lesions spoil the functional result. The use of Swanson's silastic prosthesis cannot be recommended on a single M.P. joint because it does not work in synchrony with the neighbouring M.P. joint. If the tendons are uninjured a plastic prosthesis can be used in a proximal interphalangeal joint also.

Secondary arthrodesis is more frequently indicated in interphalangeal joints. The P.I.P. joint is fixed either with a lag screw alone, with a tension-band plate, or with a compressed bridging graft. We prefer however, bone-pegging in the distal interphalangeal joint (Figs. 29 and 31).

6. Statistics about the Second to Fifth Rays

Table 3. Palmar rays (pseudarthrosis and osteotomy included)

	Number of fractures	Screw fixation	Plate fixation	Disturbed bone healing (infection or pseud-arthrosis)	Final functional result			
					A	B	C	D
Internal fixation of fractures								
Fractures of the shafts and bases of metacarpals II–V	79	44	35	8	52	19	4	4
Fractures of the heads and necks of metacarpals II–V	20	9	11	—	13	7	—	—
Fractures of the proximal phalanges of the fingers	38	28	10	4	12	10	12	4
Fractures of the middle phalanx of a finger	7	5	2	2	2	3	2	—
Pseudarthrosis and osteotomy including the thumb								
Metacarpals	16	2	14	—	10	6	—	—
Phalanges	5	1	4	—	1	3	1	—
Arthodeses								
Metacarpophalangeal Joints II–V	3	3	—	—	2	1	—	—
P.I.P. Joint II–V	22	9	13	—	15	7	—	—
D.I.P. joint II–V	14	12	2	2	10	—	4	—

A: Full function, no symptoms.
B: Slightly impaired function, no working handicap, occasional mild symptoms.
C: Considerable functional limitation, some handicap at work, permanent symptoms.
D: Functional result unknown because the patient could not be traced.

Summary of Table 3

The statistics comprise all the patients treated by us until the end of 1971. They confirm that there is a good prognosis with metacarpal fractures which are fixed with screws and plates, while the results in phalanges are significantly poorer. Disturbances in bone healing occurred in less than 10% of our cases and were not always followed by poor final function. The good final results of second operations, especially of arthrodesis, seemed to be of particular value.

7. Clinical X-Ray Examples
Figs. 85–95, pages 157–175

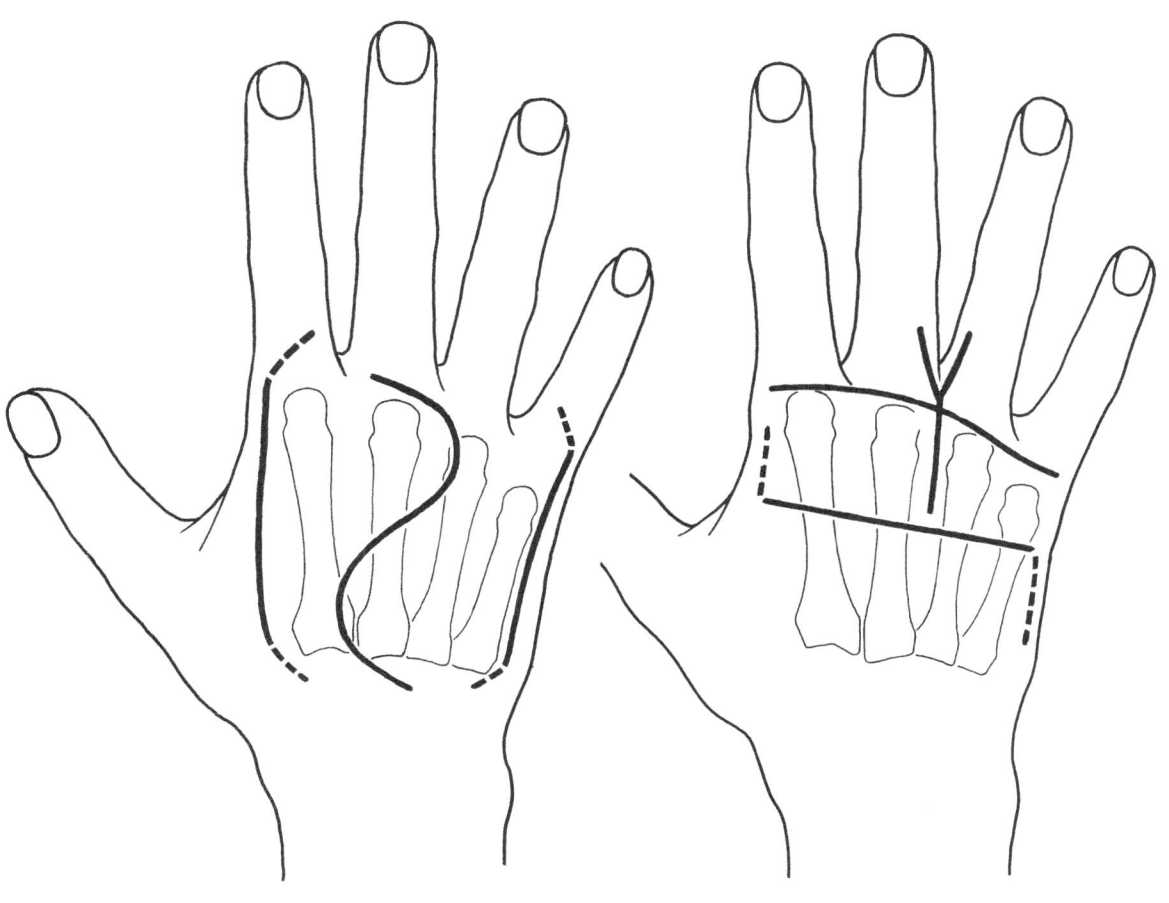

Fig. 80   Fractures of metacarpals: Incisions

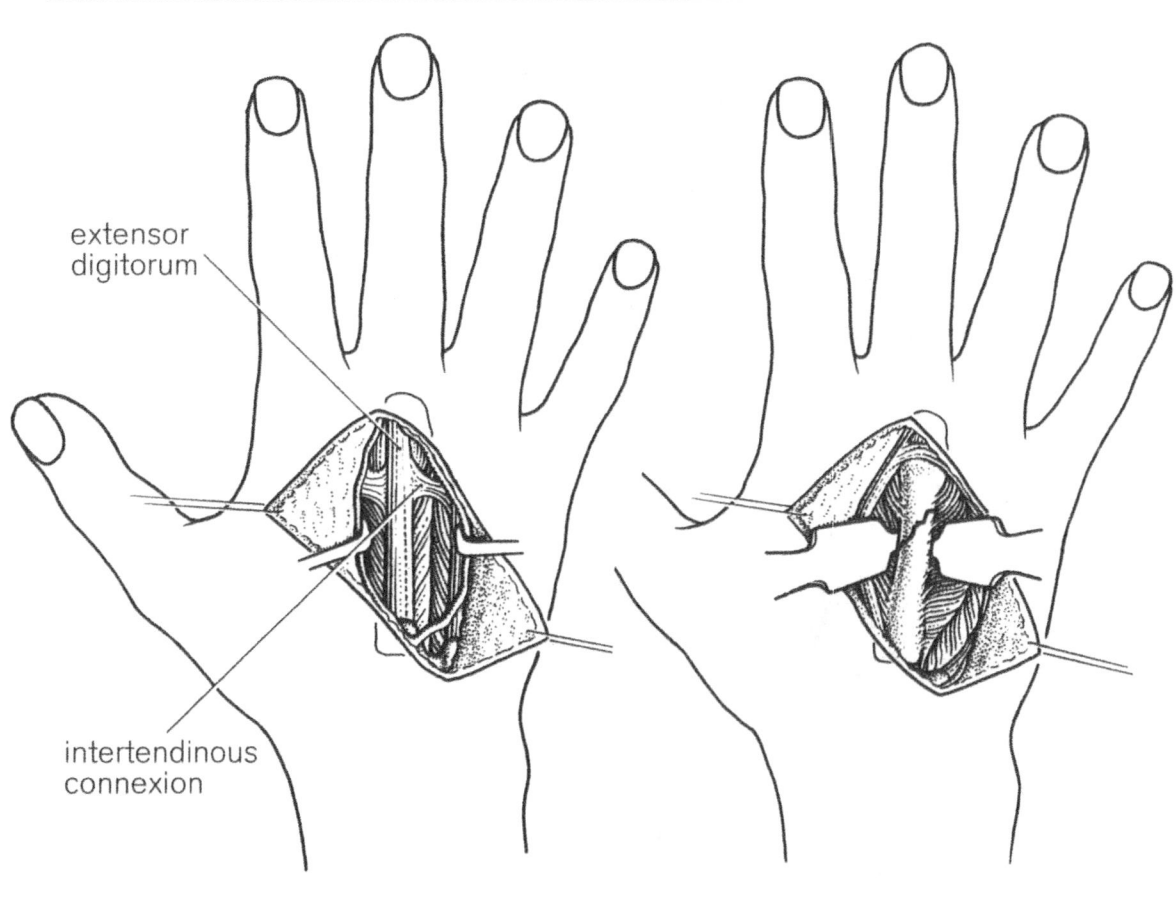

extensor
digitorum

intertendinous
connexion

Fig. 81   Fractures of metacarpals: Approach
Exposure of fracture after retraction of tendons, nerves and veins

150

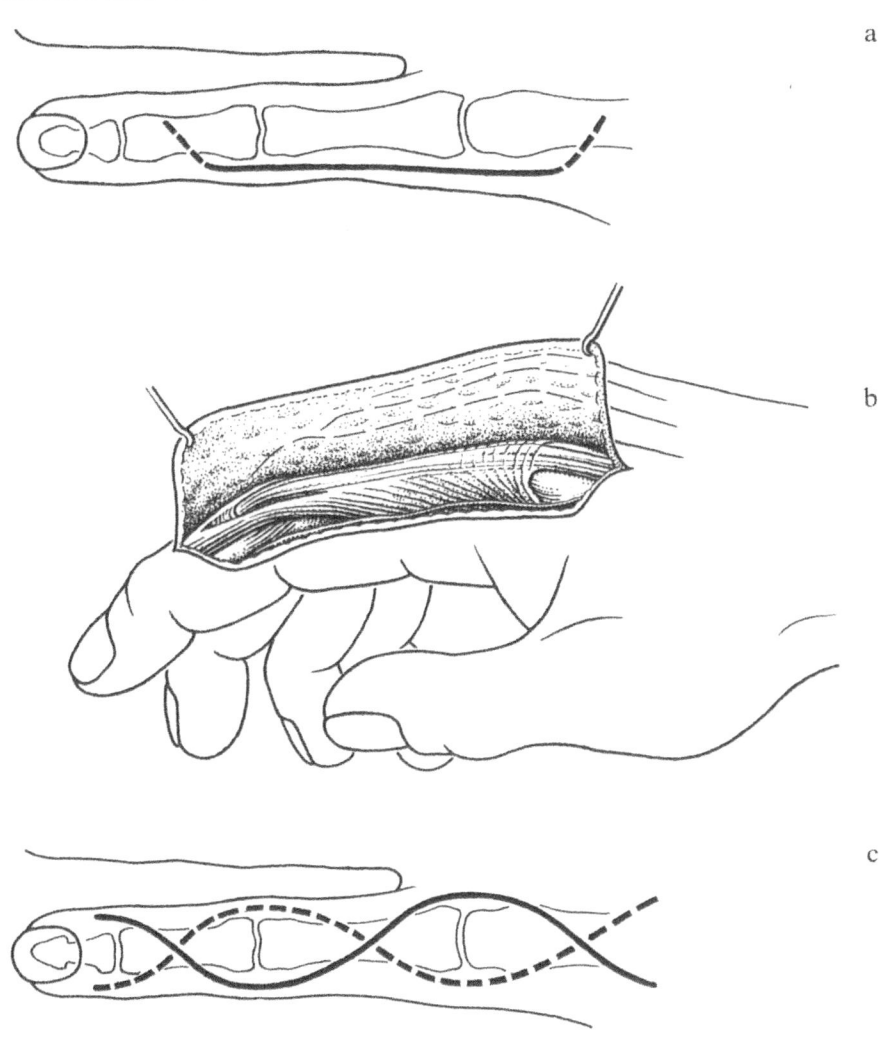

Fig. 82 **Fractures of phalanges**

   a   Postero-lateral incision

   b   Approach to the extensor apparatus

   c   Second type of incision

Fig. 83   Fractures of phalanges: Approaches and topography of the extensor mechanism

    a   Dorsal incision of the extensor aponeurosis in basal fractures of the proximal phalanx

    b   Lateral incision of the interosseous aponeurosis in fractures of the middle of the proximal phalanx

    c   Lateral approach with elevation of interosseous aponeurosis in distal fractures of the proximal phalanx

    d   Approach to articular fractures in the P.I.P. joint: opening of the flexor tendon sheath

    e   Exposure of the P.I.P. joint after division of the collateral ligament

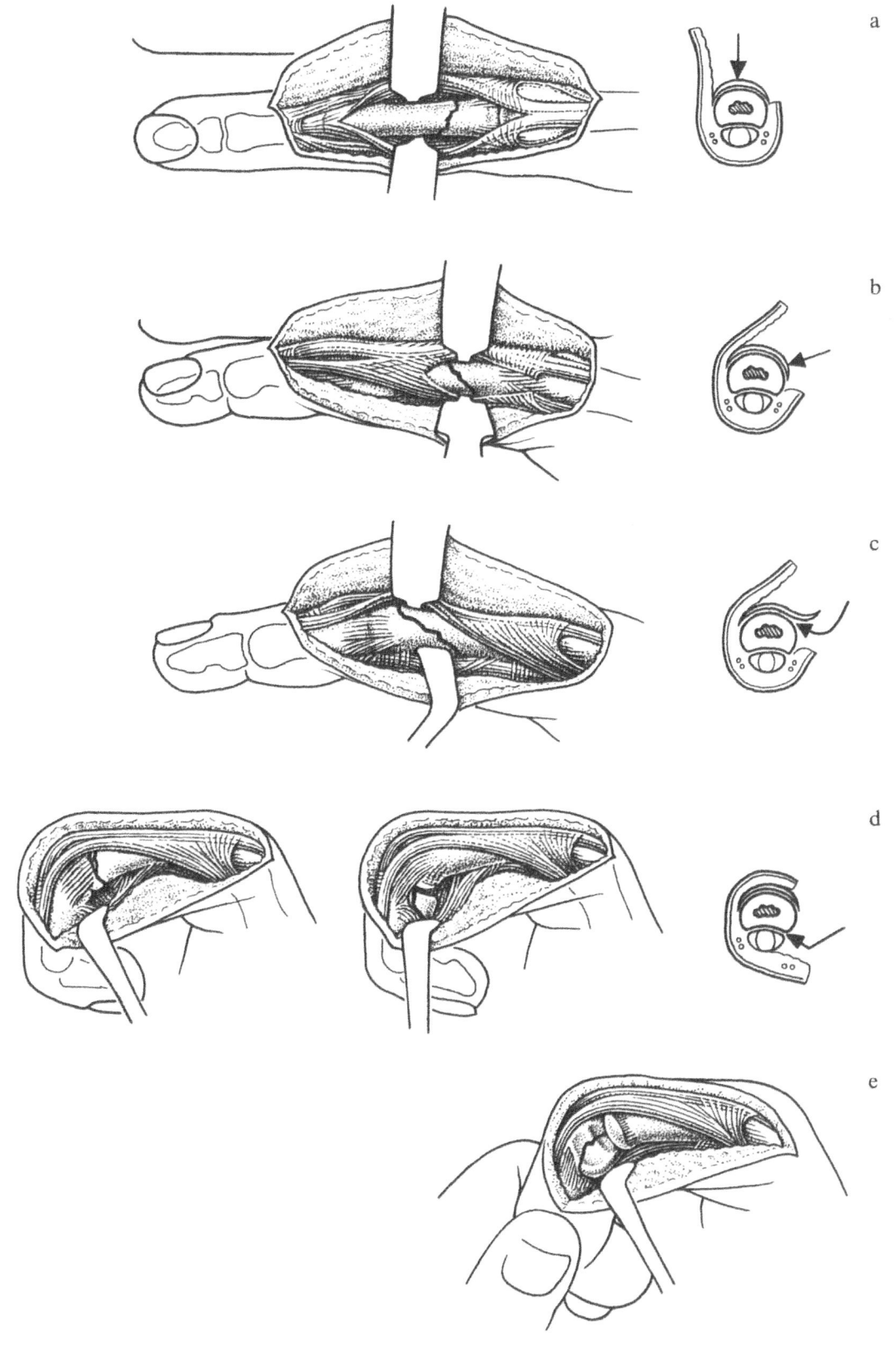

Fig. 84   Internal fixation in metacarpals and phalanges

    a   Typical fractures and internal fixation in hand bones

    b   Fracture dislocation of the P.I.P. joint. Internal fixation from the palmar side

    c   Typical malposition in a transverse fracture of the base of the proximal phalanx of the thumb. Internal fixation with a dorsal mini-plate

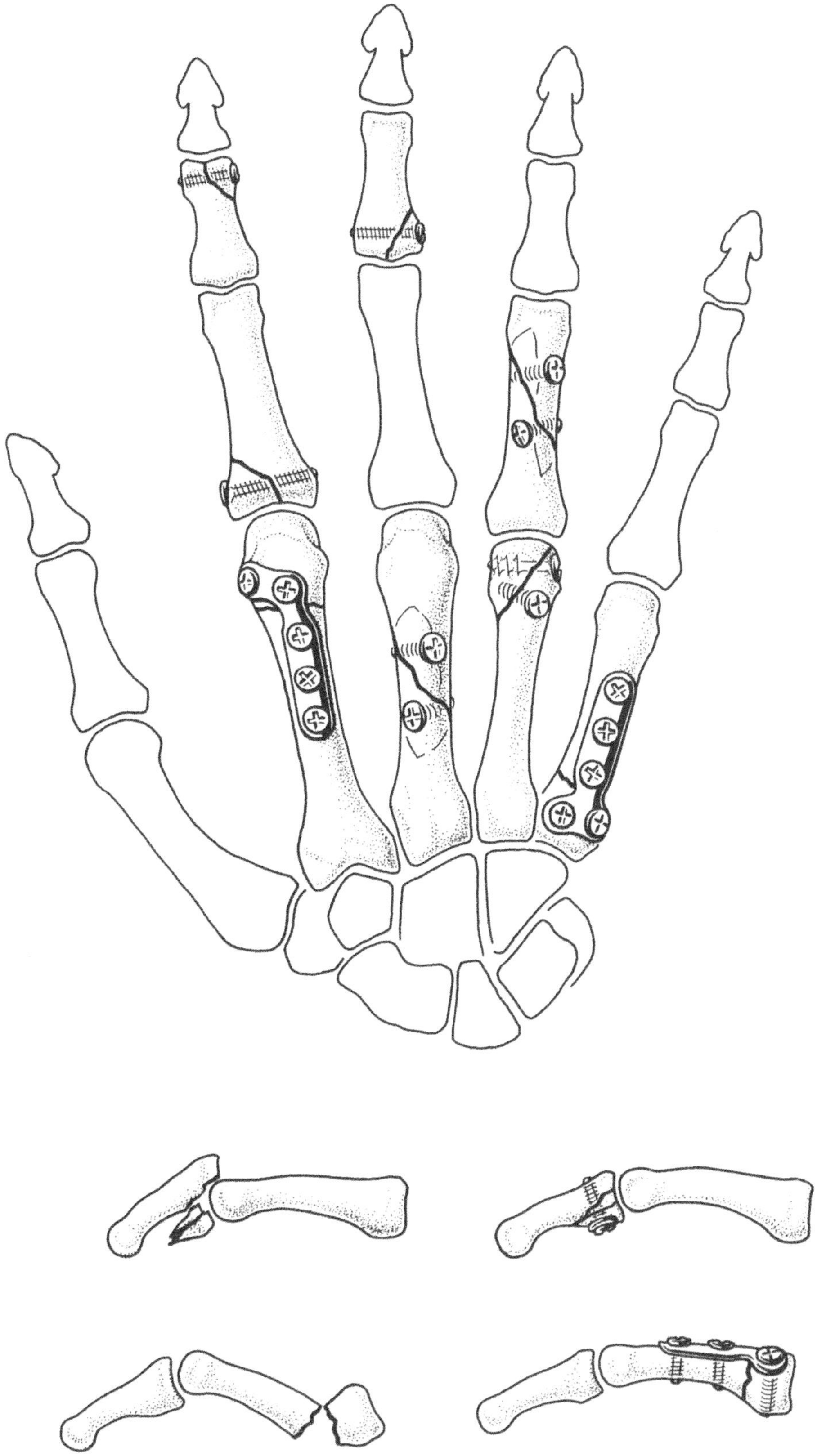

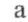

Fig. 85 **Clinical example: Shaft fracture of metacarpal**
The patient was a female student of 18, injured in a traffic accident

a Oblique fractures of the 3rd and 4th metacarpals with displacement of the fracture of the 4th into palmar flexion and shortening

b Primary internal fixation with a mini-plate to metacarpal 4, and with 2 screws of 2 mm in metacarpal 3
No complications. Consolidation of the fractures after eight weeks. Removal of the metal after four months

c Final review at 19 months: Symptom-free and full function

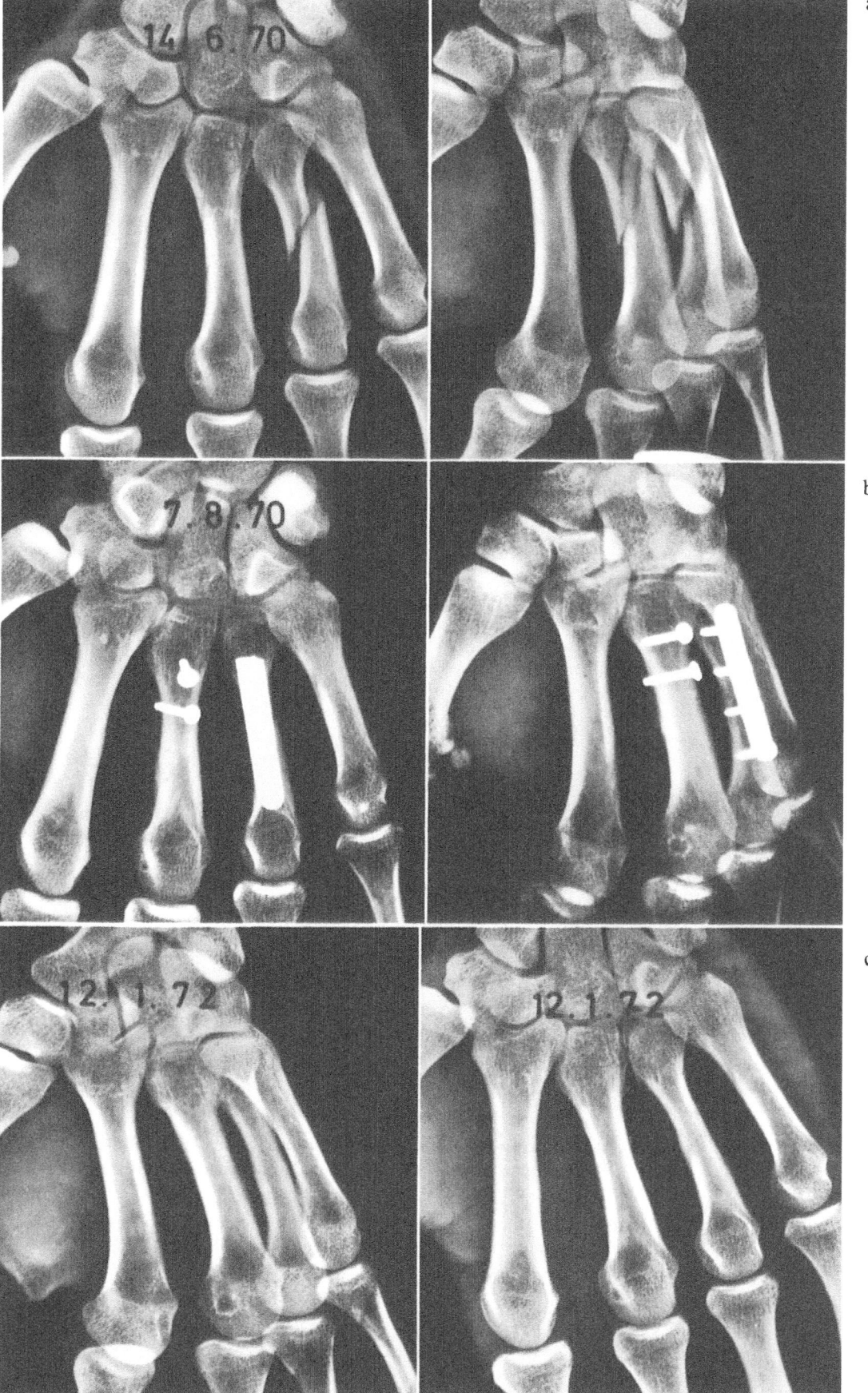

Fig. 86 **Clinical example: Oblique fracture of neck of second metacarpal**
Patient was a workman in a chemical factory, aged 36. He had his hand crushed in a conveyor belt

a   Open fracture of the neck of the second metacarpal and an additional fracture of the proximal phalanx of the thumb, and injury to the extensor tendon of the middle finger

b   Primary internal fixation of the second metacarpal with a finger plate
    Complications: Sudeck's atrophy. Removal of metal at five months

c   Final review at seven months: Symptom-free, full working capacity. Moderate loss of strength of power-grip and of flexion of the index and middle fingers. Some trophic disturbance

158

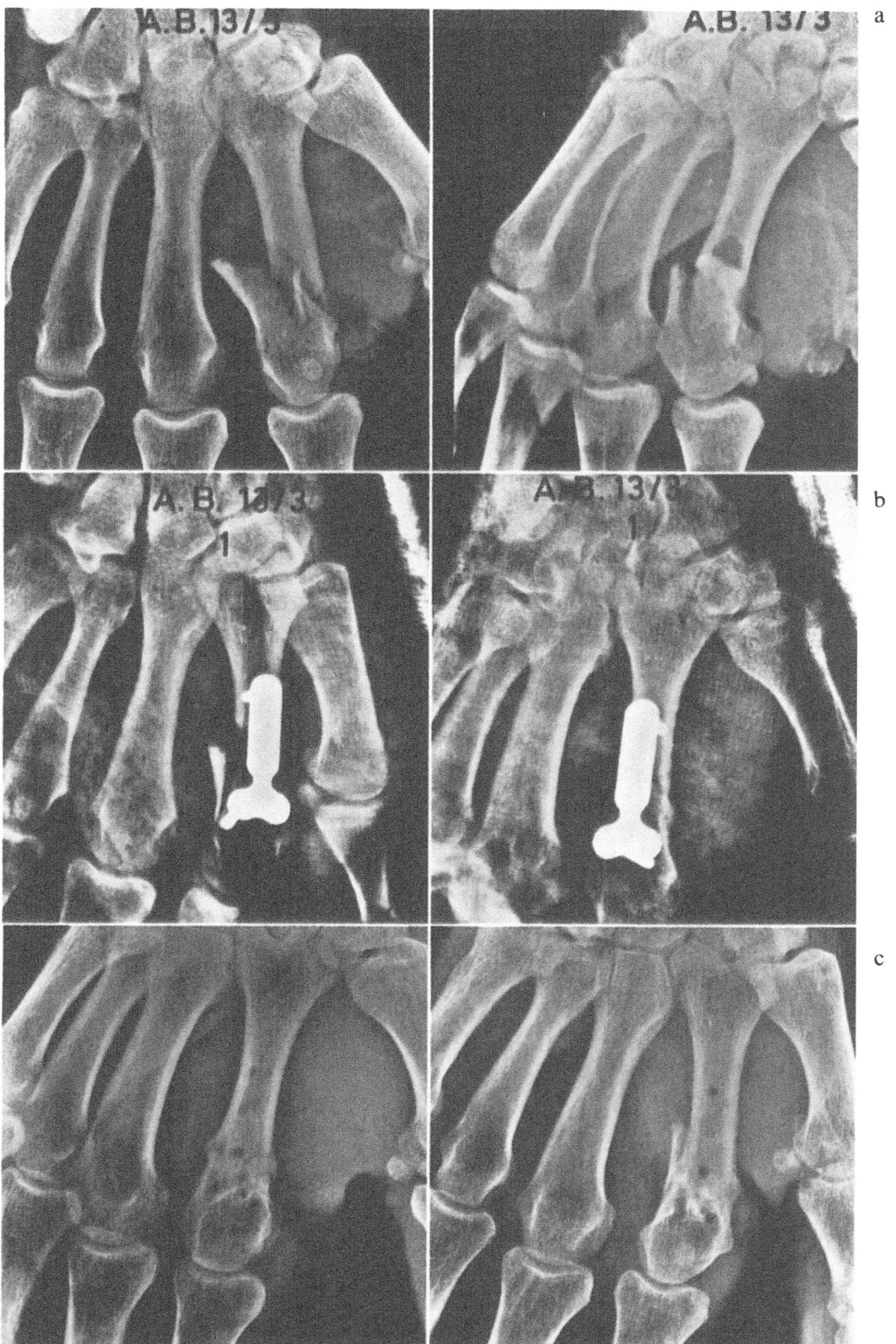

Fig. 87 **Clinical example: Fracture of the neck of the fifth metacarpal**
Patient was a male mechanic, aged 39. His hand had been crushed in a roller

a Unstable fracture of the neck of the fifth metacarpal with a palmar crack and skin damage

b Internal fixation with a finger L-plate and a free graft after four days
No complications

c Removal of metal and final review after seven months: symptom-free and full function

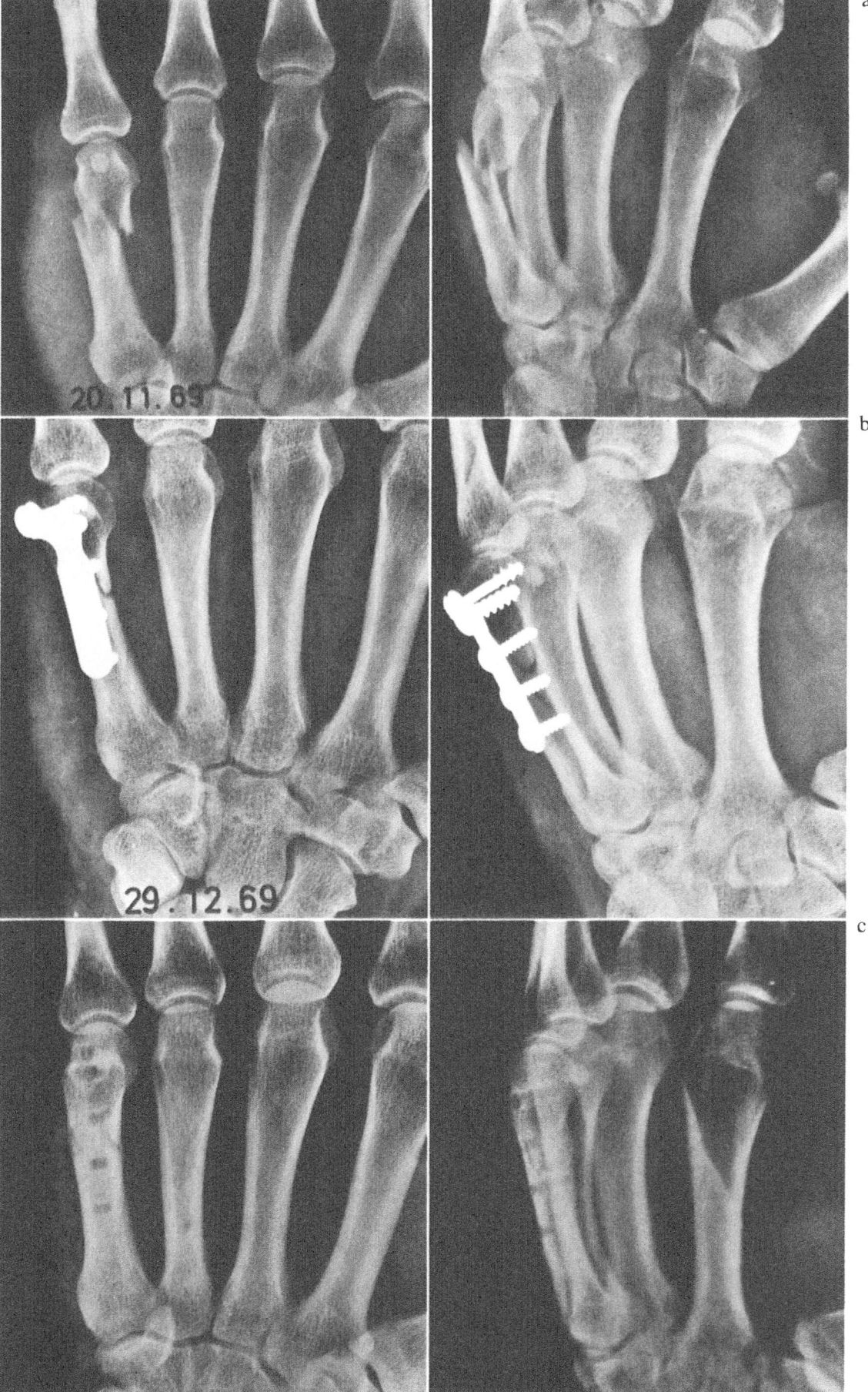

20.11.69

29.12.69

Fig. 88   Clinical example: Fracture of the base of the fifth metacarpal
Patient was an unskiled worker, aged 36. He had fallen on his hand

a   Extra-articular oblique fracture of the base of the fifth metacarpal with shortening

b   Primary internal fixation with a finger L-plate
No complications. Full working ability after 40 days

c   Removal of metal and final review at 13 months: Symptom-free, full function, strength equal
to that on the opposite side

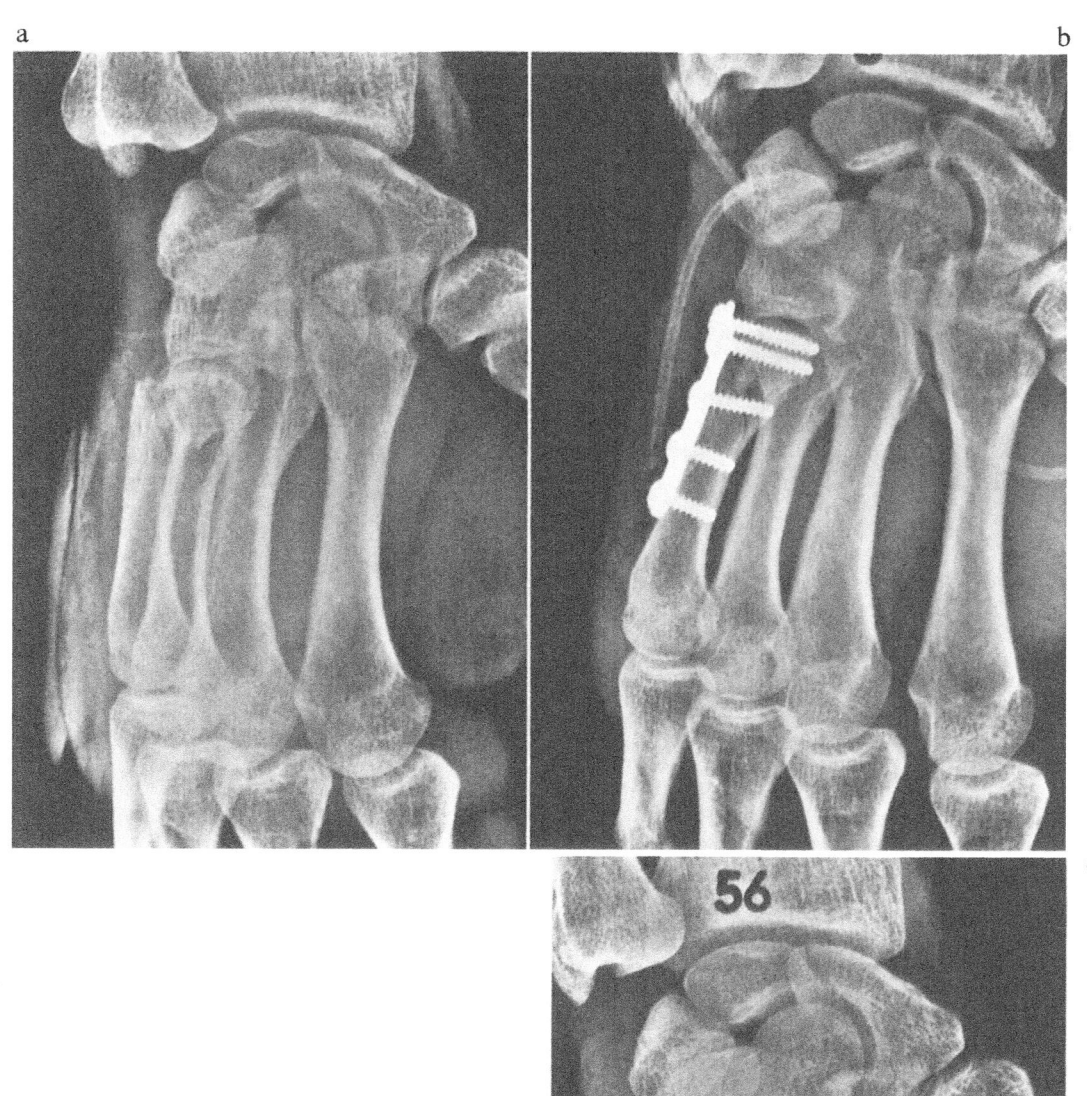

Fig. 89 **Clinical example: Spiral fracture of proximal phalanx**
Patient was a postman, aged 31. He had fallen into a crevasse

a Spiral fracture of proximal phalanx of the middle finger together with a rotational deformity. Unsuccessful treatment with splint fixation

b Internal fixation with 2 screws of 2.0 mm
No complications, functional post-operative treatment

c Removal of metal and final review after 5 months: Fracture united. Small cyst in the region of the distal screw and slight thickening of the P.I.P. joint. Flexion $-15°$, normal extension. Moderate symptoms, but full working capacity

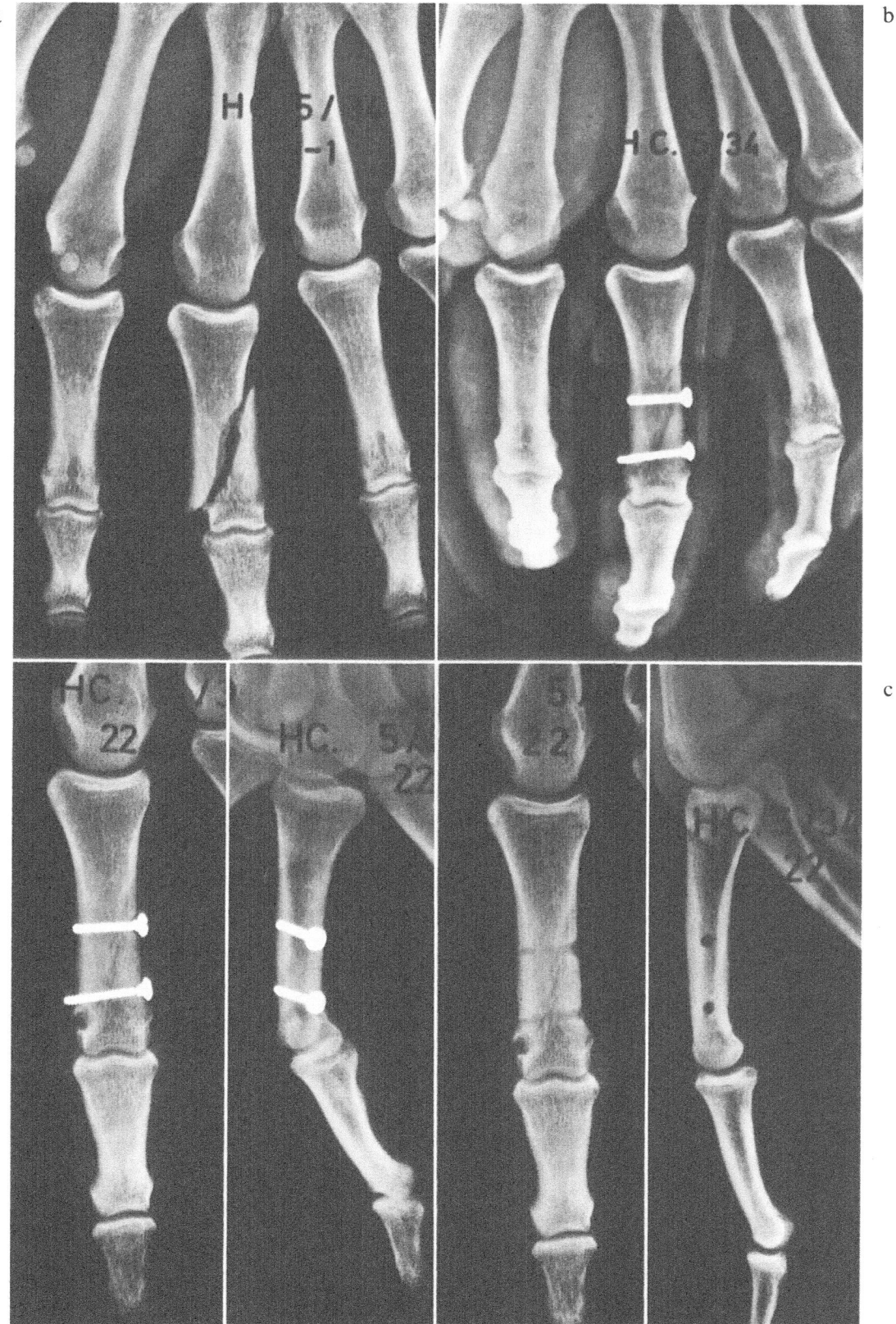

Fig. 90   Clinical example: Articular fracture of proximal phalanx
Patient was a seamstress, aged 18. Her middle finger was injured by the wheel of a sewing machine

a   Oblique fracture of the proximal phalanx of the middle finger, running into the joint. Rotational and flexion deformity

b   Closed reduction was not successful. Primary internal fixation with a Kirschner wire and a single small screw
No complications. Removal of the Kirschner wire after three weeks, and the screw after 10 months

c   Review at ten months: Symptom-free, full working ability, equal strength compared with the opposite side. Extension of the P.I.P. joint of the middle finger $-10°$

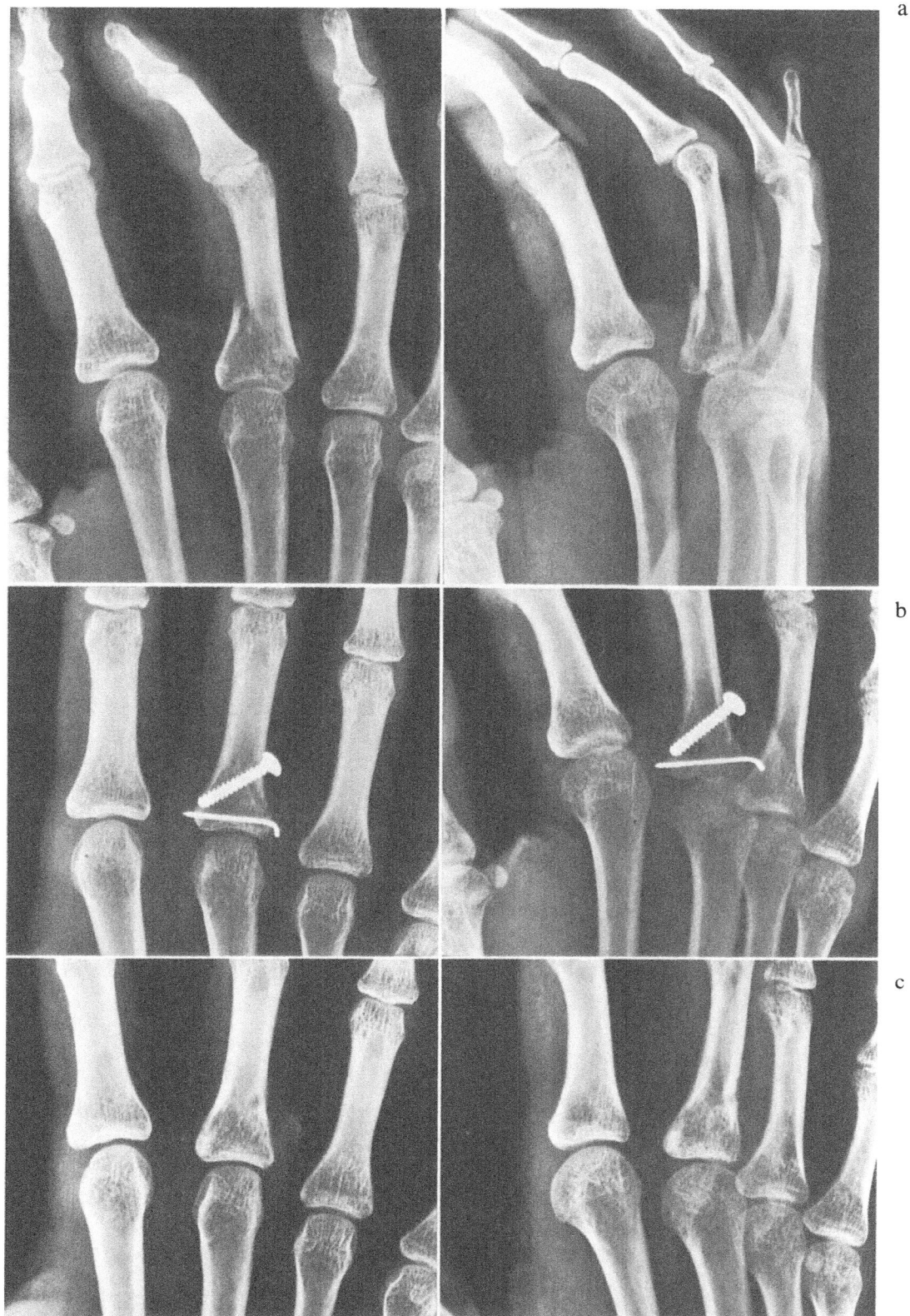

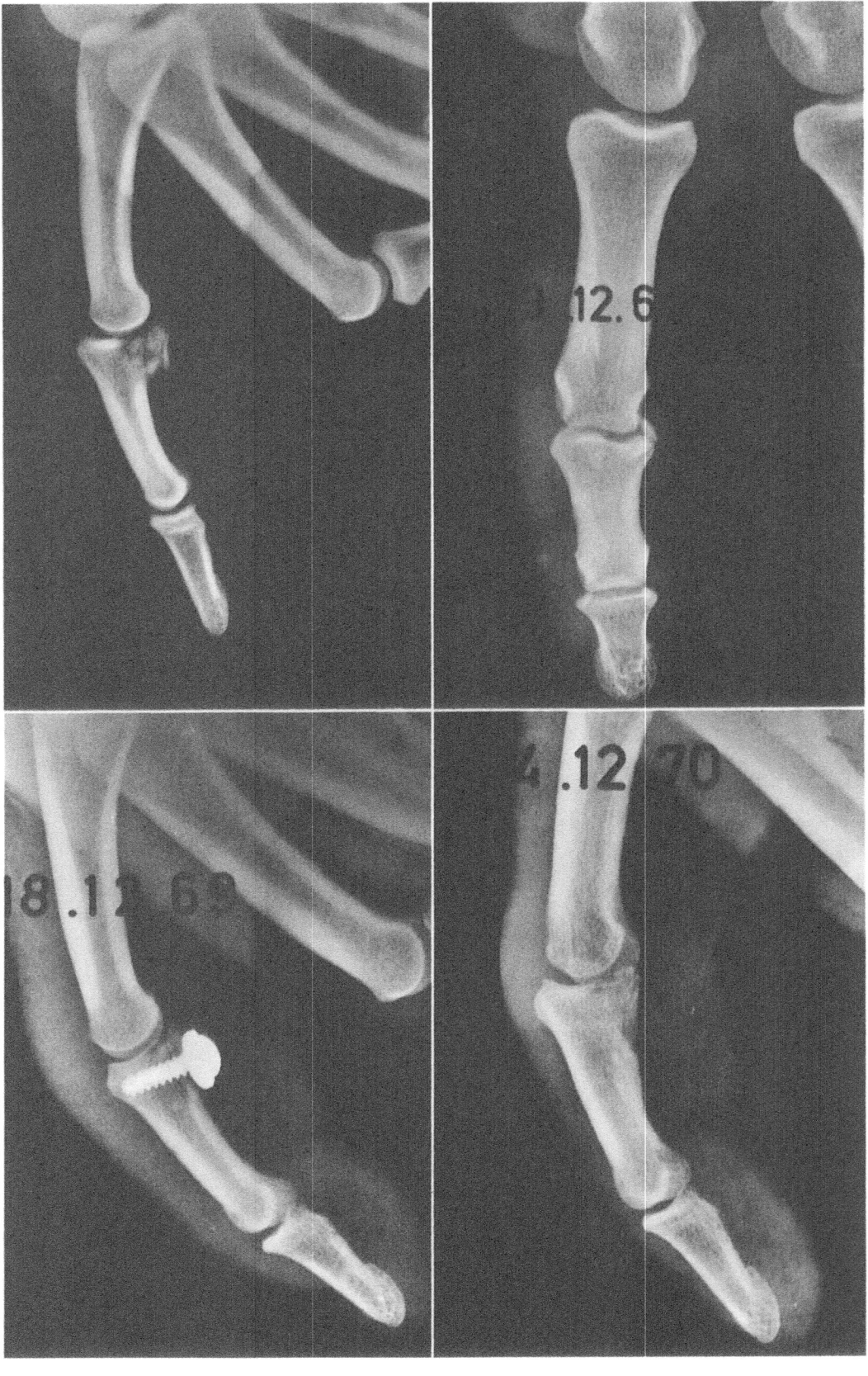

Fig. 92 **Clinical example: Small fragment avulsed from the palmar surface of the base of the middle phalanx of the middle finger**
The patient was an apprentice, aged 16. Dislocation of the P.I.P. joint of the left little finger in a ball game

a   Avulsion of the palmar fibro-cartilage at the base of the middle phalanx of the little finger with a bony fragment

b   Open reduction and fixation with a Bunnell pull-out wire
Palmar approach
No complications

c   Removal of the wire at four weeks
Final review at two months. No symptoms. Full function

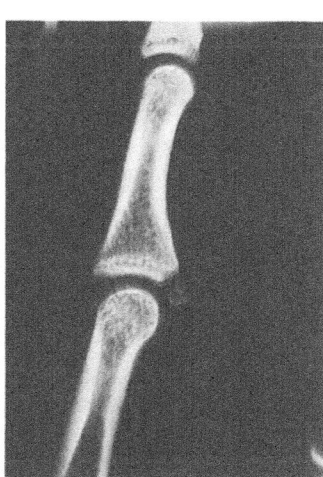

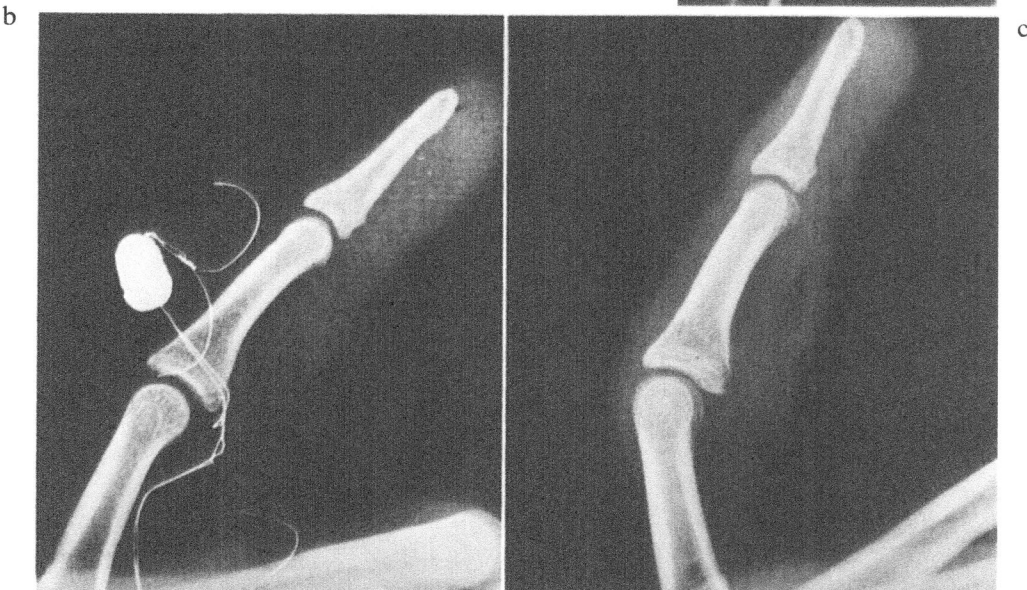

◁

Fig. 91 **Clinical example: Articular fracture of the base of the middle phalanx of the index finger**
The patient was a farmer, aged 32. He had a blow from a motor crank

a   Comminuted articular fracture of the base of the middle phalanx of the index, with partial dorsal dislocation, ulnar deviation of the finger. No improvement was obtained with closed treatment in plaster

b   After three weeks, internal fixation with a small screw and washer: palmar approach
No complications. Removal of the metal at four months

c   Final review at twelve months: moderate symptoms, full working capacity in farming and is able to milk, moderate arthrosis, the subluxation was fully corrected, and the mal-alignment improved

a

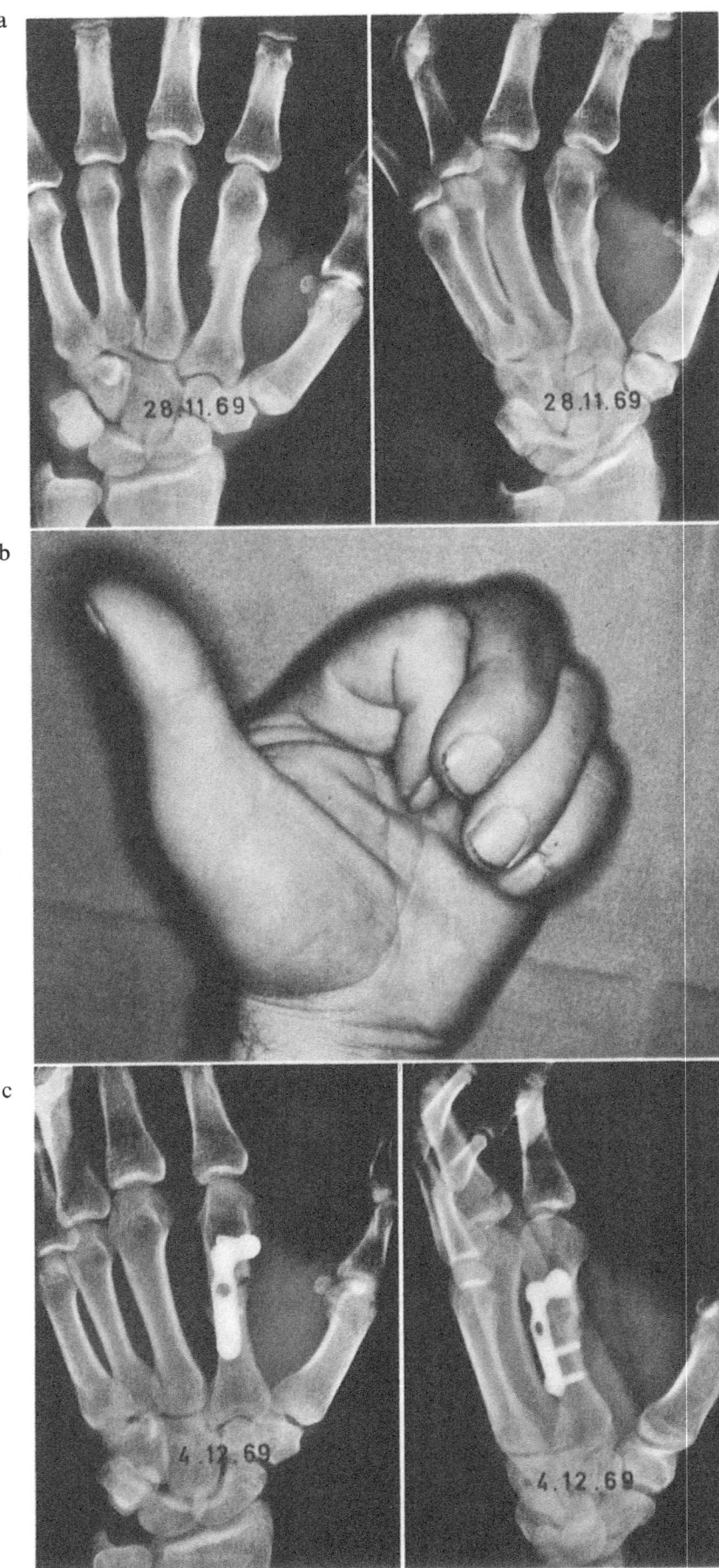

b

c

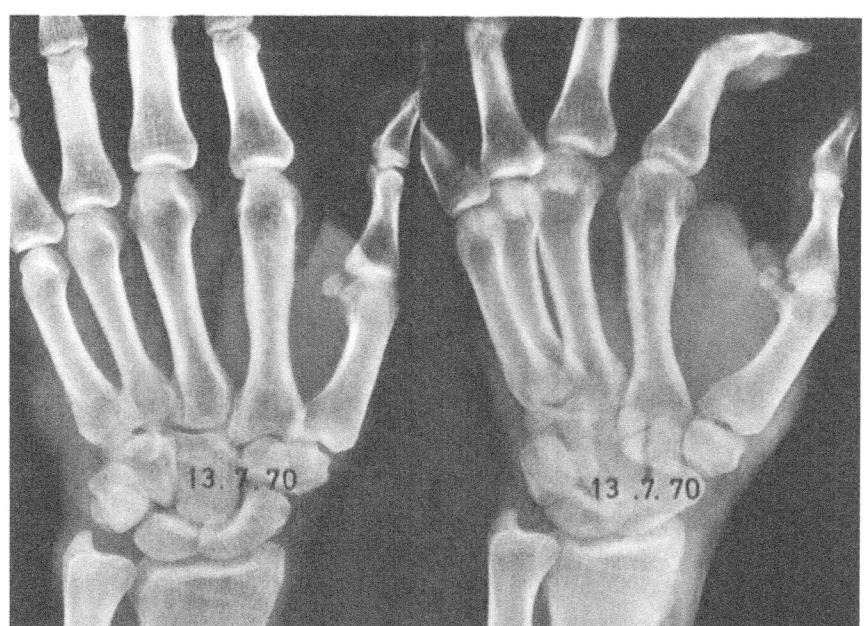

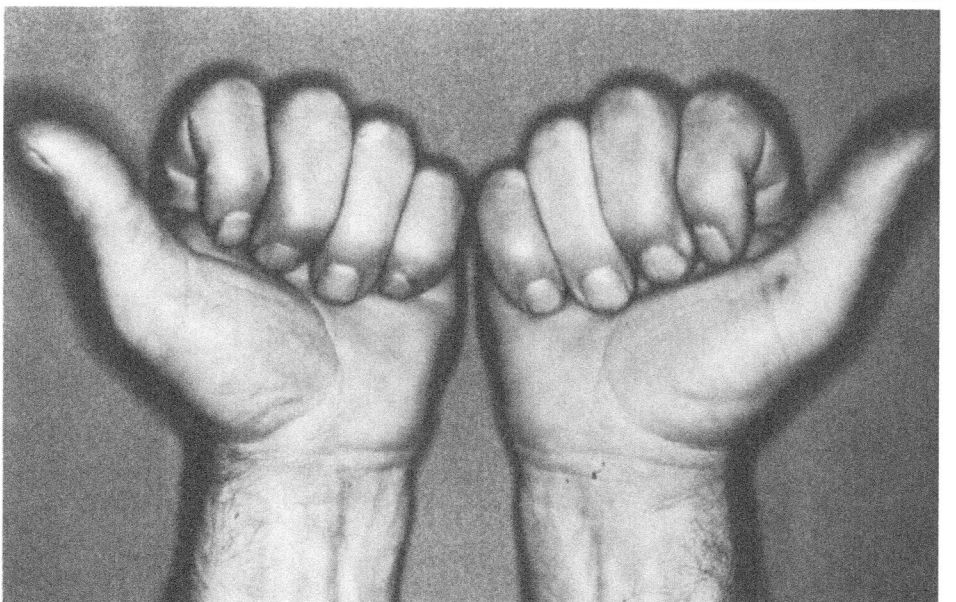

Fig. 93   Clinical example: Osteotomy of the second metacarpal
Patient was a lathe-hand, aged 29. He had a crushed finger. Transverse fracture of the shaft of the second metacarpal

a   Fracture was splinted in almost full extension. A tight pseudarthrosis developed

b   There was a rotational deformity

c   Rotation osteotomy with bone peg and tension-band plate applied four months after the accident No complications. Active post-operative treatment without external support. Full working capacity at three months

d   Removal of metal at eight months

e   Final review at ten months: Symptom-free, full function, flexed position identical on both sides

171

Fig. 94   **Clinical example: Arthrodesis of the P.I.P. joint**
Patient was a carpenter, aged 26. He had been injured in a milling machine

a   Open fracture of the index, middle and ring fingers. Partial amputation of the middle finger. Articular fracture with some loss of bone at the P.I.P. joint of the index finger, resulting in a painful rotational deformity and loss of pinch between thumb and index

b   Arthrodesis with compressed bridging graft and mini-plate nine months after the accident. At the request of the patient it was put up in almost full extension to suit his work

c   No complications. Active post-operative movement without any external support. Able to carry out part of his work after six weeks. The arthrodesis was consolidated after four months. He was booked for metal removal

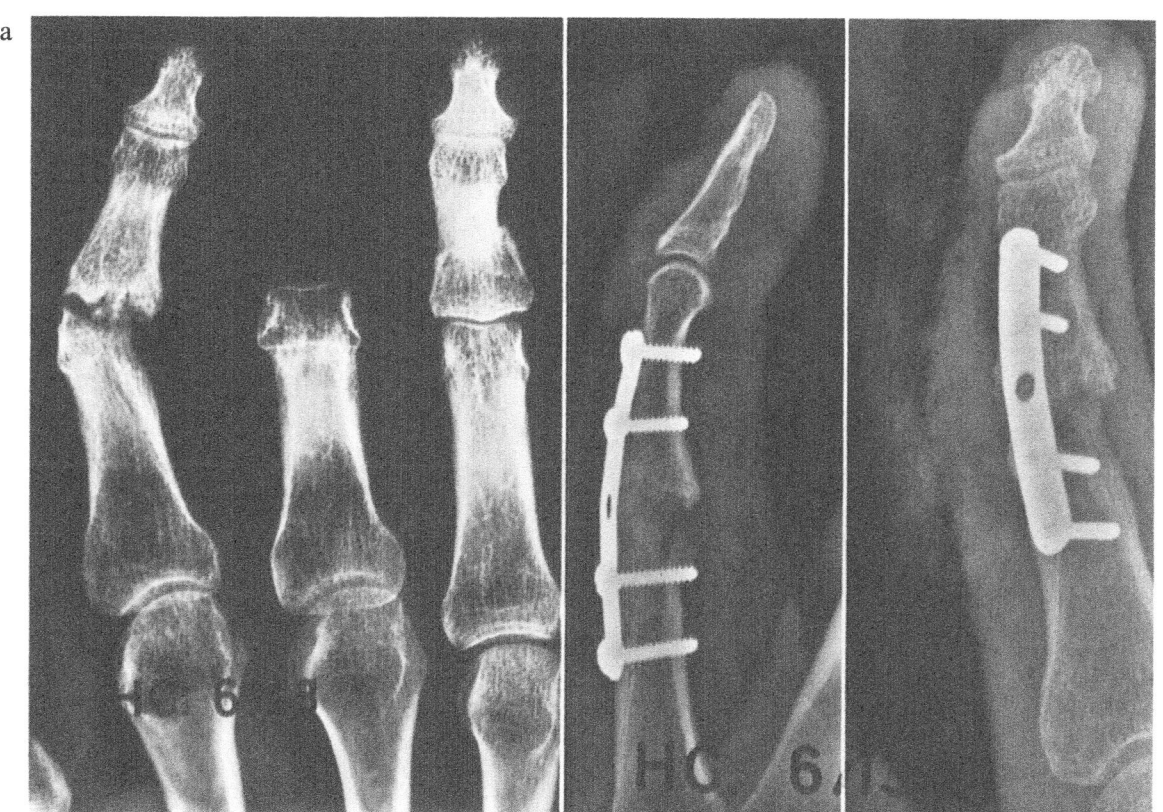

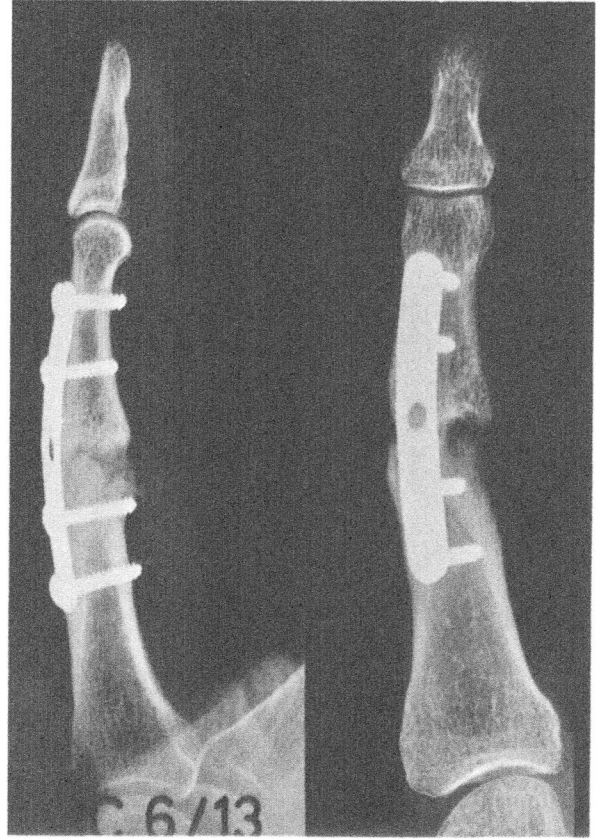

Fig. 95   Clinical example: Arthrodesis with a screw at the P.I.P. joint of the ring finger
The patient was a designer constructor, aged 33. He was injured in a sawing mill

a   Open comminuted fracture of the ringer finger at the level of the P.I.P. joint with damage to the extensor apparatus

b   Primary closure of the wound and stabilization with a Kirschner wire

c   Secondary arthrodesis with a screw at seven weeks
No complications. Removal of the metal at 13 months

d   Final review at $1\frac{1}{2}$ years. Slight occupational handicap. Bony union of the arthrodesis. Some loss of flexion of the D.I.P. joint caused by the scarring of the extensor apparatus

a

b

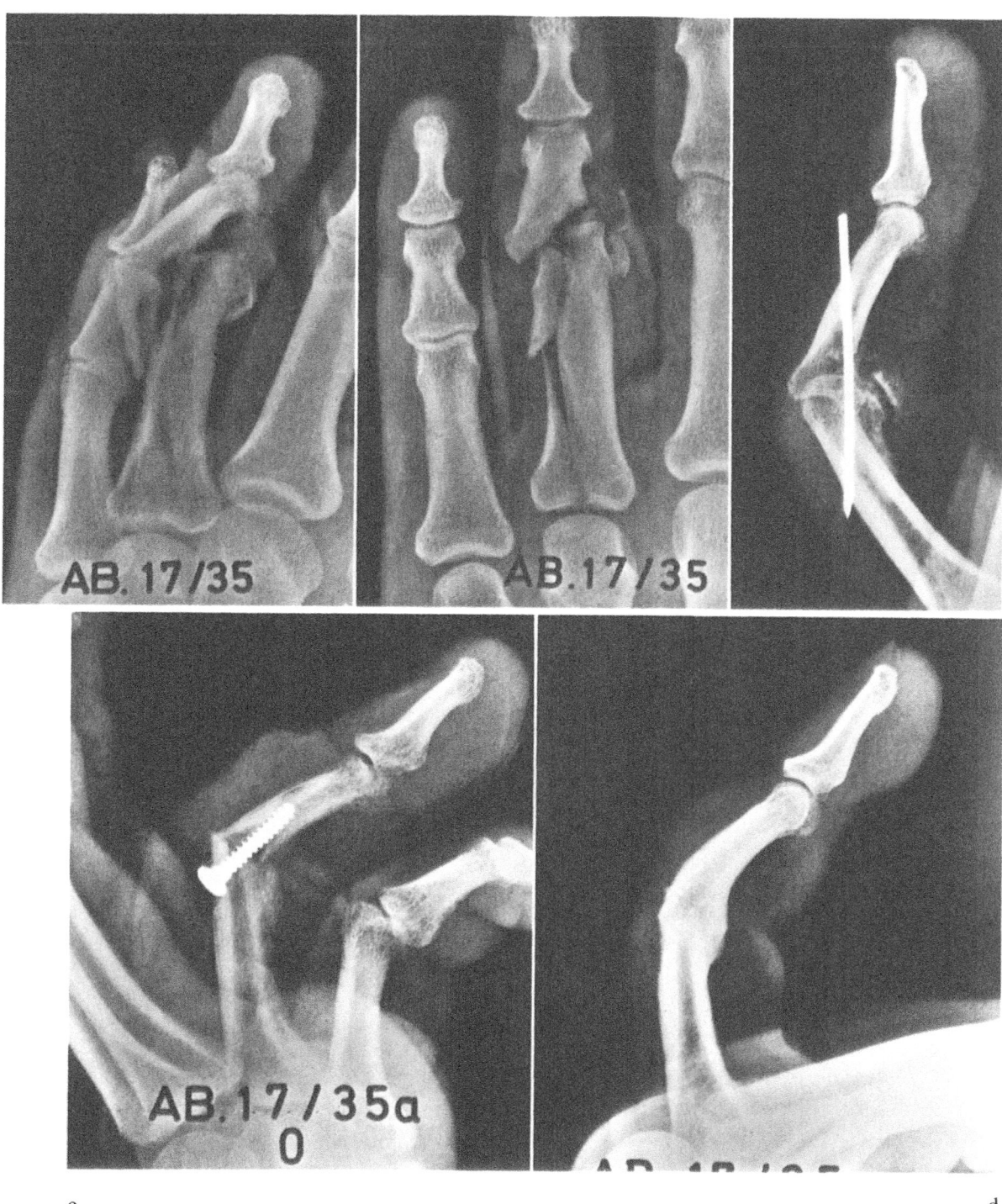

AB. 17/35

AB. 17/35

AB. 17/35a
0

c

d

175

XI. The Ankle Joint

The use of the SFS in the region of the ankle joint is steadily increasing. This is true for the many types of malleolar fracture as well as for distal articular fractures of the tibia, and sometimes for those of the talus.

Since the beginning of the ASIF group, most of these fractures have been treated by internal fixation. Though the indications for operation have remained unchanged, the method of using the small implants now available has led to recent modifications. Medullary nailing of the fibula and the use of large cancellous screws are now uncommon, and the small cancellous screw has largely replaced the malleolar screw. Small plates, which spare the tissues and occupy little space, are increasingly coming to the fore. The use of these implants in the neighbourhood of joints calls for special descriptions of the technical details.

A. Lower Tibia

1. Comminuted Fractures of the Lower Tibial Epiphysis

Simple fractures without cancellous bone involvement occasionally occur in juvenile patients. They can usually be repaired with one or more small cancellous screws (Fig. 96).

2. Depressed Comminuted Fracture

In recent years this type of fracture has become more common. Since problems of diagnosis and treatment differ from those of other tibial fractures (Bandi, Decoulx, Gay, Müller, Tru-

chet), a special discussion seems to be necessary.

a) Definition and Signs

Depressed comminuted fractures are characterized by impaction of the distal articular surface of the tibia. This results on the one hand in shortening and broadening of the epiphysis, and on the other in loss of substance of epiphyseal and metaphyseal cancellous bone. Here we are nearly always faced with comminuted fractures, of which the fragments and surfaces are hardly discernible on X-rays since they are concealed by cancellous and thin cortical bones.

Operation confirms the presence of the following typical components, listed in order of frequency (Fig. 97a):

— A large medial malleolar fragment resembling that in an adduction fracture. This is present *in all cases.*

— A defect of cancellous bone of variable extent.

— An anterior impaction of the articular surface of the tibia, consisting of one to three independent fragments which are displaced proximally.

— An antero-lateral fragment of the tibia, consisting of the tubercle of Chaput.

— A malleolar fracture of type C. Because the anterior tibio-fibular syndesmosis is intact, it is attached to the antero-lateral tibial fragment. Where there is no fracture of the fibula, which is in about 10% of all cases, the syndesmosis and lateral ligament are always ruptured as a result of the impaction (Fig. 97b).

— A backward angulation together with dorsal supra-malleolar fracture.

b) Indications for, and Technique of Operation

Ideas about treatment have changed in recent years (Burnett, Maurer, Müller, Rüedi, Weber). Despite the considerable technical difficulties, operative treatment is gaining ground since only the anatomical reconstruction of the joint can prevent post-traumatic arthrosis.

The basic principles of the operative techniques were laid down by Rüedi, Matter, and Allgöwer in 1968. They comprise:

— Internal fixation of the fibula.
— Reconstruction of the articular surface of the tibia.
— Autogenous cancellous bone graft.
— Internal fixation of the tibia with a buttress plate.

Since 1968, the clover-leaf plate (Fig. 6b) has become available for this difficult type of internal fixation. This malleable plate, particularly in its broad distal part, can be accurately contoured to fit the fracture site. The stability obtained usually allows active post-operative movement. Below we present an abbreviated account of the operative technique which has stood the test in over 80 cases (Heim).

c) Approach

To obtain precise reconstruction, all the elements of the comminuted fracture listed above must be exposed. Long bilateral incisions and wide access to the depth are indispensable.

Medial Incision (Fig. 98a): This runs in a curve from the anterior border of the lower tibia, in front of the medial malleolus to the foot, and permits a wide opening of the ankle joint immediately in front of the deltoid ligament. Exposure is thus obtained of the large medial malleolar fragment, of the depressed antero-medial articular surface, of the immediately adjacent epiphyseal depression or defect of cancellous bone, as well as of the medial aspect of the upper surface of the talus. In order to correct or avoid recurvation, the medio-dorsal border of the tibial fracture, which lies just proximal to the groove for the tendon of tibialis posterior, must be exposed.

Lateral Incision (Fig. 98b): A slightly S-haped incision runs from the posterior border of the distal shaft of the fibula beyond the anterior edge of the lateral malleolus distally. The superficial branch of the lateral popliteal nerve must be protected. The exposure must extend to the frequently complex fracture of the lateral malleolus and to the antero-lateral fragment of the tibia. The lateral aspect of the articular surface of the tibia and the upper surface of the talus must be just as fully exposed as the anterior tibio-fibular syndesmosis and the fibulo-talar ligaments. Where the latter are ruptured a suture must be inserted.

The skin bridge between both incisions must have a width of at least 5 cm to preserve an adequate blood supply (Fig. 98c).

d) Reduction of the Fractures

We begin with *internal fixation of the fibula,* since its correct length and position provide landmarks and partial support for the subsequent precise reduction and reconstruction of the depressed tibia (valgus or varus deformity, recurvation or rotational deformity). We usually apply a long narrow semi-tubular plate with 6–8 holes (Fig. 99a), which also provides rigid fixation of the comminuted fractures. For technical details, see the paragraph dealing with the malleolar fractures of the C type (pages 195).

Reduction and *reconstruction of the articular surface of the tibia* presents some difficulty. It may either involve a medial or lateral approach, but more often both procedures are combined for correction as well as reconstruction of depressions and defects. The surgeon must choose his approach according to the findings.

In order to improve the exposure of anterior articular steps, the medial malleolar fragment must sometimes be temporarily retracted (Fig. 99b–d). Provisional fixation is obtained by Kirschner wires which stabilize articular fragments and in addition fix the epiphysis to the shaft (Fig. 100).

178

e) Autogenous Cancellous Bone Graft

When the articular surface has been restored attention is turned to the area of impacted cancellous defect. This gap must be completely filled in with autogenous cancellous bone graft to prevent subsequent collapse. This graft has both a supporting and biological function however and it also contributes to early fracture healing. The usual donor site is the iliac fossa, but sometimes the greater trochanter (Fig. 101 a).

The operation for *obtaining cancellous bone* should be carried out as a *separate procedure* before the actual internal fixation. This is imperative as the internal fixation in itself is time-consuming and safe tourniquet time must not be exceeded. The volume of the cancellous bone needed is estimated from the x-rays taken after the accident. Where the amount of graft proves to be insufficient for filling the defect, an *extra amount can be obtained from the tibial condyle*. This donor area is of advantage as it is close to the operation site and easily accessible. The procedure is simple and time saving. Make a small incision above the upper end of the medial subcutaneous surface of the tibia. Incise and reflect the periosteum. Open the thin cortex with a curved osteotome. Soft cancellous bone is then obtained with a sharp spoon (Fig. 101 b). The *defect is usually filled in with graft* after reduction or temporary fixation, through a cortical gap in the antero-medial area of the fracture zone.

f) Internal Fixation of the Tibia

We usually begin with screw fixation of the lateral fragment of the tibia. Then the clover leaf plate is contoured and fixed medially. It may be necessary to cut off the posterior end of the plate lest the tendinous canal of the tibialis posterior should be compressed. Rigid fixation of a comminuted fracture can only be achieved if the metal gains a grip at all levels. Therefore, an "epiphyseal block" must first be established in sagittal and transverse planes (Fig. 102). Once this stage of the reduction is reached, the fracture can be buttressed proximally to obtain axial stability (Fig. 102).

The clover-leaf plate is first fixed to the distal tibia. Here special attention must be paid to the stability of individual parts and any malposition must be immediately corrected. The plate is then fixed temporarily to the proximal shaft-fragment by means of forceps. Separate individual fragments can be fixed with additional single screws. It is not necessary to insert screws into every hole of the plate but solid fixation of the large medial malleolar fragment is of utmost importance. At this point temporary Kirschner wires are successively removed, and the plate is then screwed to the main proximal fragment (Fig. 102). Valgus deformity can be corrected by applying tension to the plate from above.

The operation is completed by suturing the periosteum and by inserting Redon drains on both sides. The closure of the soft parts above the flat clover-leaf plate presents no difficulty, as it scarcely alters the outer contour of the foot, and the patient can subsequently use normal shoes.

g) Post-Operative Treatment

It has proved to be satisfactory to hold the foot elevated at 90° with a plaster splint and to avoid active movement until the swelling has completely subsided. Hospital treatment for these patients, therefore, lasts a few days longer than in the case of the usual internal fixation of the tibia. Weight-bearing should not be begun before the 16th week.

The clover-leaf plate is left in place until the 14th month. The large number of screws does not seem to be detrimental and as the contact surfaces are very small, corrosion between screws and plate has so far not been observed.

3. Secondary Surgery

In the presence of pseudarthrosis or malposition, operative correction must sometimes be carried out in the distal epiphyseal area of the tibia. Malpositions are either due to varus deformity often combined with recurvation and rotational deformity, to valgus position, or to rotational deformity alone. Osteotomy of the fibula is not necessary in all instances. Double plate fixation may be used for such an operation on the tibia. The small tissue-protecting plates which require little space are particularly appropriate here. For anatomical reasons, the main plate must be applied medially where it can obtain a purchase on the medial malleolus. The broad clover-leaf plate gives more rigidity than the long narrow semitubular plate. Axial compression is a pre-requisite for early consolidation

a) Varus Deformity

Correction is indicated where the mal-alignment exceeds 8°. Osteotomy of the fibula may usually be dispensed with, but it is advisable to make a small lateral incision to fix a small semi-tubular plate with two holes which is adequate for the coaption of the distal and proximal fragments with one screw in each. Thus rupture and splitting of the lateral cortex is avoided (Fig. 103a and b.).
Reconstruction or opening of the pseudarthrosis and osteotomy are carried out medially. A wedge-shaped defect is produced and this is filled with cancellous bone graft. Axial correction is controlled by X-ray. The medial buttress plate is applied and fixed distally and if necessary the plate can be placed under tension from the upper end. A primary slight over-correction of the mal-alignment may sometimes be advisable, since the plate then compresses the graft and this promotes early healing.

b) Valgus Deformity

Correction is indicated where the mal-alignment exeeds 14°. It is achieved by simple oblique osteotomy about 3 cm above the articular surface. Fixation is obtained with a medial plate and axial compression. Osteotomy of the fibula is not usually necessary (Fig. 104).

c) Rotational Deformity

Rotational deformity is often combined with the deformities described under a and b. Combined osteotomy of the tibia and fibula is required for correction. Fixation of the tibia is obtained with either two small semi-tubular plates or with a clover-leaf plate (Fig. 105).

d) Post-Operative Treatment

The rigidity achieved by this type of osteotomy allows post-operative active movement without any external support in almost every case. Joint movement is quickly regained during the healing process of the bone and this has an advantageous effect on the blood supply. Consolidation of the bone and the ability to bear weight are achieved within 8–12 weeks.

Fig. 96   **Comminuted fractures of the lower tibial epiphysis**   ▷

Internal fixation with cancellous screws

Fig. 97   **Impacted comminuted fracture**

a   Appearance of the fracture, viewed from the front and from the side: Impaction of the articular surface of the tibia together with broadening of the epiphysis. Large medial malleolar fragment. Comminuted zone of the cancellous bone of the epiphysis. Anterior joint fragment. Anterolateral fragment of the tibia. Fracture of the fibula. Posterior fracture with backward angulation

b   When the fibula is intact, impaction leads to rupture of the antero-lateral ligaments

180

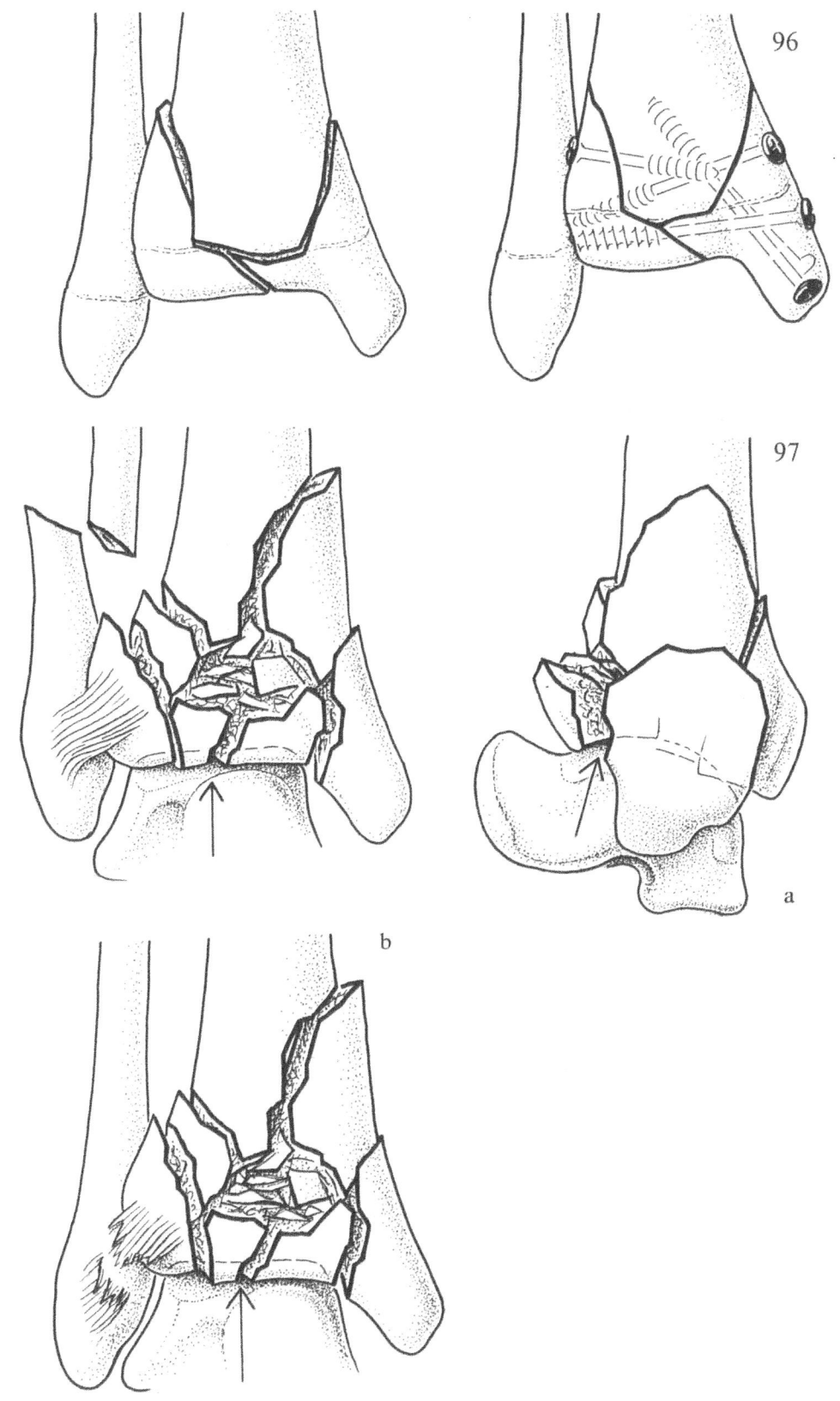

a

b

Fig. 98 **Incisions and approaches**

a   A medial incision allows exposure of the ankle joint. The arrows mark the critical points to be observed in this approach

b   A lateral incision to expose the ankle joint. The arrows mark the critical points for this approach

c   Anterior view of both incisions. The minimum distance between the two incisions is 5 cm. The arrow marks the exposure of the anterior part of the ankle joint obtained by the combined approaches

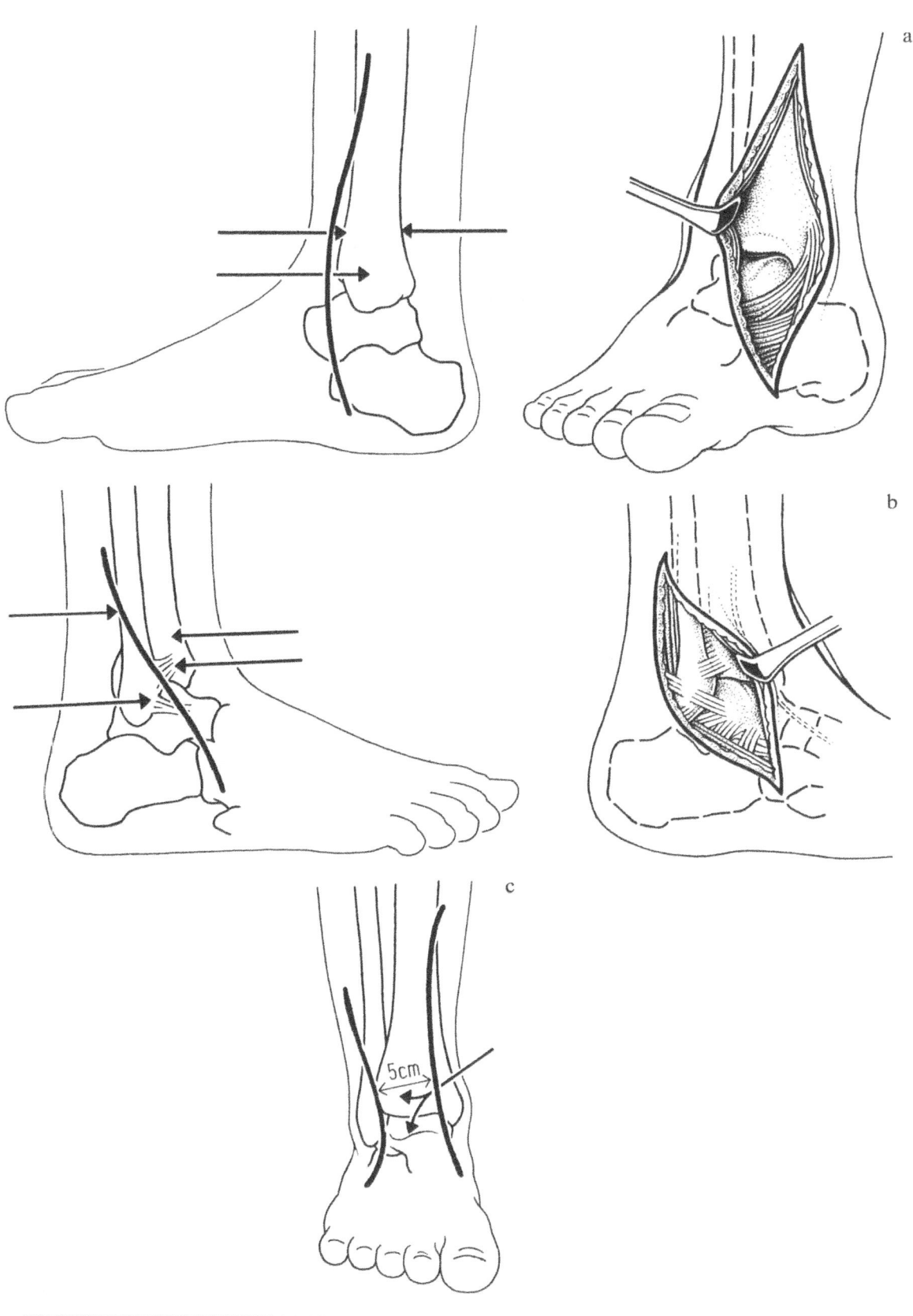

Fig. 99   Reduction of the fracture

    a   The fibula is fixed with a small semi-tubular plate

b–d   Reduction and reconstruction of the articular surface using the antero-medial approach. A large medial malleolar fragment is temporarily retracted. Provisional fixation with Kirschner wires. A wide gap develops at the site of impaction

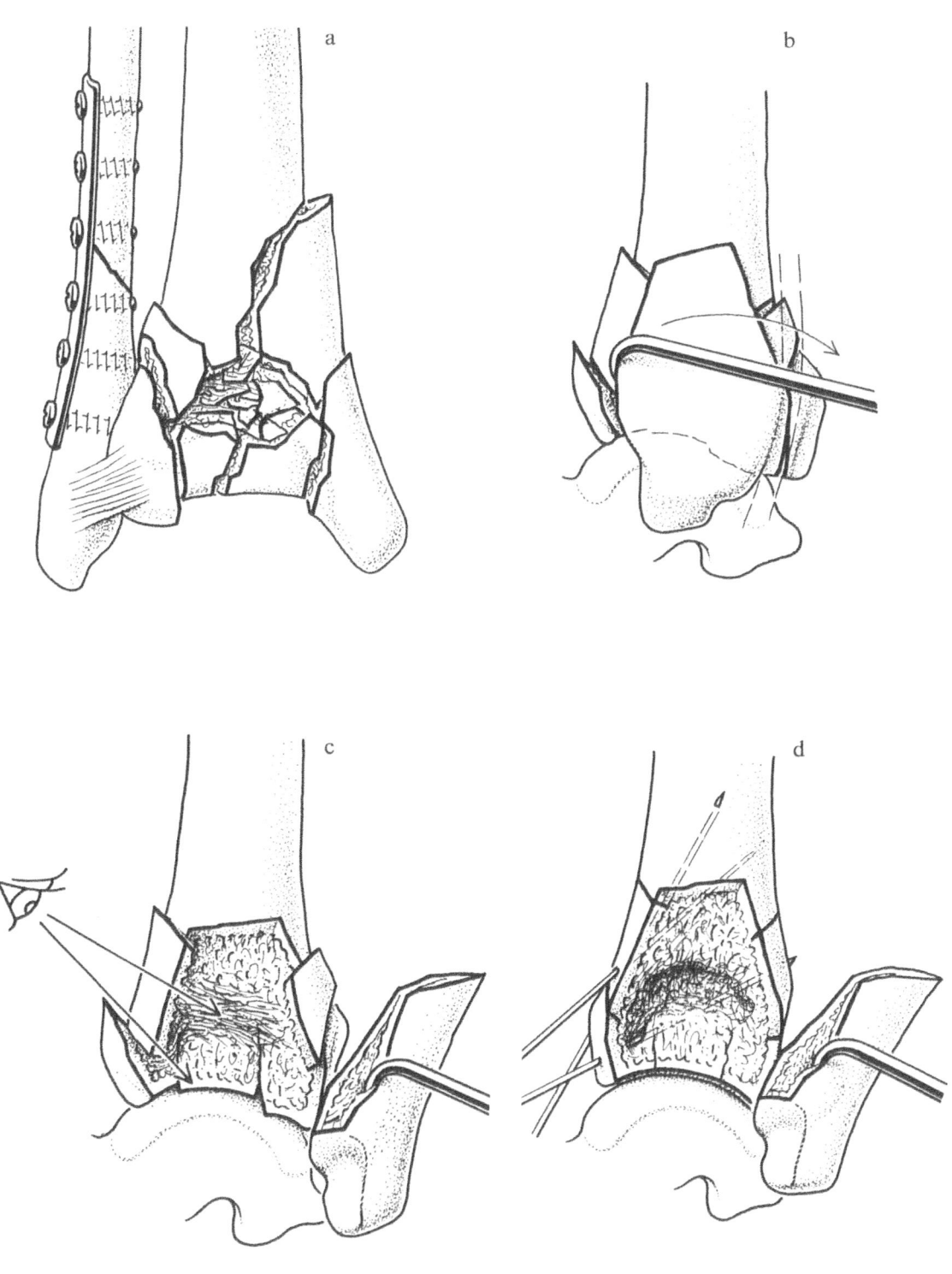

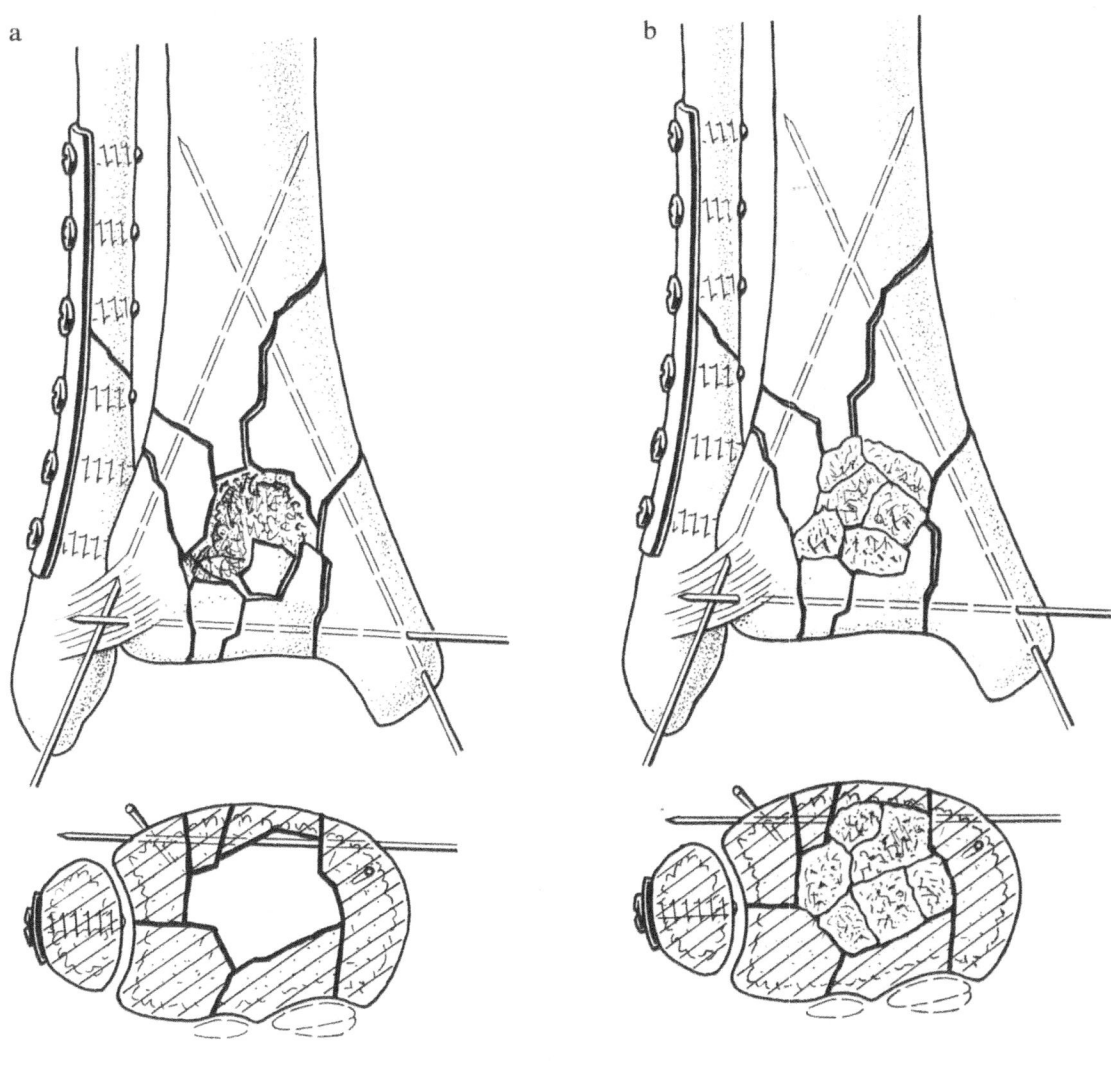

Fig. 100 Autogenous cancellous bone graft

   a Anterior view and section through the reduced and temporarily fixed fracture. The defect in the cancellous bone is shown

   b The defect is filled in with cancellous bone

186

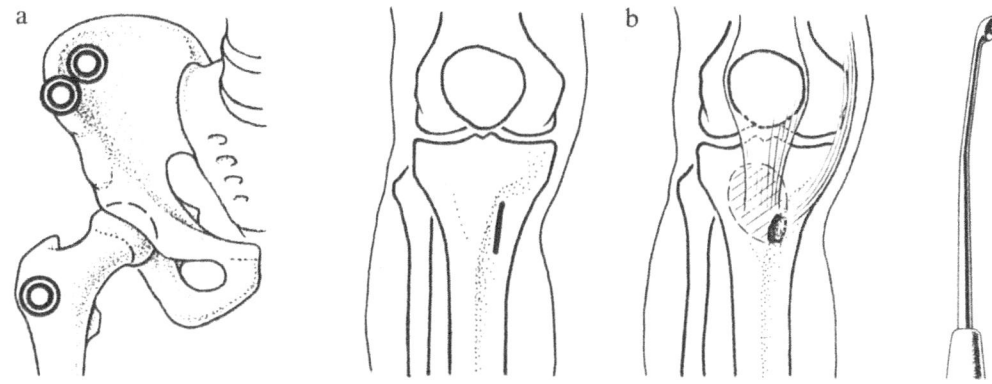

Fig. 101   Donor sites for the cancellouse bone

    a The anterior superior spine and the iliac crest, and the greater trochanter are the best sites. The graft is obtained in a separate preliminary operation

    b If the amount of graft is insufficient or if an unexpected amount is required, cancellous bone may be obtained from the upper end of the tibia. Through a small longitudinal incision graft is taken, using a sharp spoon

Fig. 102 Internal fixation of the tibia

   a Screw fixation of the antero-lateral fragment and of the medial aspect of the tibia holding the plate with small screws to the epiphysis

   b Completed internal fixation of the tibia. Clover-leaf plate is fixed on the shaft fragment with 4.5 mm cortex screws

   c Section through the epiphyseal area of the fracture: the whole width of the clover-leaf plate is in contact. Screws obtain a powerful grip

   d Section through the epiphyseal area of the fracture: the posterior end of the plate has been cut off in order to protect the canal for the tibialis posterior tendon. The plate is, therefore, shorter on the anterior surface and the effect is less rigid

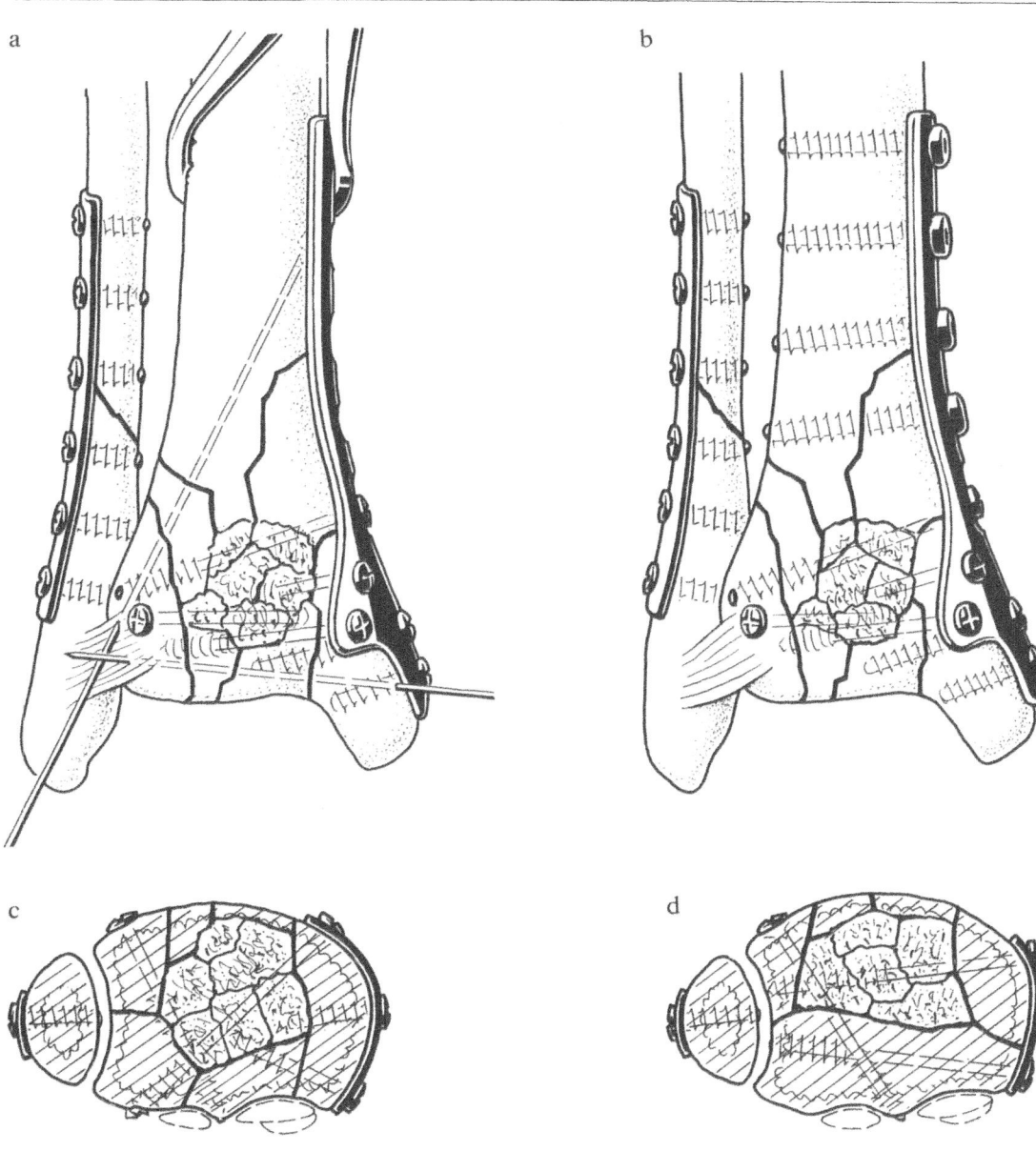

a

b

c

d

189

Fig. 103 Correction of a varus deformity

   a   Lateral fixation with a small plate

   b   Medial osteotomy and over-correction with cancellous bone in the gap

   c   Positioning and distal fixation of the clover-leaf plate

   d   Plate is placed under tension until the over-correction is removed. The graft is then under compression

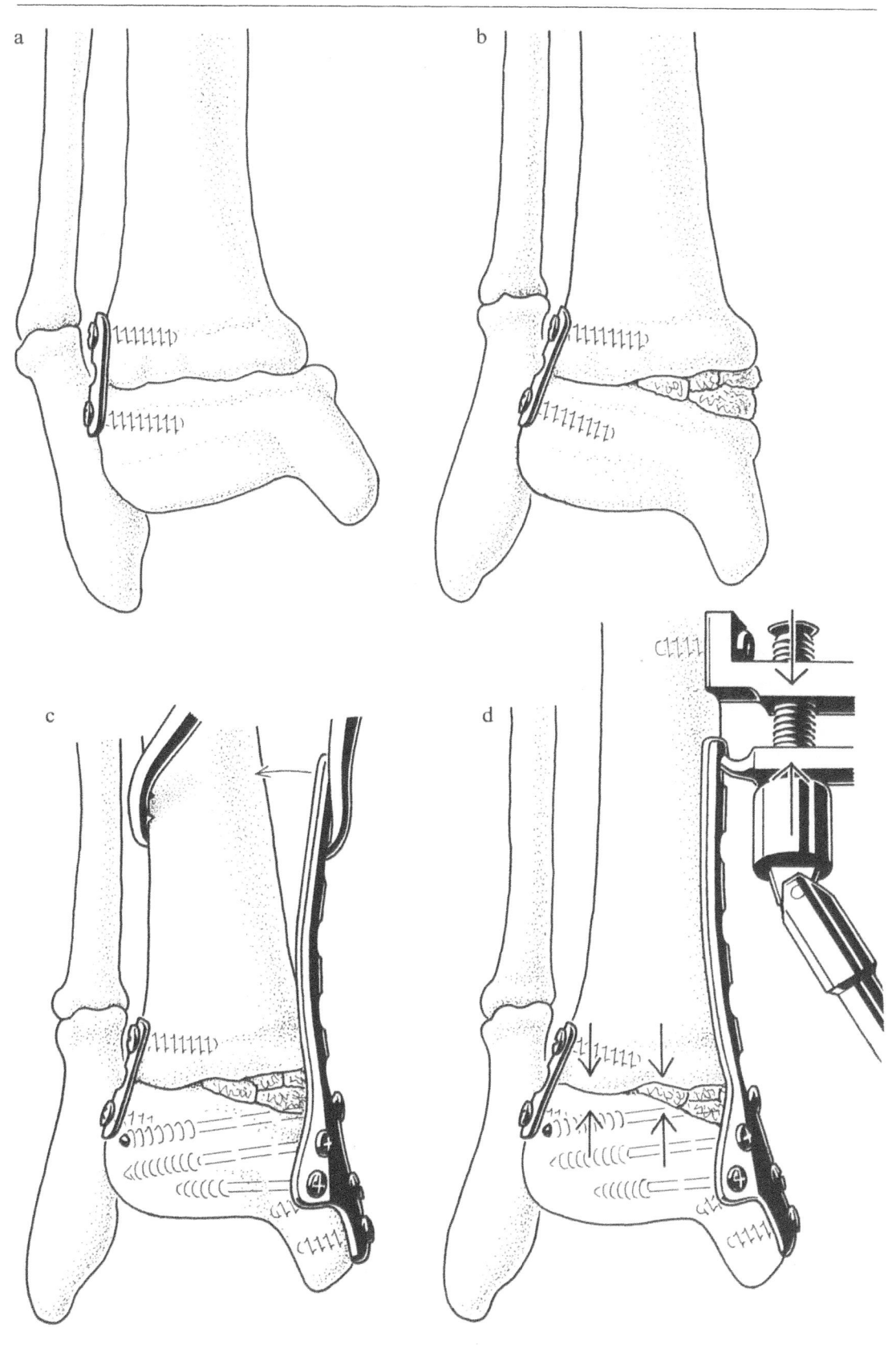

Fig. 104   Correction of a valgus deformity with a clover-leaf plate

Fig. 105   Correction of a rotational deformity with two small semi-tubular plates

192

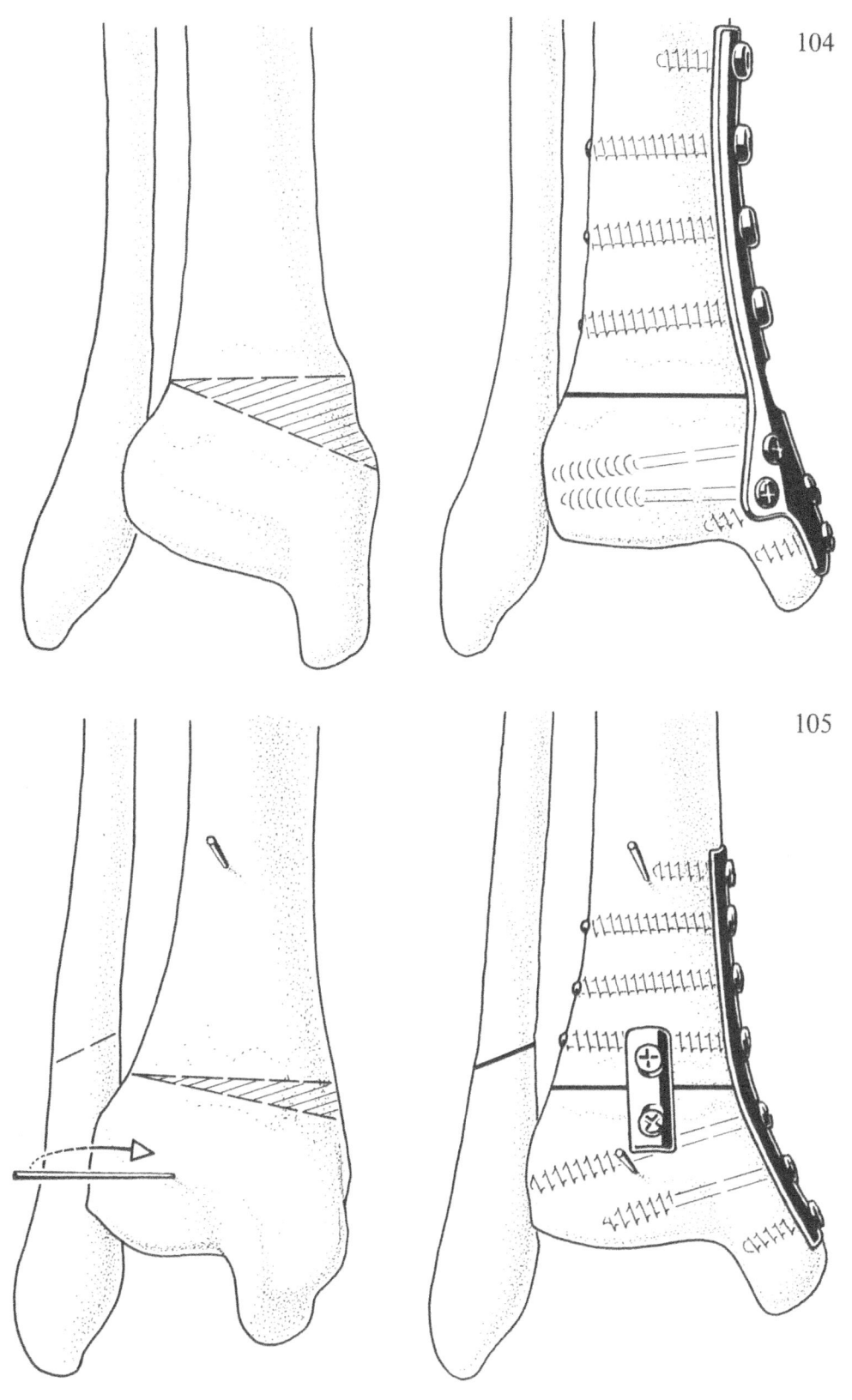

B. Malleolar Fractures

1. Introductions and Indication

Malleolar fractures are some of the most common injuries to the human skeleton. They are characterized by an extraordinary variety of lesions and have been a continuous subject of aetiological, clinical and therapeutic studies. Developments over recent years have led to operative treatment predominating. Here the credit is mainly due to H. Willenegger and B. G. Weber who have developed a clear and useful classification of the fracture types based on Danis' and Bonnin's studies. This scheme has rapidly gained ground and the surgical as well as the technical principles derived therefrom are now widely applied. A second edition of "Verletzungen des oberen Sprunggelenkes" by Weber has recently been published.

Attention now focuses on the pathology of the tibio-fibular syndesmosis and the following classification deals with the fracture dislocation of the ankle joint (Fig. 106):

Type A: Fractures of the fibula either at the level of, or distal to the tibio-talar joint.

Type B: Fracture of the fibula at the level of the sydesmosis.

Type C: Fracture of the fibula proximal to the syndesmosis, which is always associated with rupture of the interosseous ligament.

In type A the tibio-fibular syndesmosis remains intact. In type B it is often ruptured while in type C it is invariably torn and must be repaired.

The chief aim in operation is to reconstruct exactly and stably the fibula and this must be done if active post-operative treatment is to be carried out.

We shall now discuss the range of applications of small implants, as systematic trials have only been completed during recent years. There are still types of malleolar fracture which cannot be fixed by these implants in isolation. It is quite often necessary to combine items of the small fragment set with Kirschner wires and tension wires. We shall also deal with the very important repair of the syndesmosis as this is closely related to the use of the SFS.

Internal fixation of the medial malleolus will be dealt with separately from that of the lateral malleolus.

2. Lateral Internal Fixations

Lateral internal fixation is required in fractures of the lower fibula associated with spiral fractures of the tibia, in type C malleolar fractures with its different varieties, for type B and A malleolar fractures, in fractures of the triangular posterior fragment of the tibia (Volkmann), and in those of the anterior tibial triangle (Tillaux-Chaput).

a Anatomy and Topography of the Lower Fibula

The shape and structure of the lower fibula must be considered when using the SFS for fixation. On the outer side it is suitable for placing a plate, as there are no muscular insertions here.

Level with its articular surface, the fibula widens considerably and has a double bend which requires special attention. Small plates must be contoured into this S-shape (Fig. 107a).

In this region, the bony structure changes from hard cortical to softer cancellous bone (Fig. 107b). As the latter gives a less firm grip, small cortex screws of 3.5 mm or cancellous screws of 4.0 mm should be used as both these have sufficiently wide threads. 2–3 cm above the ankle joint the fibula has a lateral prominence which widens proximally (Fig. 107, marked with an arrow). This accounts for the lateral surface rotating increasingly in a dorsal direction. Plates must, therefore, be twisted to fit this surface to avoid any rotational deformity (Fig. 107d).

At this level the fibula is more posterior to the tibia so that screws must be aimed more forward towards the tibia. This may be helpful when a screw is required to transfix the fibula at right angles into the tibia, and using the 2.0 mm bit the cortex can be penetrated without a crack occurring (Fig. 107 c).

b) Associated Fracture of the Lower Fibula with Fractures of the Lower Leg

Most of these fractures are of the "vassal" type. Internal fixation of the tibia results in a spontaneous reduction of the fibula which then requires no further treatment (Fig. 23). This, however, does not always hold true; about 7% of fractures of the tibial shaft treated by us required additional operative fixation of the lower fibula. This occurs in two situations:

Irreducible axial deformity of the lower fibular fragment may occur after internal fixation of the tibia has been completed. Open reduction of the fibula is required to prevent any disturbance of the mobility of the ankle mortice (Fig. 108 a).
The short longitudinal incision directly above the fracture usually gives sufficient access. Oblique fractures are first reduced and then fixed with a cerclage wire or a small cortex screw. Where there is an indented transverse fracture or small fragment present, a small short semi-tubular plate may sometimes be applied (Fig. 108 b–d).

Instability of the ankle mortice after internal fixation of the tibia. Here the fibular fracture is associated with rupture of the anterior tibiofibular syndesmosis. The looseness of the ankle joint cannot for certain be diagnosed before the tibia has been fixed. After this the mortice must be carefully examined either clinically or with the image intensifier which is more reliable. If there is movement, the fibula must then be fixed by a long narrow semi-tubular plate and the ligaments must be repaired following the principles which apply to type C (Fig. 108 e).

c) Internal Fixation of the Fibula in Type C

The fracture is proximal to the syndesmosis which is always ruptured. These fractures are usually fixed with neutralization plates. The small semi-tubular plate has almost completely replaced medullary nailing of the fibula as the latter method offers very little resistance to rotation and can sometimes damage the bone badly. Two special conditions are now discussed in detail:

Comminuted Fractures of Type C

The fibula must be restored to its normal length, axial alignment and rotation, and this can often be difficult. In addition to the special forceps, temporary cerclage wiring may occasionally be necessary for the reduction. Long narrow semi-tubular plates with 6–8 holes are suitable for fixation. To prevent rotational deformity plates must be bent and twisted so that they exactly fit the shape of the lower fibula (Fig. 109). Small defects of cortical bone which are often present heal early and require no cancellous bone graft.
The next step is the repair of the syndesmosis including the interosseous membrane. Where the anterior and posterior ligaments are ruptured or where a small Volkmann triangle has been avulsed, the stability of the ankle mortice may be impaired despite the exact internal fixation of the fibula and repair of the syndesmosis. The fibula must then be fixed in place against, the tibia.

Transfixation to the Tibia

This is carried out with a screw which is placed 3–5 cm above the ankle joint and thus proximal to the syndesmosis. The screw should provide stability without actually compressing the syndesmosis. A cortex screw is therefore used rather than a cancellous or malleolar screw. The thread in the fibula should be retained and no gliding hole made. The screw gets a grip of three layers of cortical bone consisting of two cortices in the fibula and one in the tibia so that an elastic fixation is achieved which does not impede the mobility of the ankle mortice. This transfixtion screw can usually be inserted through one of the holes in the plate. When the internal fixation of the fibula and repair of the syndesmosis has been completed, one screw may be removed from the plate at a suitable point for its replacement with the transfixtion screw, and the drill hole is then extended into the tibia. After tapping the thread, a long 3.5 mm cortex screw is inserted in the empty plate hole and anchored in the distal tibial metaphysis (Fig. 110a and b).

The *internal fixation of a high fibular fracture*. A transfixtion screw can be inserted below the end of the plate simply joining the tibia to the fibula (Fig. 110c).

From our experience early removal of a transfixation screw inserted by this technique is unnecessary. Because no compressive effect has been achieved, there is no danger of limiting the ankle joint movement nor of calcification or ossification in the syndesmosis. Areas of bone resorption can sometimes be seen at the tip of the screw where very small degrees of movement have been required.

High Fibular Fractures in Type C Cases

Here special surgical techniques are required, of which one is *direct internal fixation*; rigid fixation of fractures of the shaft of the fibula can be obtained either by screw fixation or by a neutralization plate. After repair of the ligaments we must again check the stability of the ankle mortice. Where this is adequate, transfixation can be omitted but it must be undertaken when there is unsatisfactory stability.

The second method is to use *indirect fixation:* while direct fixation is possible in the middle of the shaft of the fibula, above this it is more difficult and may endanger the lateral popliteal nerve. Weber's technique may then be used:

— The lower end of the fibula is reduced under tension into the notch of the tibia.

— Temporary transfixion of the fibula to the tibia near to the joint with a transverse Kirschner wire.

— X-ray comparison with the normal side is used to confirm that full length of the fibula has been restored and the films will also show whether the higher fibular fracture has been reduced by this method.

— Final fixation is carried out by inserting one or two transverse screws between the fibula and the tibia, proximal to the syndesmosis.

The following procedures are then used:

— Repair of the syndesmosis must be done *before* final fixation and must involve the anterior tibio-fibular ligament as well as the interosseous membrane. Sutures inserted into the bone are often necessary (see below).

— Because of the posterior position of the fibula, holes for positioning screws must be drilled obliquely from a posterior position in the fibula in an antero-medial direction. It is important to prevent the screws causing a rotational deformity in the lower fibula (Fig. 107).

— For transfixion, we use long cortex screws of 4.5 mm or sometimes of 3.5 mm, and they must obtain a grip with four threads in both tibial cortices. The fibula too should be tapped so that screws threads can obtain a bite here as compression of the syndesmosis must be avoided (Fig. 110d).

— *Maisonneuve's fracture* provides the extraordinary type of C fracture. Here the fibula is fractured at its head, near the knee and is often overlooked. The whole length of the interosseous membrane is then torn and fixation of the fibula can only be indirectly effected, as described above.

d) Internal Fixation of the Fibula in a Type B Case

The fracture of the fibula is on a level with the syndesmosis which itself is often ruptured.

This fracture can usually be reduced and fixed with small cortex or small cancellous screws. In a short oblique fracture or where there are multiple fragments additional support is needed. Here we often use a well contoured small semi-tubular plate with 5–6 holes applied as a neutralization plate (Fig. 111 a–c). Since the positioning of this plate is rather time-consuming, it is sometimes replaced by oblique or axial Kirschner wires. An obliquely placed transfixion Kirschner wire at a proximal level has no detrimental effect on the ankle joint (Willenegger). Sometimes tension-wiring alone is suitable for this type of fracture (Fig. 111c).

e) Internal Fixation of Fibula in Type A

The fibular fracture is situated at the joint line and the syndesmosis is intact.

Here there is usually a short oblique or transverse fracture which can seldom be reduced by screws. Some cases are suitable for neutralization plates, but most are fixable with Kirschner or cerclage wires (Fig. 111f). We have altogether given up the use of screws inserted into the tip of the malleolus running vertically upwards. It is difficult to achieve an exact point of insertion, and tightening such a screw often causes secondary displacement of the fracture (Fig. 111d). Special attention must be paid to the associated rupture of ligaments distal to the syndesmosis, namely the anterior fibulo-talar and the fibulo-calcaneal ligaments which must be sutured to give a stable joint.

f) The Technique of Repairing the Syndesmosis in the Ankle Joint

Weber especially stresses the importance of repairing ruptured ligaments which is necessary for the reconstruction of the ankle joint. Here we enumerate the lesions which need to be sutured.

Anterior Tibio-Fibular Syndesmosis:

— Avulsion of the ligament from the tibia with or without a small cortical bone fragment.
— Rupture of the substance of the ligament which is often Z-shaped.
— Avulsion from the fibula with or without a small cortical bone fragment.

Interosseous Membrane:

— Avulsion from the tibia predominates.

Fibulo-Talar and Fibulo-Calcaneal Ligament:

— Avulsion from the fibula predominates.

Deltoid Ligament:

— Talar avulsion.
— Tibial avulsion.

Where surgical repair of such ruptures is advocated, one often encounters the argument that torn tendons cannot be properly sutured. Transfixion screws are then often used between the tibia and the fibula — *much too frequently* in our opinion. As the technique for the repair of the syndesmosis in the ankle joint is not yet well understood and since it is closely connected with the use of small implants, we now describe the *basic principles* involved:

— Ligament ruptures with tibial or fibular fragments of large enough size are repaired by *screw fixation* (Figs. 111c, 114).
— Periosteal tears or ligaments ruptured in their substance are repaired by means of *transosseous suture*. Tunnels can be drilled on either side with a drill bit, with Kirschner wires or with a small hand drill (Fig. 112b and c).
— Fibular sutures are best *anchored in metal*, which may be a small plate, a cerclage or tension wire, or a Kirschner wire (Fig. 112d).
— The choice of suture material is of less importance. We use Dexon of calibre 0 or 00. As this material is absorbable, disturbances in wound healing are minimised while it ensures fixation until fibrous tissue has regenerated. Its elasticity allows the necessary small degree of movement in the syndesmosis.
— Where an extensive repair of the syndesmosis has been required, post-operative treatment must not force active mobilization of the ankle joint. When the wound has healed, the ankle joint is held at 90° with an external splint which is left in place until the end of the sixth or eighth week. By that time, fibrous tissue has usually regenerated and subsequent post-operative treatment depends on the healing of the fracture.

g) Posterior Triangle Fragment of the Tibia (Volkmann)

Although this is a lateral fracture, a medial approach is used for its reduction. Internal fixation of the tibia produces a lateral stabilizing effect.

Reduction of the lateral malleolus produces a spontaneous setting of small fragments. The intact posterior syndesmosis restores the small triangle to its normal position.

When a lateral X-ray shows that the fragment carries one third or more of the articular surface (between 0.8 and 1 cm in width), internal fixation is indicated. Reduction is achieved *from the medial side* using Weber's method, with the help of the reduction forceps which he has designed. Two small cancellous screws are inserted at slightly different levels. When the first screw has been fixed nearest to the joint, the reduction forceps are removed and replaced by a second screw inserted in the same direction (Fig. 113). The stability thus achieved exceeds that obtained with a single screw. The short thread on the cancellous screw guarantees appropriate interfragmentary compression. The second screw counteracts any shearing forces which are particularly prone to fall on the posterolateral end of the tibial articular surface when post-operative movement begins (Weber).

We seldom use the *posterior approach* though it does allow an exact open reduction. Posterior screw fixation can also achieve better interfragmentary compression (Fig. 113e). On the other hand, reduction of the fragments and especially repair of the anterior syndesmosis often requires re-positioning the patient and sometimes a third incision, which lengthens the operating time and the risk of the procedure.

h) The Antero-Lateral Triangle of the Tibia (Tillaux-Chaput)

It is sometimes difficult to discern this fracture on the X-ray. When this is the case, additional oblique projections should be made. The size of the fragment varies from a very small avulsed chip at the insertion of the syndesmosis, to a wedge-shaped fragment. Stabilization is imperative because of the connection with the anterior tibio-fibular syndesmosis, but can usually be obtained with a small cancellous screw. When the fracture is exposed, the cutaneous branch of the fibular nerve must be carefully protected (Fig. 114).

3. Medial Malleolar Fixation

From the bio-mechanical aspect, fractures of the lateral malleolus are of much greater importance than those of the medial side of the ankle joint. Because of this, technical problems about the reduction of the medial side of the ankle joint have been somewhat neglected. These fractures must, however, also be accurately reduced and rigidly fixed. The special shape of the medial malleolus, consisting of a double curve must be taken into special consideration. Particular attention must be paid to the area of the tibial epiphysis as well as to the posterior tendinous canal of the tibialis posterior, and the long flexors of the toes with their strong synovial sheaths.

Besides the typical medial malleolar fracture there are other injuries on the medial side: a long spiral fracture of the tibia may reach the malleolus, there may be impaction of the anterior articular surface in adduction fractures, and finally there are the epiphysial fractures of the posterior tibia.

a) Associated Malleolar Fracture in Fracture of the Tibial Shaft

This fracture is quite common. Our statistics show that in over 10% of spiral fractures of the tibia, the fracture reaches the medial side of the ankle joint, involving the medial malleolus. Since some crack fractures are invisible on standard X-rays, they may only be discovered during the operation for fixation. They may be found anteriorly, laterally or posteriorly, and must all be fixed to allow active post-operative movement. Reduction of mobile fractures involving the articular surface of the ankle must be given priority over the main tibial fractures. Where simple fissures are concerned, this procedure may be reversed.

Approach: The slightly curved elongation of the standard incision for internal fixation of the tibia; incision should run along the anterior edge of the medial malleolus to its tip. Here the long saphenous vein is encountered and often needs to be divided between ligatures. The ankle joint is exposed just in front of the deltoid ligament (Fig. 115). The accuracy of the reduction and its stability should be confirmed by direct vision.

Internal Fixation: three different methods of fixing these associated fractures have proved to be effective: The *long semi-tubular plate* is used to neutralize the fracture of the lower tibia while extending far enough to fix the malleolar fracture as well. Its relative flatness and ease with which it can be contoured are an advantage. The wide oval screw holes allow the most distal cancellous screw to be placed parallel to the ankle joint and the head is well enough recessed (Fig. 116c). The standard straight ASIF plate is less suitable for this purpose as the distal screw could enter the joint. It is also somewhat too bulky and occupies much space.

Where internal fixation must extend to the very tip of the malleolus, an *additional small semi-tubular plate* can be used to extend the fixation (Fig. 116b).

In fractures where the proximal tibia is involved, and a long crack extends to the medial malleolus it is better to avoid the use of a very long plate. Crack fractures in the ankle should be reduced by *separate screw fixation* while the tibial fracture is held with a neutralization plate. In other words, both fractures should be reduced according to the methods used in fractures at two levels (Fig. 116c).

In the *typical fracture* of the medial malleolus, fixation with small cancellous screws is clearly indicated. Comminuted fractures are often reduced by a combination of Kirschner wires and tension-band wiring. The screw, however, is usually the basic requirement in open reduction here.

Where there is a large malleolar fragment, this should be reduced with two screws inserted in different directions according to the stabilization rule 1 (p. 24). Shearing forces are thus counteracted and interfragmentary compression is improved as the screws get a bite at several levels of the fracture surface, which is often irregular (Fig. 117a).

Where the condition of the soft tissues is poor, a single screw inserted through a stab incision can provide sufficient stability.

We distinguished four fractures types:

b) The Small Avulsion Fracture,

which lies either at the edge of the articular surface or more distally. This is reduced by screw fixation or tension wiring. Ruptures of neighbouring ligaments must also be repaired (Fig. 117c).

c) Larger Anterior Fractures,

which may consist of several fragments (Fig. 117b and c).

d) Posterior Semi-Circular Fractures,

of which the boat-shaped fragment extends well backward into the posterior articular surface of the tibia. Inadequate reduction of such a fracture leads to arthrosis. Here a wide exposure of the posterior synovial sheath is indispensable and the standard incision has to be extended both distally and proximally. The tibialis posterior tendon must be retracted with a blunt hook. After reduction and temporary fixation with Kirschner wires, screws are inserted in such a manner that their heads lie on the edge of the synovial sheath to prevent any rubbing effect. As the cortical bone is stronger in this area, it gives a sufficient grip for the screws. When screwing has been completed, the synovial sheaths are closed with a few sutures (Fig. 117e).

e) Adduction Fractures

are those in which the fracture surface extends to the medial proximal cortex of the tibia. Fixation is obtained with two cancellous screws inserted in a direction roughly parallel to the articular surface. Special attention must be paid to any impaction of the antero-medial articular surface of the tibia which can be small though rather dense. Exact adaptation of fracture surfaces can then be difficult. There are also wider impactions approaching those found in the comminuted tibial fracture (Fig. 118a). Before reduction, these impacted areas must be carefully identified, while the major malleolar fragment is retracted with a hook. Reduc-

200

tion of the articular surface is obtained with a suitable lever. If a cancellous bone defect develops, it must be filled with autogenous bone graft. Where only a small graft is needed, it can be obtained from the adjoining tibial epiphysis if this is intact. That may be termed "a local shift of cancellous bone" (Fig. 118 b). Screw fixation thus compresses the reconstructed articular surface and prevents any further breakage.

4. Secondary Intervention after Malleolar Fractures

a) Delayed Internal Fixation

Non-union occurring after the conservative treatment of fractures requires secondary open reduction. In the presence of instability or where easily visible callus can be removed, the reduction is carried out according to the principles of primary treatment. This is often feasible even if several months have passed since the accident. The same implants are used as those for primary internal fixation.

b) Pseudarthroses

Pseudarthroses occur very rarely after primary surgery in malleolar fractures. After conservative treatment they are commoner in the medial than lateral malleolus. They are reduced either by compression alone with two small screws, or combined with autogenous cancellous bone graft in the form of a compressed bridging graft. In some cases, a figure-of-8 tension wire will obtain better compression than a screw (Fig. 28 c)

c) Osteotomy

Shortening of the lateral malleolus combined with neglected ligament ruptures are the most frequent indications for osteotomy in the ankle joint. Weber and Willenegger have especially stressed the importance of these conditions, and investigated feasible procedures for their surgical correction. The lengthening osteotomy of the fibula can be easily fixed with the small semi-tubular plate. It is appropriate to fill the defect with cancellous bone in the graft interposition manner (Fig. 27). This peg is axially compressed by the main fragments and also fixed by the plate. Skin strips inserted transosseously are recommended for the reconstruction of the syndesmotic ligament.

C. Fractures of the Talus

The rare indications for internal fixation of fractures of the talus include the dislocated fracture which requires open reduction as well as cases where there are defects in cancellous bone. Small cancellous screws inserted obliquely from the medial side in a proximal direction are very suitable. Weight relief by the use of a walking caliper for several months is a vital part of the post-operative management (Fig. 128).

D. Clinical X-Ray Examples

Figs. 119–128, pages 222–239

Fig. 106 Classification of malleolar fractures
(see also Müller *et al.*, Manual of Internal Fixation, 1970, p. 196)

Type A Transverse fractures of the fibula, either at the level of, or distal to the joint. Possible shear fracture of the medial malleolus

Type B Spiral fracture, level with the syndesmosis, together with rupture of the anterior tibio-fibular ligament. Rupture of the deltoid ligament or avulsion fracture of the medial malleolus

Type C Oblique fracture of the fibula immediately above the syndesmosis. Rupture of the syndesmotic ligaments, possible avulsion of the posterior margin of the tibia
High fracture of the fibula with tearing of the interosseous membrane and both ligaments of the syndesmosis

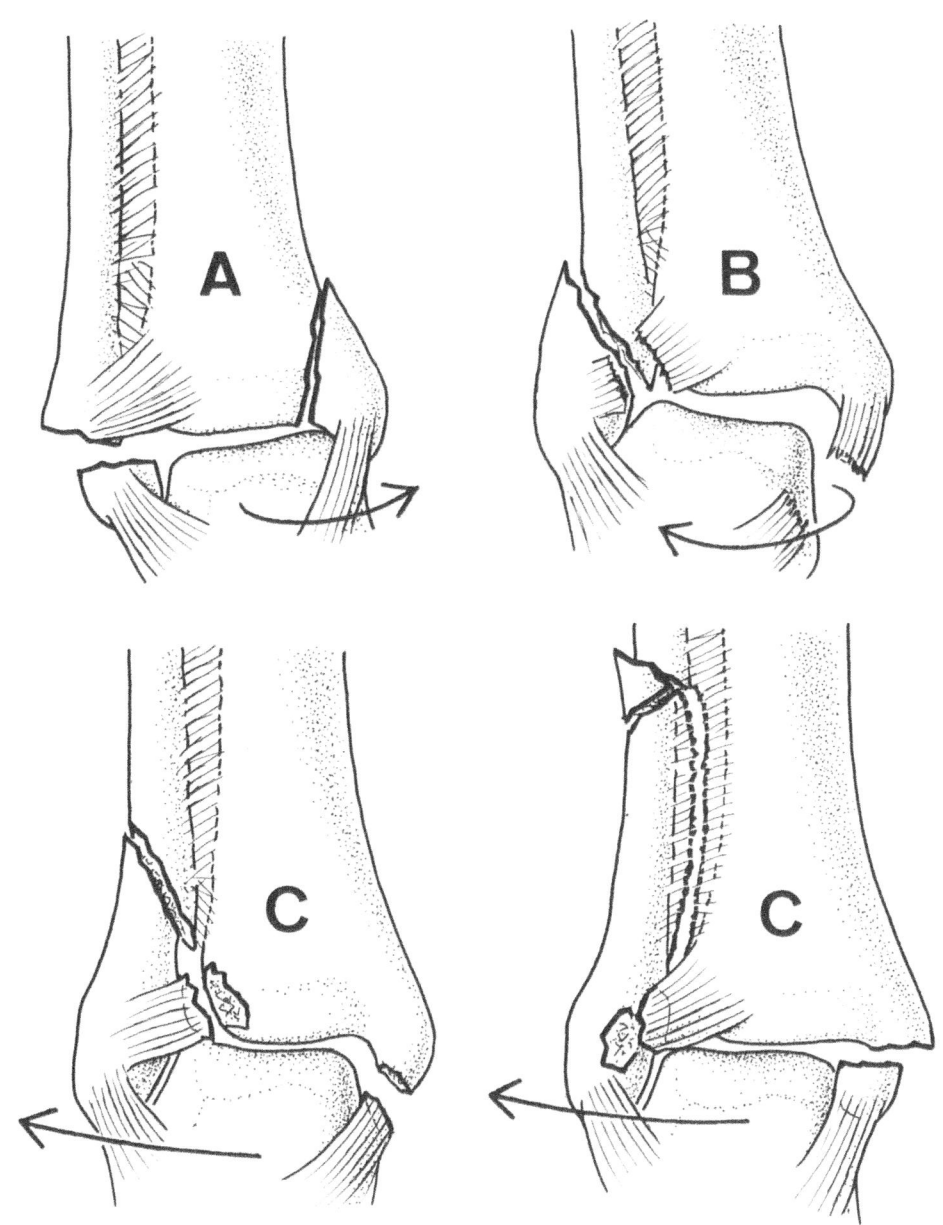

Fig. 107 Anatomy of the lower fibula

a Lower fibula seen from the front with an accurately contoured small semi-tubular plate, and a lateral view

b Cross sections of the lower fibula at different levels: Changes in the bony structure. Lateral spur marked with arrow

c Topographical relations between the fibula and tibia: the dorsal position of the fibula in relation to the tibia. Posterior inclination of the lateral surface of the fibula in the area above the malleolus

d The slope of the lateral fibular surface requires a twist to be applied to the small semi-tubular plate

e Cross section at different levels to show the situation of the small semi-tubular plate. Plate screws above the malleolus are also inserted in a direction towards the tibia and this allows one to be used for transfixion

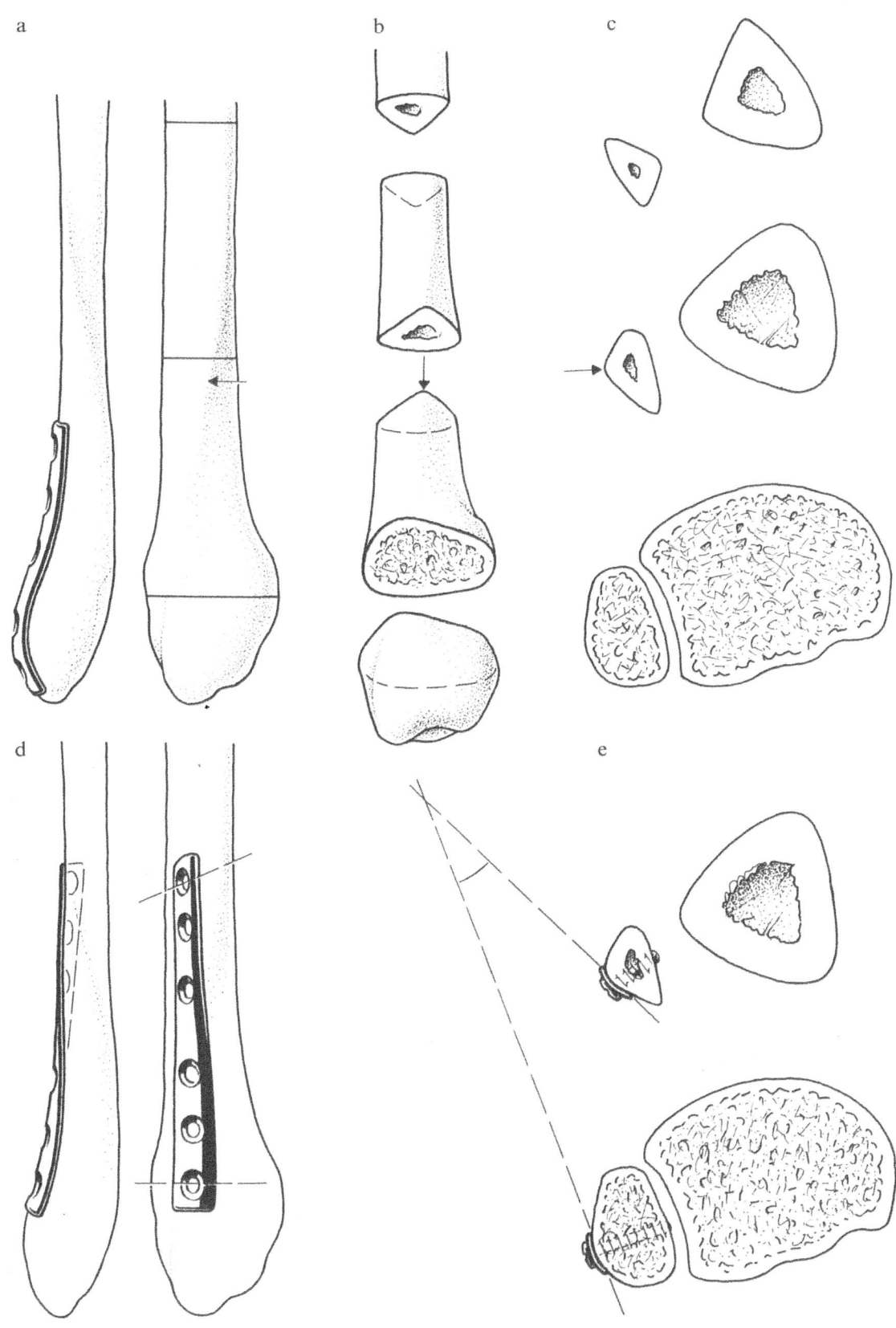

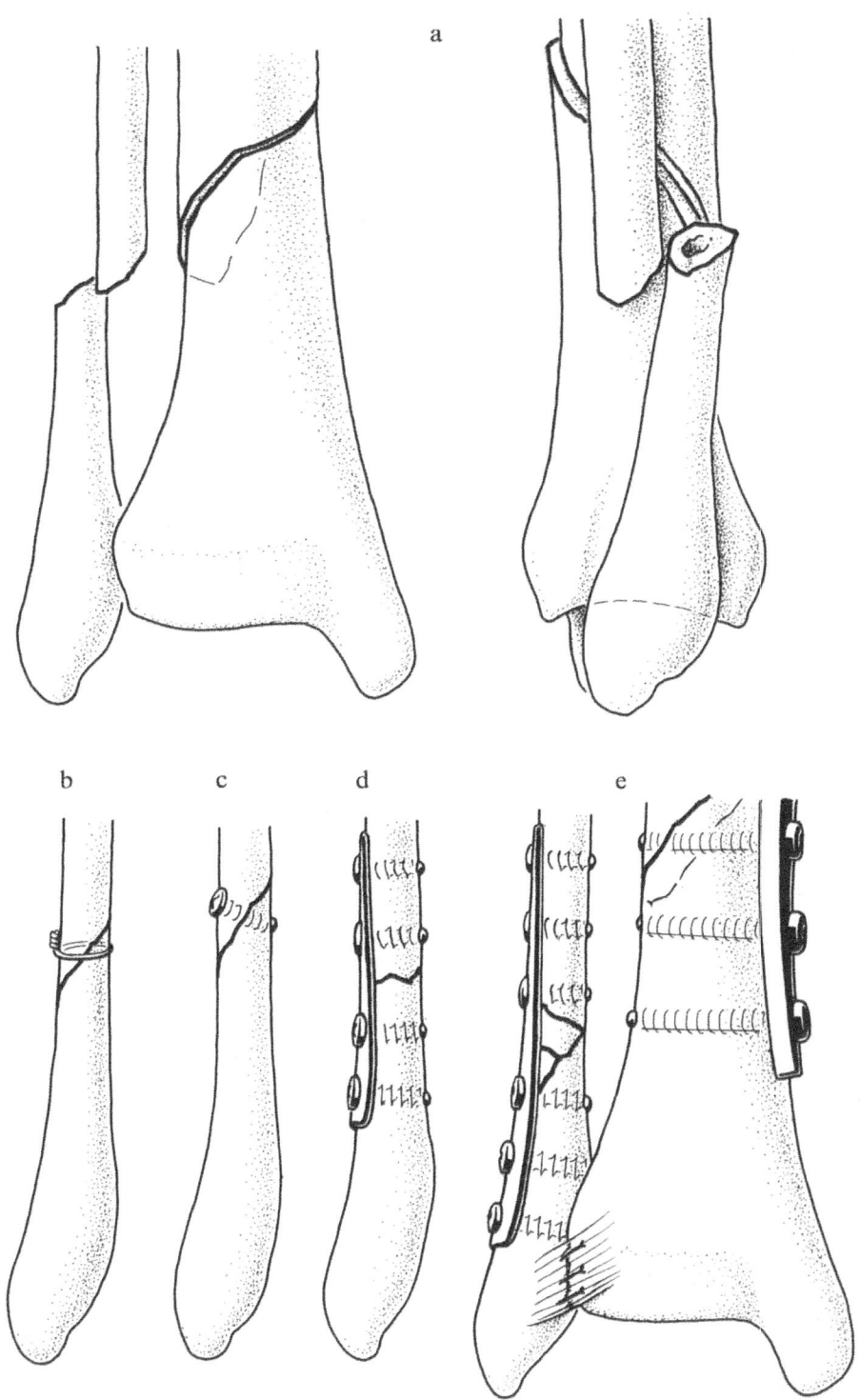

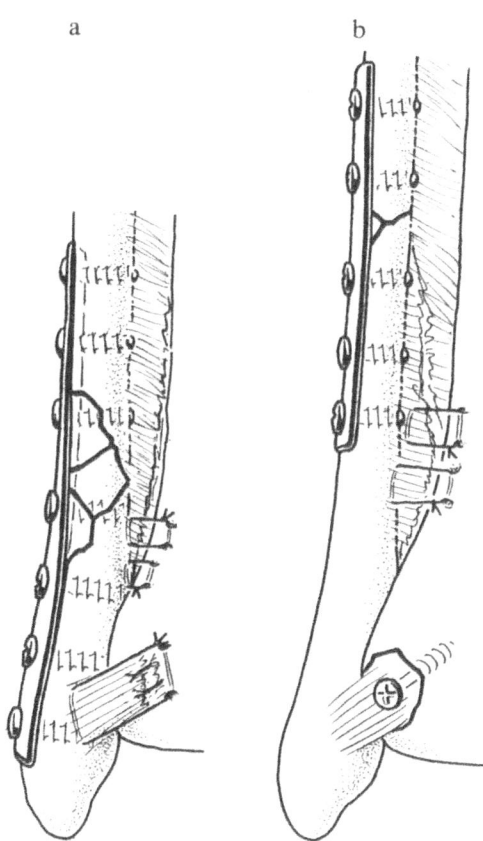

a   b

Fig. 109   Internal fixation of the fibula in type C

    a   Comminuted fracture: Long narrow semi-tubular plate and repair of the syndesmosis including the interosseous membrane

    b   High fracture of type C: Small semi-tubular plate and repair of the syndesmosis or screw fixation of a small antero-lateral fragment of the tibia

◁

Fig. 108   Associated fracture of the lower fibula with fracture of the lower leg

    a   Persistent displacement of the lower fibula in internal fixation of the tibia

  b–d   Procedure in the "vassal" fracture: Open reduction and fixation with cerclage wire, a single screw or a short semi-tubular plate

    e   Procedure in the presence of instability of the ankle mortice: A long narrow semi-tubular plate and repair of the syndesmosis

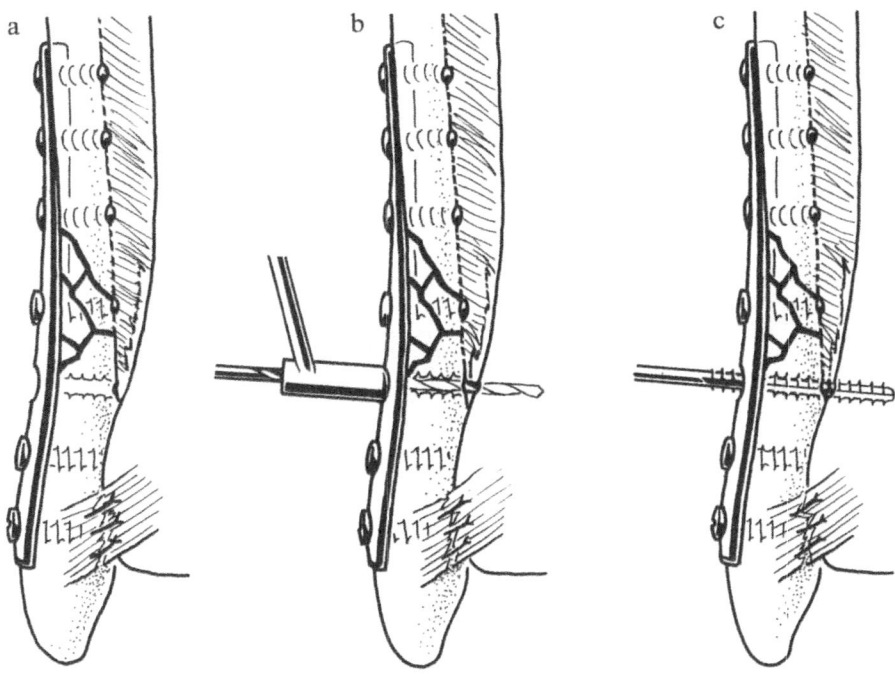

Fig. 110 Transfixion of the fibula and tibia: to be carried out after completion of internal fixation and ligament repair

Technique:

a Removal of one plate screw 3–5 cm above the ankle joint

b Drill-hole in the fibula is extended to the lateral tibial cortex with a 2.0 mm drill bit. No gliding hole is made in the fibula

c A hole in the lateral tibial cortex is tapped

Principle of stabilization without compression:

d Since the transfixion screw is anchored in three cortices, compression is avoided

e Incorrect procedure: If the hole in the fibula is converted into a gliding hole, the transfixing screw is anchored in only one layer of cortical bone, that is in the lateral tibia, and this results in compression between the fibula and tibia

f Where the transfixion screw is anchored in four cortices (1–2–3–4) proximal displacement of the lower fibula is prevented. This applies to high fibula fractures

Different types of transfixion:

g Supramalleolar comminuted fractures: fixation by the lowest plate screw but two

h High fracture of the fibula: transfixion via the lower end of the plate

i Transfixion with a screw inserted independently from the plate when the latter is placed at a higher level

k Position of screws in Maisonneuve's fracture: Screws are biting on four cortices. For the sake of stability, 4.5 mm screws are used as a rule

208

d

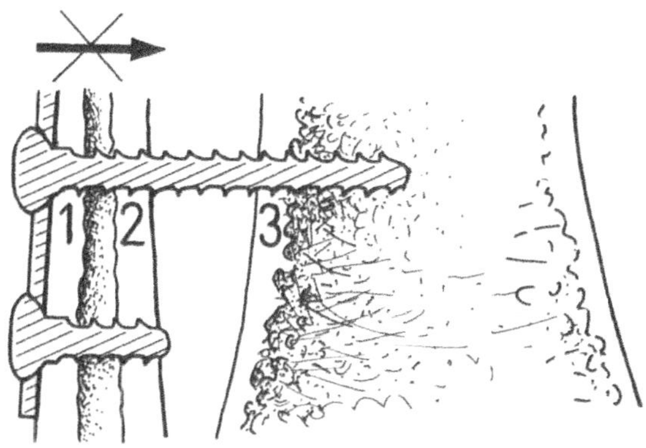

e

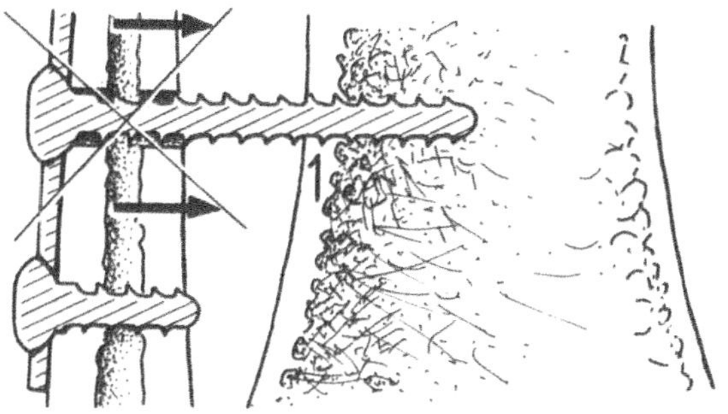

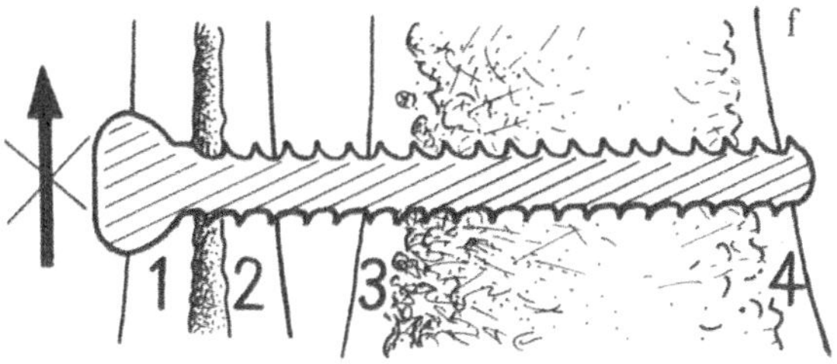

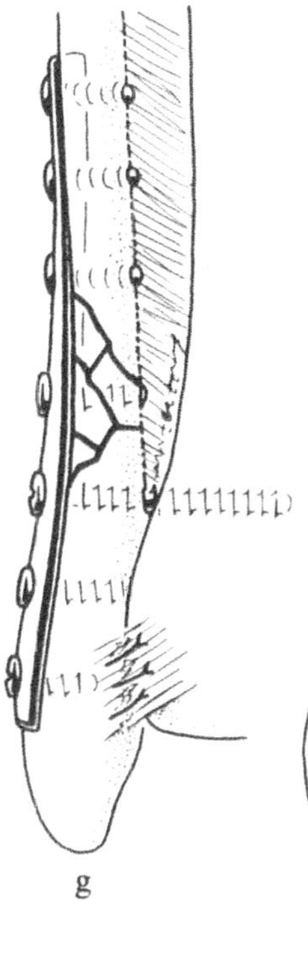

g

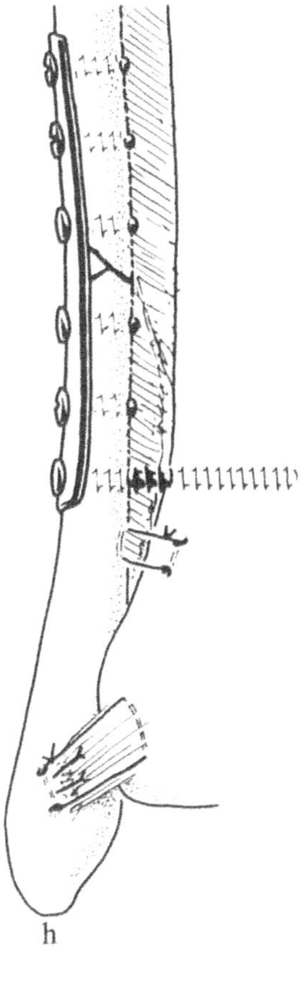

h

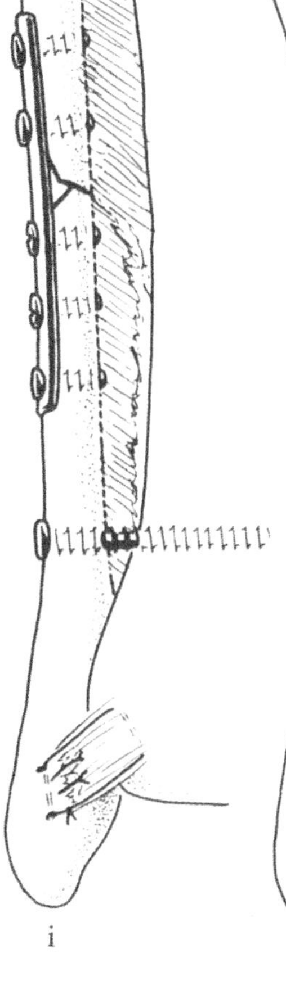

i

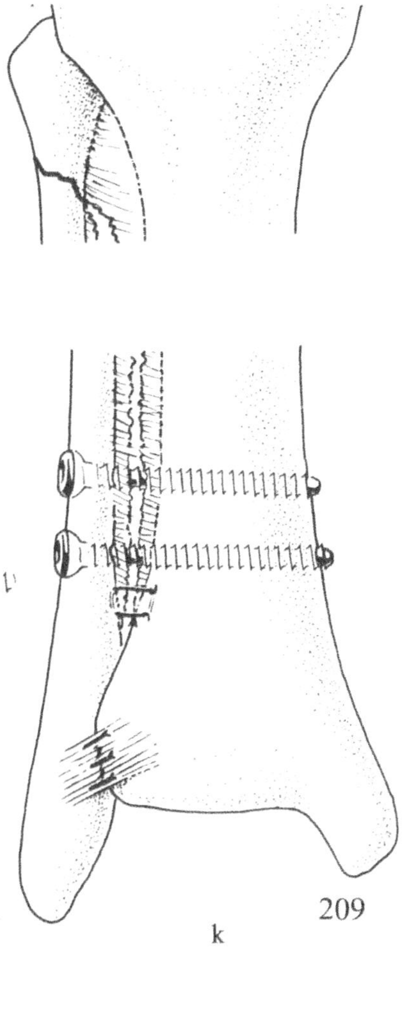

k

Fig. 111 Internal fixation of fibula in fracture type A and B

a Screw fixation of a long fracture of type B and repair of the ligament

b Screw fixation and neutralization plate as well as suture of the ligament

c Neutralization plate and screw fixation of an avulsion fracture of the fibular cortical bone at the insertion of the anterior tibio-fibular ligament

d Two methods of internal fixation, recently discontinued: Medullary nailing and cerclage wiring, axial screw fixation

e Modified internal fixation: Reduction with Kirschner wires and oblique transfixtion wires possibly combined with tension-band wiring

f Internal fixation by tension-band wiring in a fracture type A

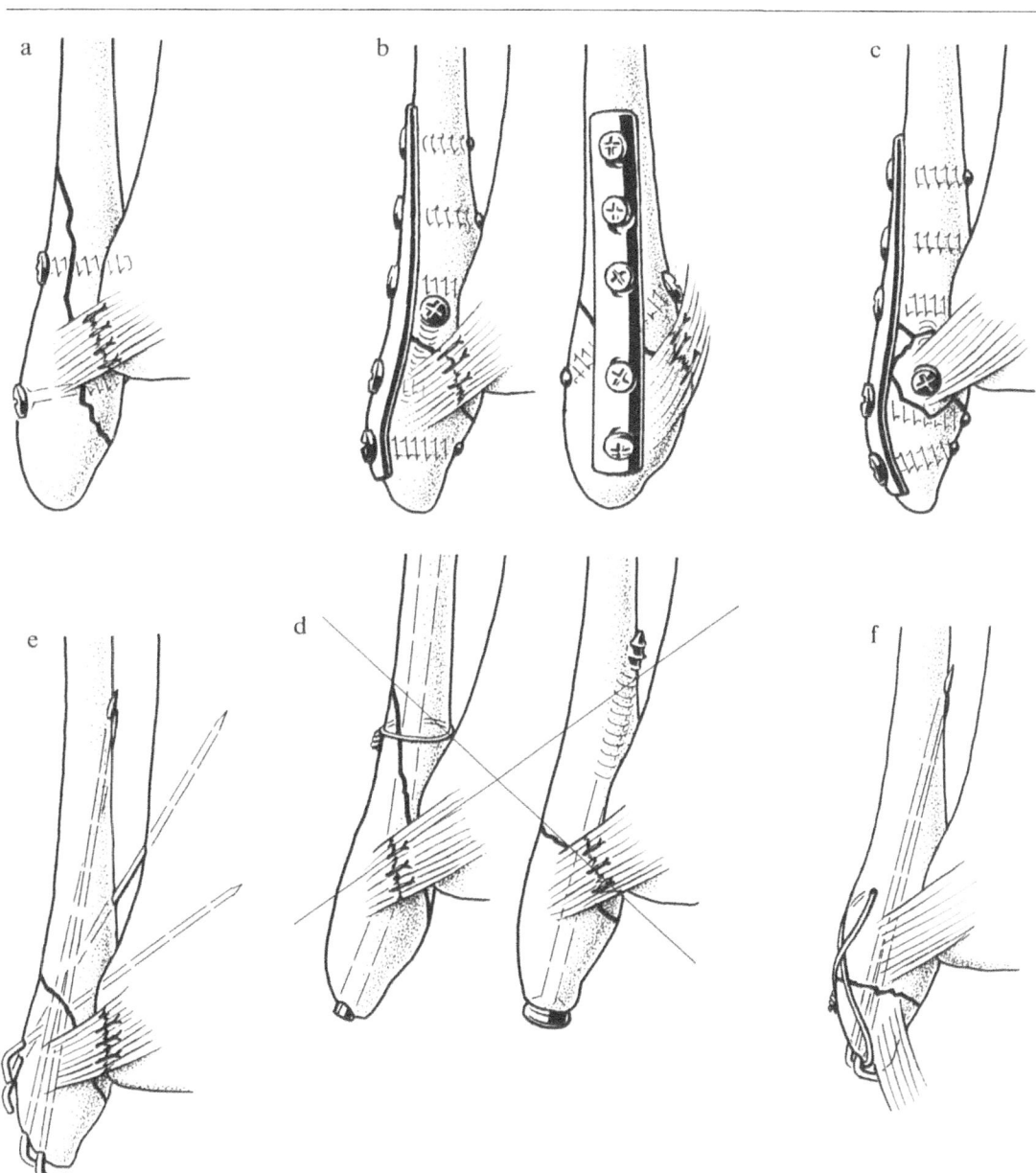

Fig. 112 The technique of ligament repair in the ankle

   a   Usual suture of rupture of the substance of the anterior syndesmotic ligament

   b   Supplementary interosseous reinforcing suture of a torn anterior syndesmotic ligament (site is framed)

   c   Sutures inserted through holes in one bone in the following ligament ruptures: sutures are inserted through holes in the tibia for ruptures of interosseous membrane and the syndesmotic ligament, but in the fibula for fibulo-talar ligament. Interosseous reinforcing sutures are passed twice through the drill holes

   d   Supplementary sutures may be anchored in different ways in the material used for internal fixation: around a small semi-tubular plate, around a tension-band wire, and around the projecting ends of Kirschner wires whether these have been inserted from the tibia to the fibula or vice versa

   e   Intraosseous suture: Oblique holes are made with a drill and a curved needle can then pass through these holes

212

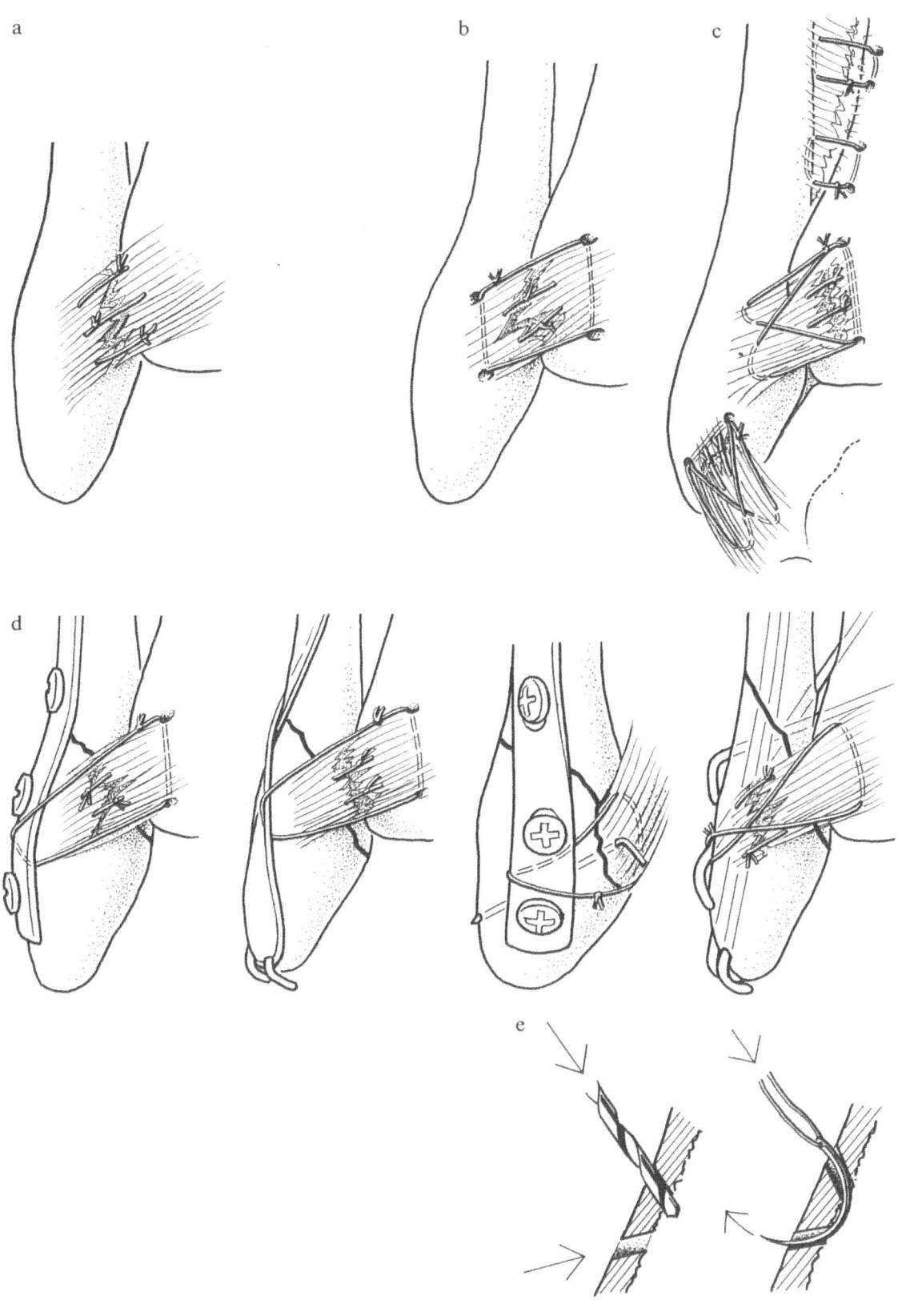

Fig. 113 **Internal fixation of the postero-lateral triangle (Volkmann)**

  a Initial position

  b Reduction with the special forceps designed by Weber. The first drill hole is made near the joint

  c Insertion of the first screw and removal of forceps

  d Second screw is inserted in exactly the line of the forceps which have just been removed

  e Posterior screw fixation

Fig. 114 **Fracture of the antero-lateral triangle of the tibia:** Screw fixation

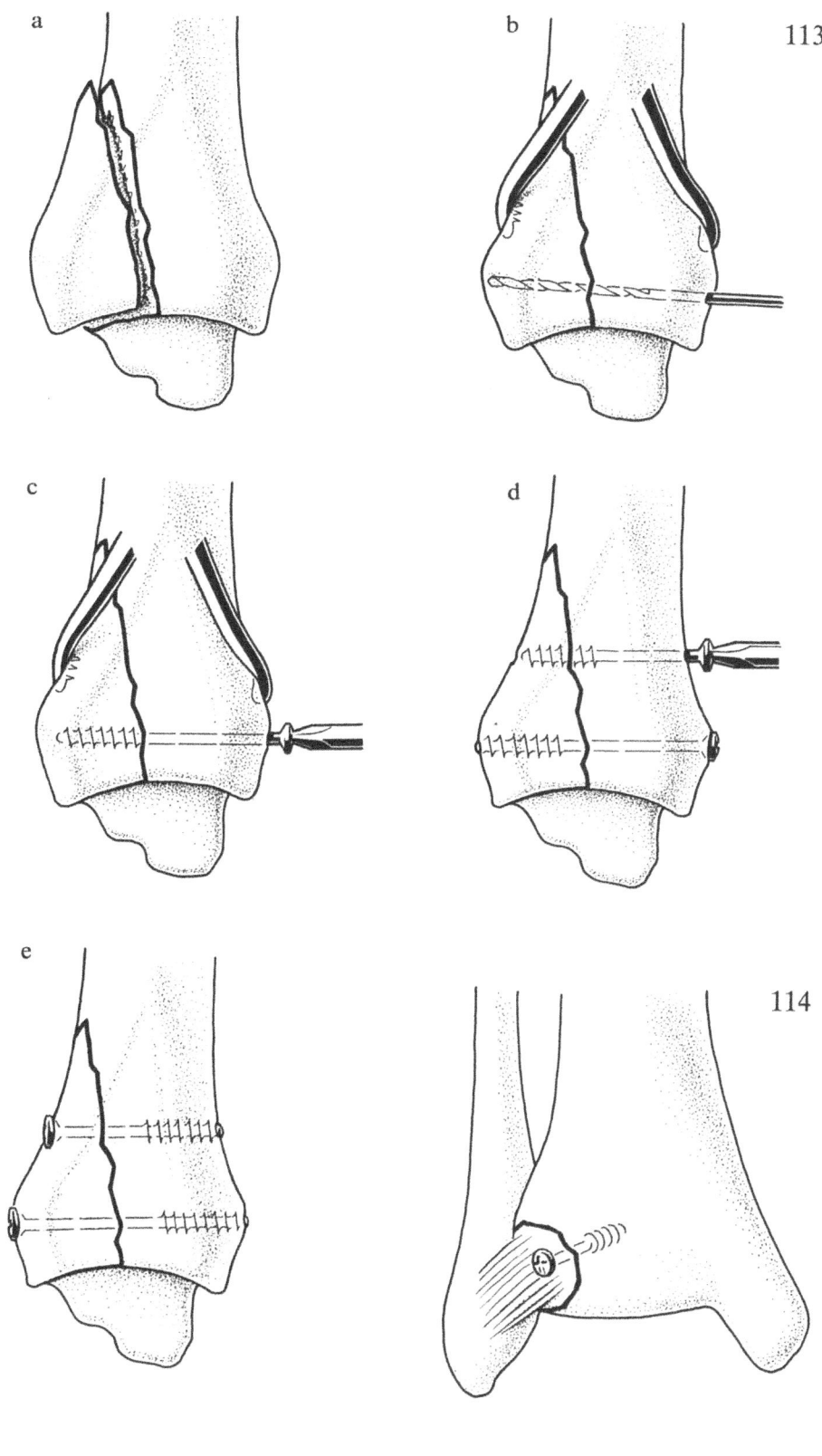

Fig. 115 Malleolar fracture combined with a fracture of the tibial shaft: Incision and approach

Curved extension of the standard incision running along the anterior crest of the medial malleolus. Exposure of the ankle joint after division and ligation of the long saphenous vein

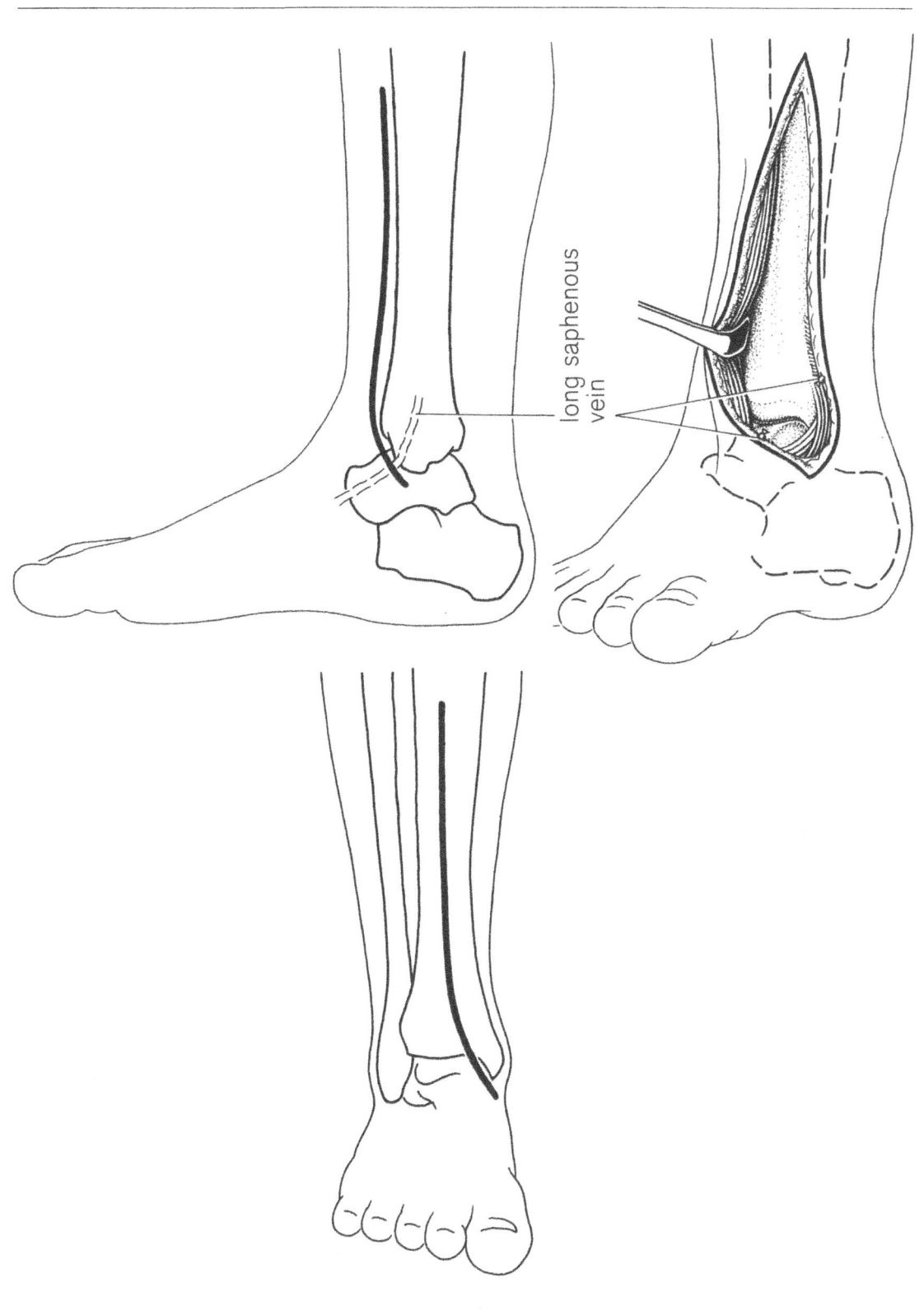

long saphenous
vein

Fig. 116 Internal fixation of fracture of the medial malleolus combined with a fracture of the tibial shaft

a The semi-tubular neutralization plate extends down to the articular fragment, while the bottom cancellous screw inserted parallel to the articular surface, fixes and compresses the malleolar fracture

b Extending the effect of the semi-tubular plate by adding the small semi-tubular plate to fix the malleolus

c Independent fixation of a fracture of the tibial plateau with a narrow straight ASIF plate, while the distal fracture is reduced and held by screws

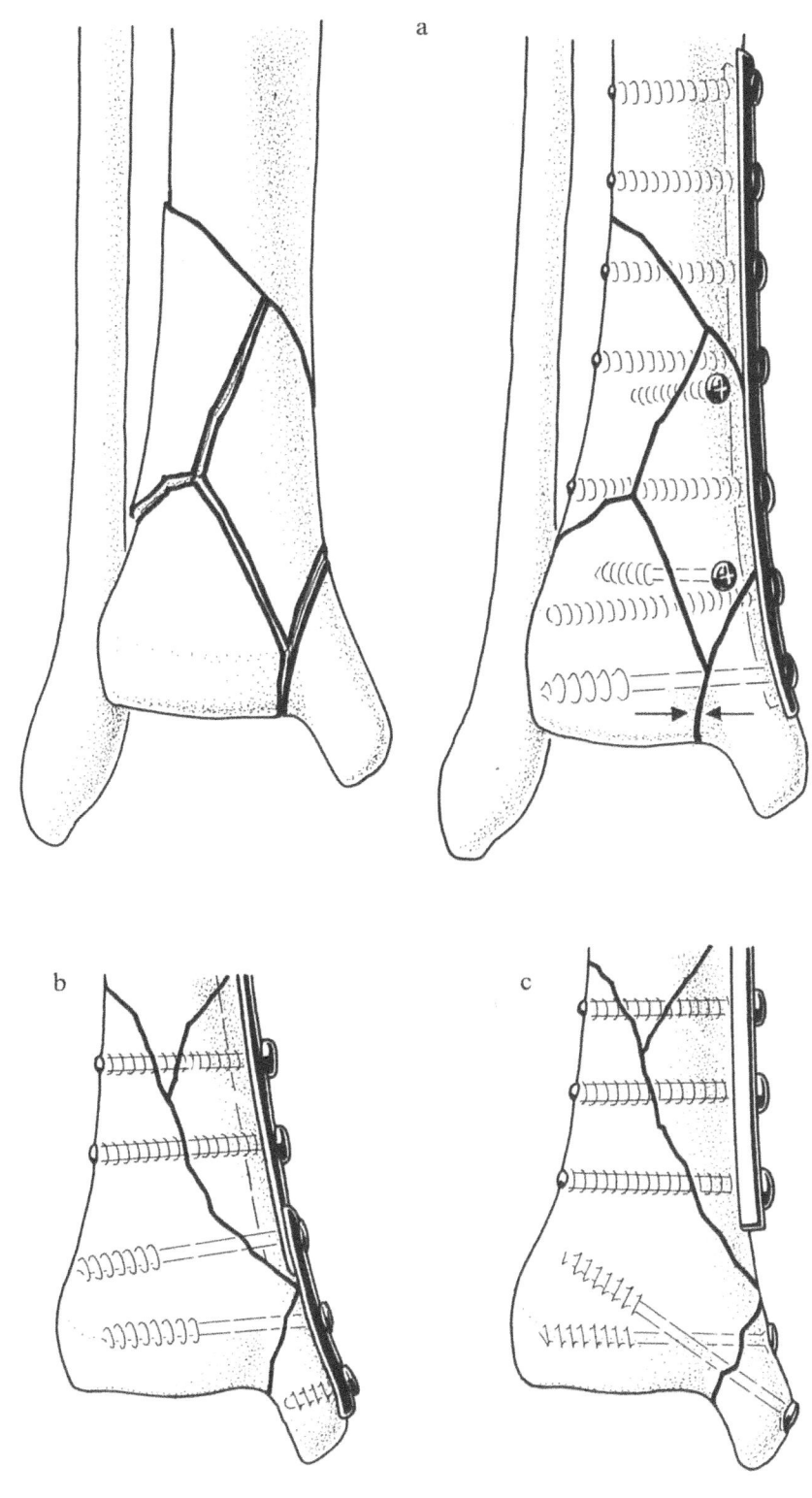

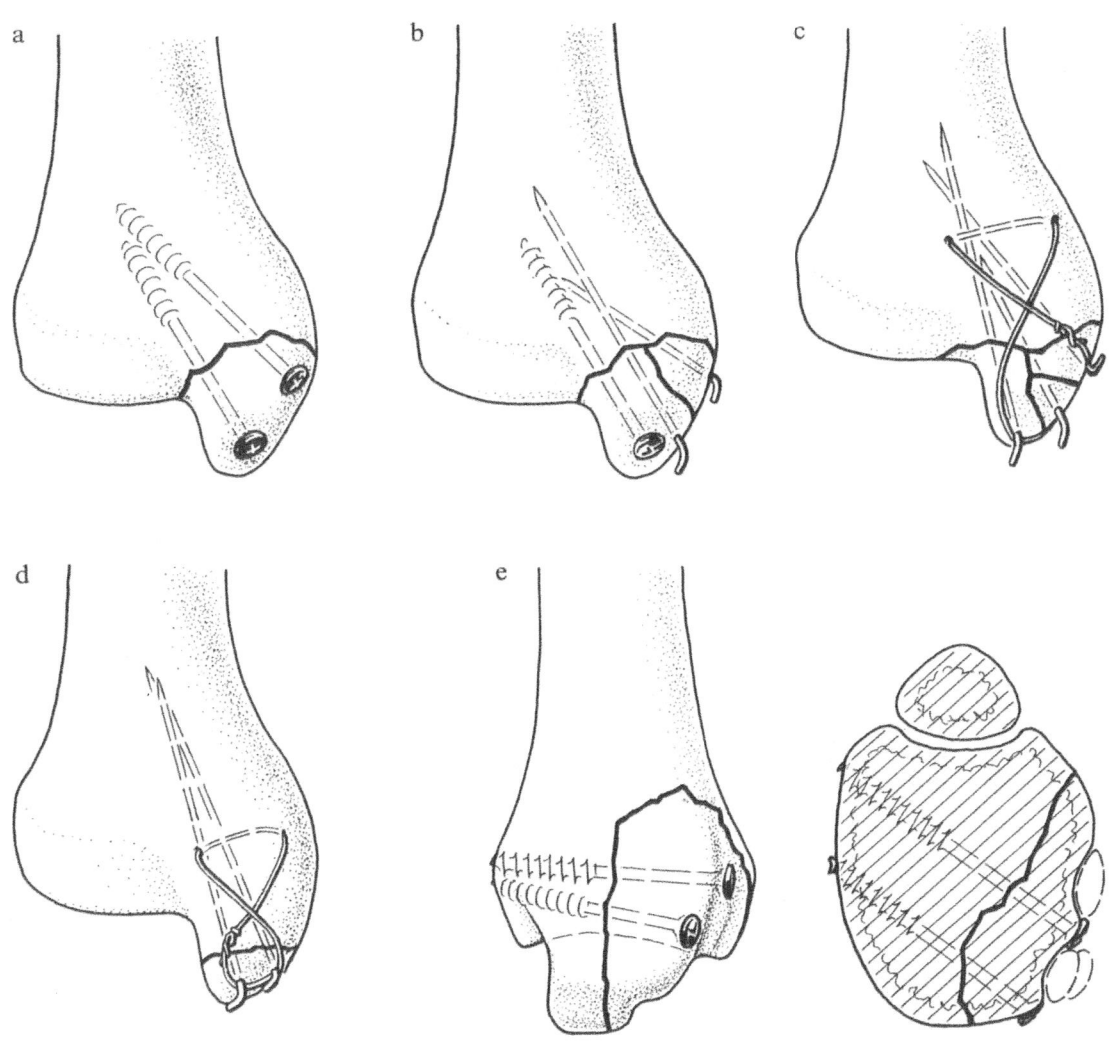

Fig. 117   Various methods of internal fixation of the medial malleolus

   a   Screw fixation of a large anterior fracture

   b   Multiple fragments are reduced by screws and Kirschner wires

   c   Reduction of comminuted fracture with tension-band wiring

   d   Tension-band wiring in small avulsed fracture

   e   Screw fixation of postero-medial fragments. Screws are inserted between the grooves for the tibialis posterior and the toe flexors

220

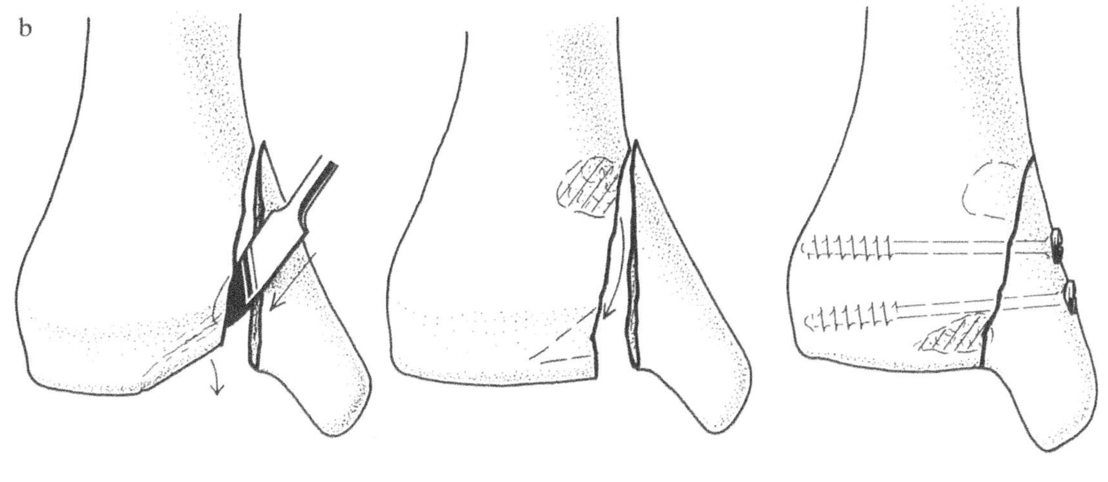

Fig. 118 Adduction fractures

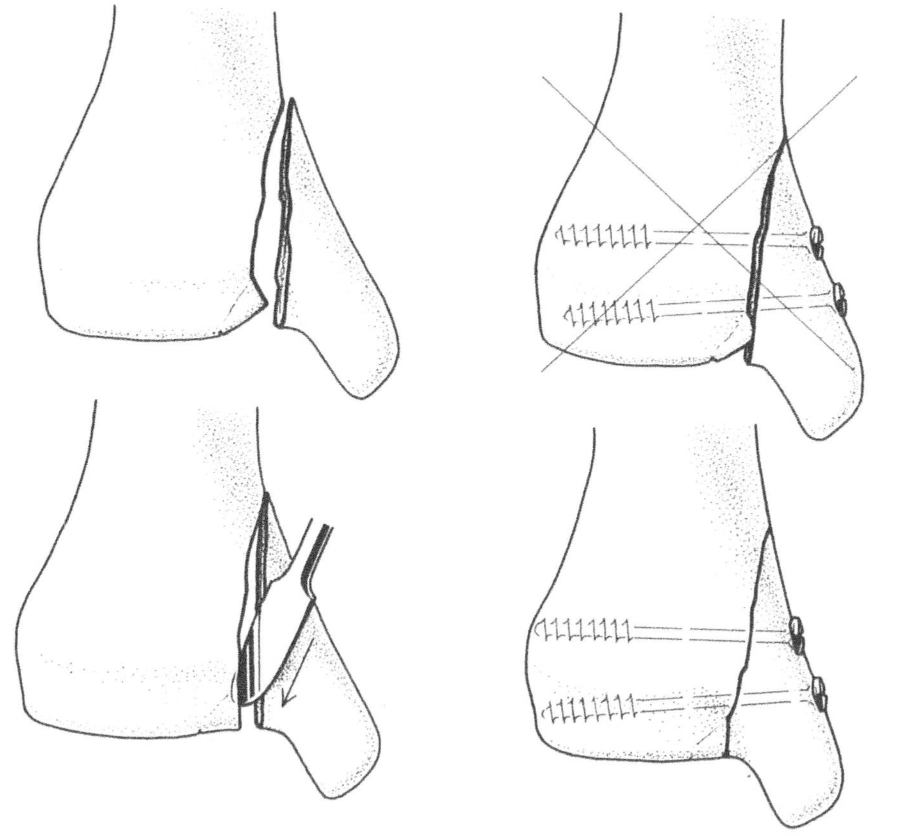

  a The small impacted area at the medial articular border of the tibia impedes exact reduction. The impacted area must be lifted up with an elevator

  b In the presence of larger impacted areas, the defect is filled with cancellous bone taken from the adjoining tibial epiphysis

a

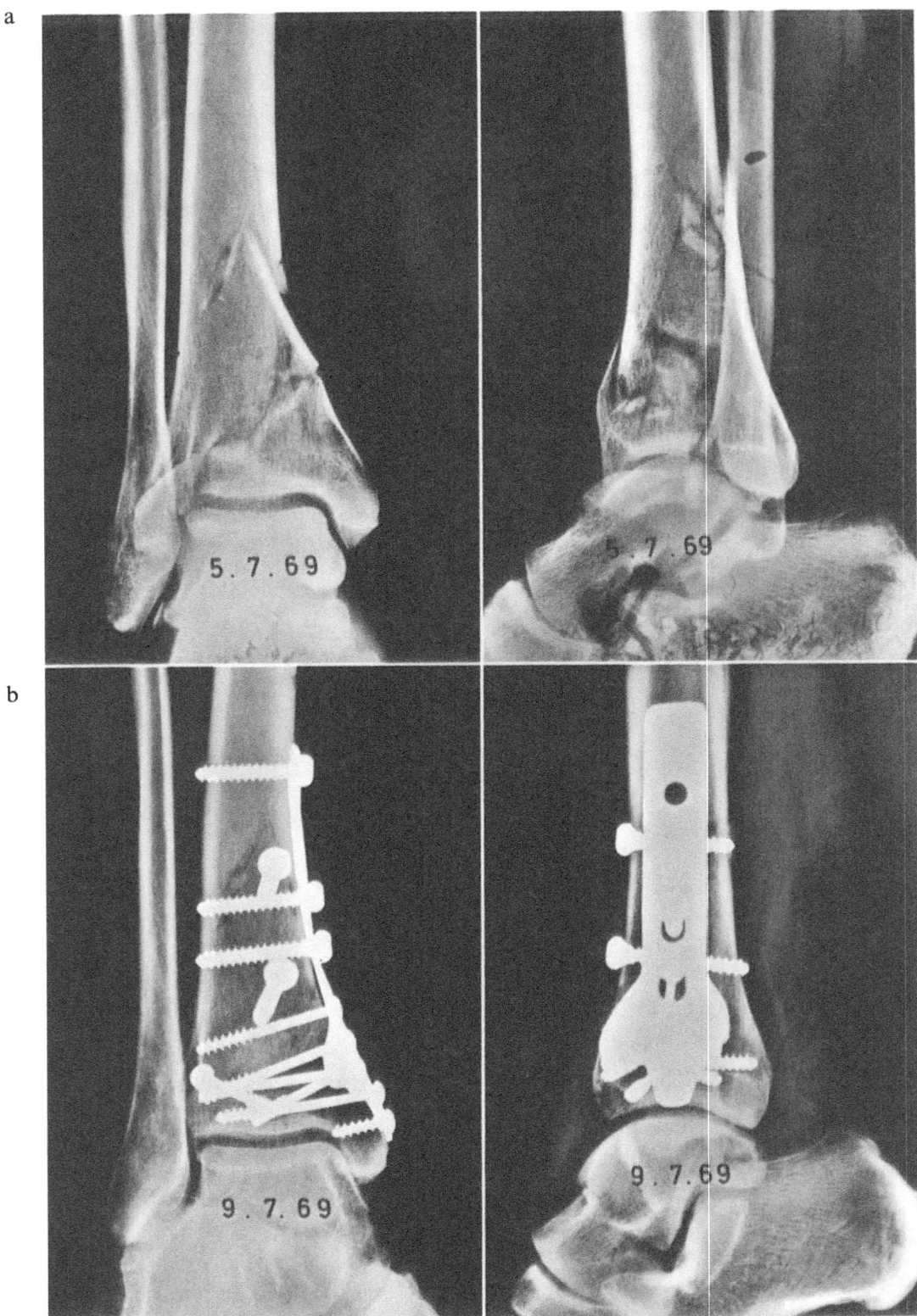

b

222

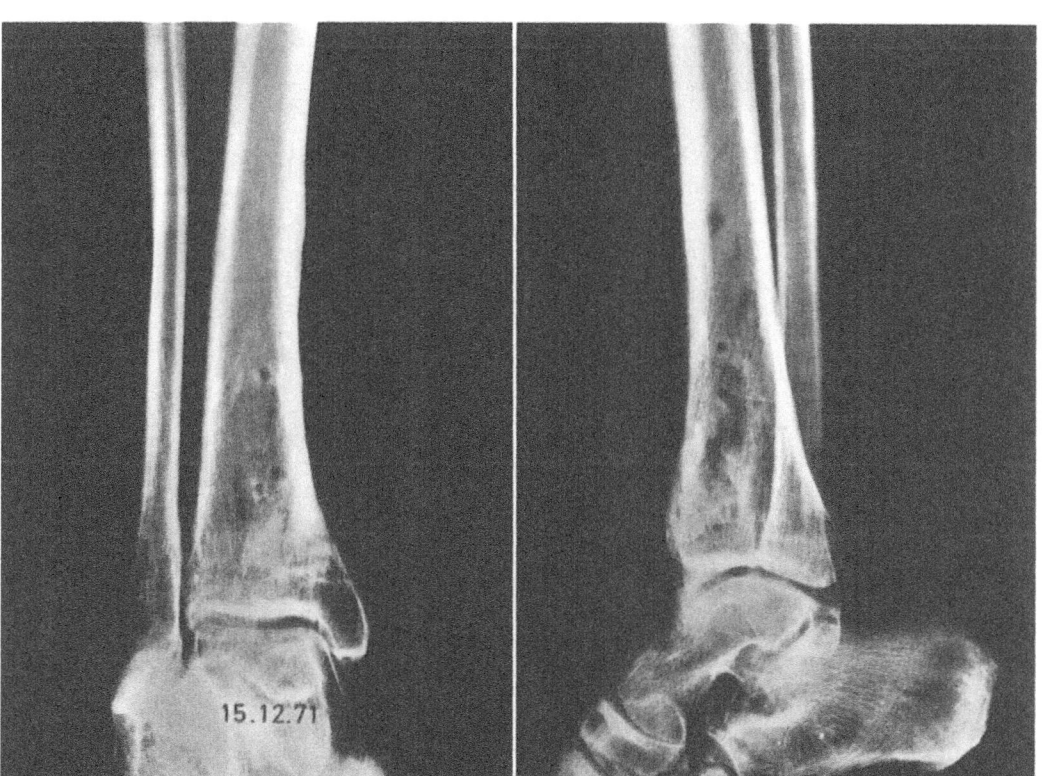

Fig. 119 Clinical example: Intra-articular impacted fracture of the lower tibia (pilon tibial)
A housewife, aged 52. Fall in the mountains

a Impacted articular fracture of the lower end of the tibia with an intact fibula. Os calcis traction and elevation until the swelling had subsided

b Internal fixation after four days: Clover-leaf plate, screw fixation of the antero-lateral tibial fragment. Cancellous bone graft taken from the upper tibia. Anterior tibio-fibular ligament, the fibulo-talar and the fibulo-calcaneal ligaments all sutured
No complications. Plaster-free post-operative treatment. Weight-bearing from the sixteenth week. Removal of metal at the end of 15 months

c Final review at $2^1/_2$ years: occasional mild symptoms, full mobility, no sign of atrophy. X-ray shows slight arthrosis

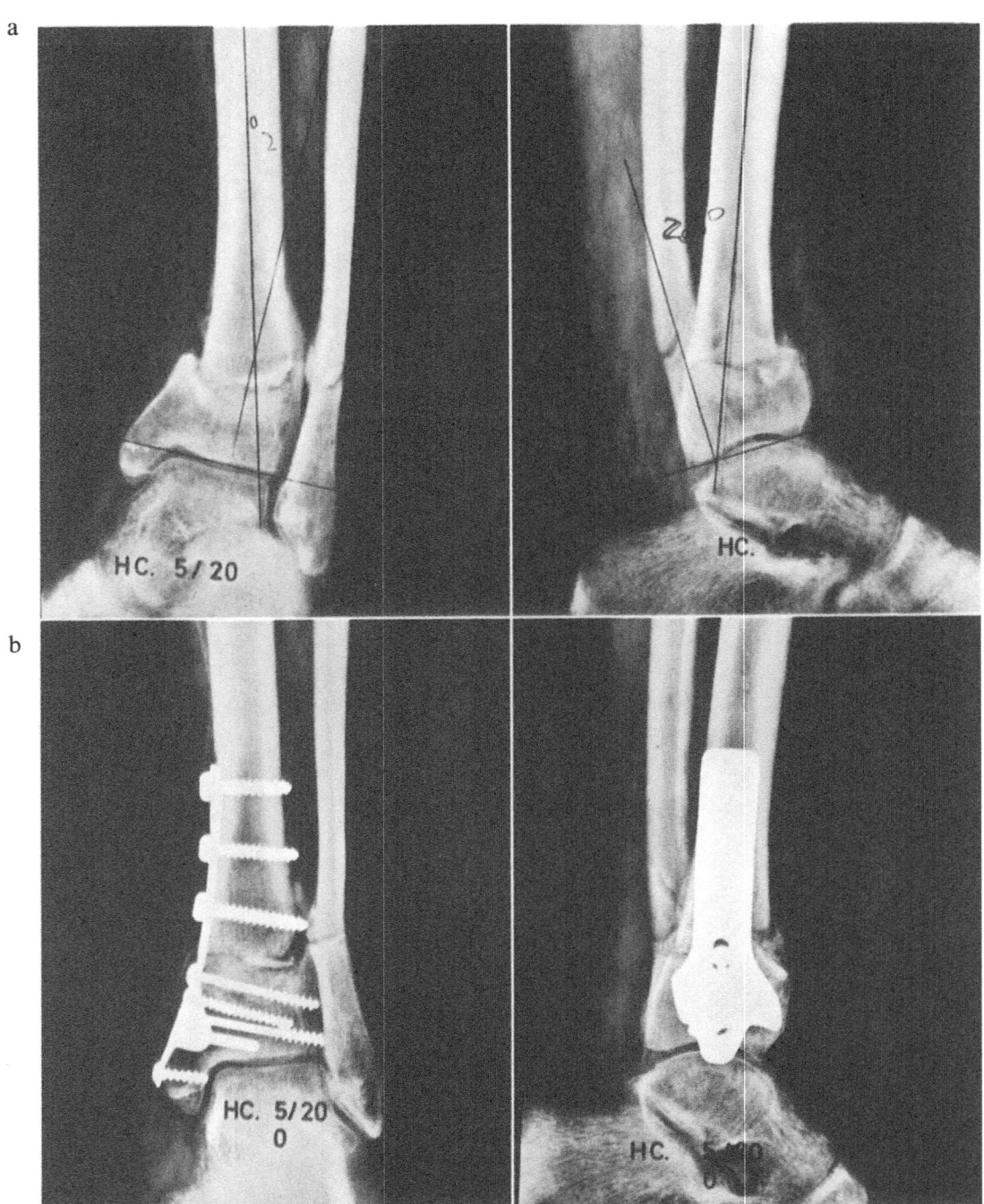

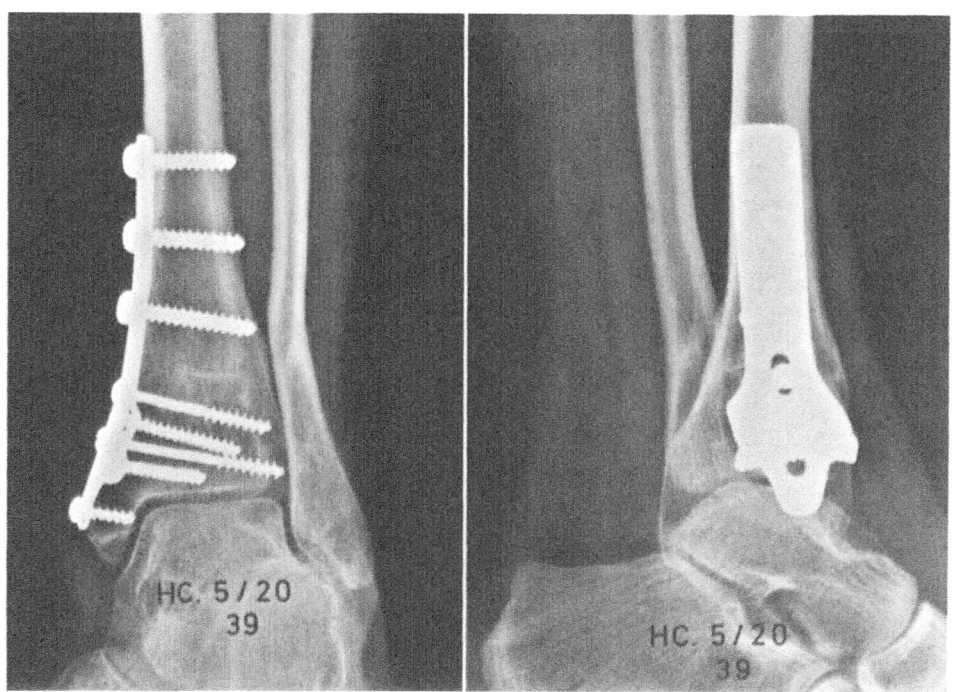

Fig. 120   Clinical example: A supra-malleolar varus deformity

The patient was a girl of 16 who is a pupil at commercial school. Skiing accident. Supra-malleolar transverse fracture of the lower leg. Primary treatment by extension, followed by plaster cast resulted in icreased deformity. The patient was referred to us three months after the accident

a   A firm pseudarthrosis in the lower leg. Varus deformity of 20°, backward angulation of 20°

b   Medial osteotomy. A cancellous bone graft taken from the iliac crest. Compressive internal fixation using a clover-leaf plate on the medial side. Plaster-free post-operative treatment. Full movement and consolidation at the end of 8 weeks. Full weight bearing at the end of 10 weeks

c   At review after 9 months: No handicap, full mobility, booked for metal removal

225

Fig. 121 Technical example: Internal fixation of lower fibula in fracture of the lower leg
Patient was a male injured in a skiing accident

a   Multiple distal fractures in the lower leg with soft tissue damage suspected
Emergency internal fixation: Stabilization of the tibia with a neutralization plate and lag screws, two of which were small screws fixing thin fragment tips or displaced fragments. After reduction of the tibia, clear mobility of the ankle mortice was discovered by examination with the image intensifier. Therefore, additional

b   internal fixation of a fibular fracture with a small semi-tubular plate (6 holes) and small lag screw. Subsequent repair of the ruptured anterior ligament

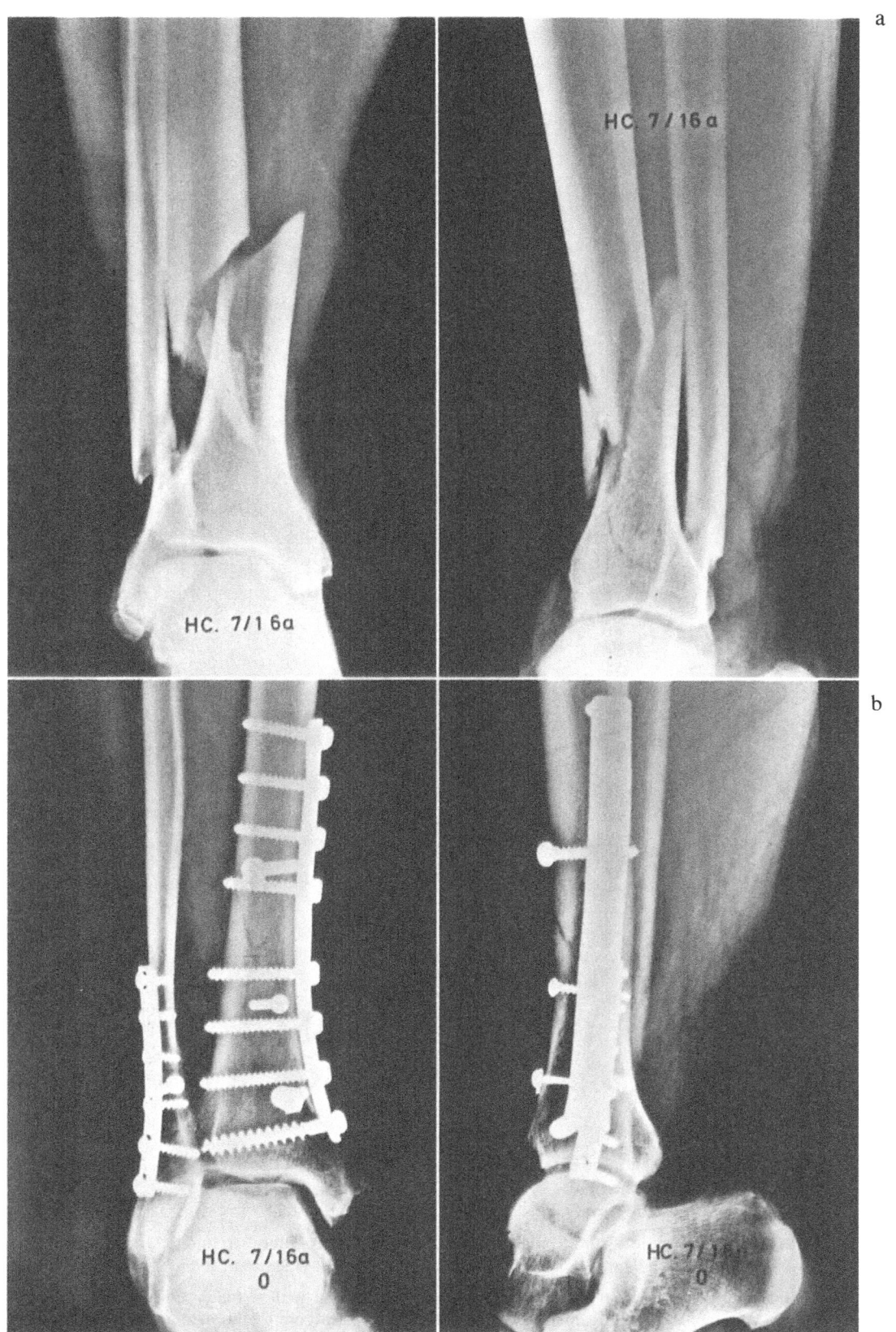

227

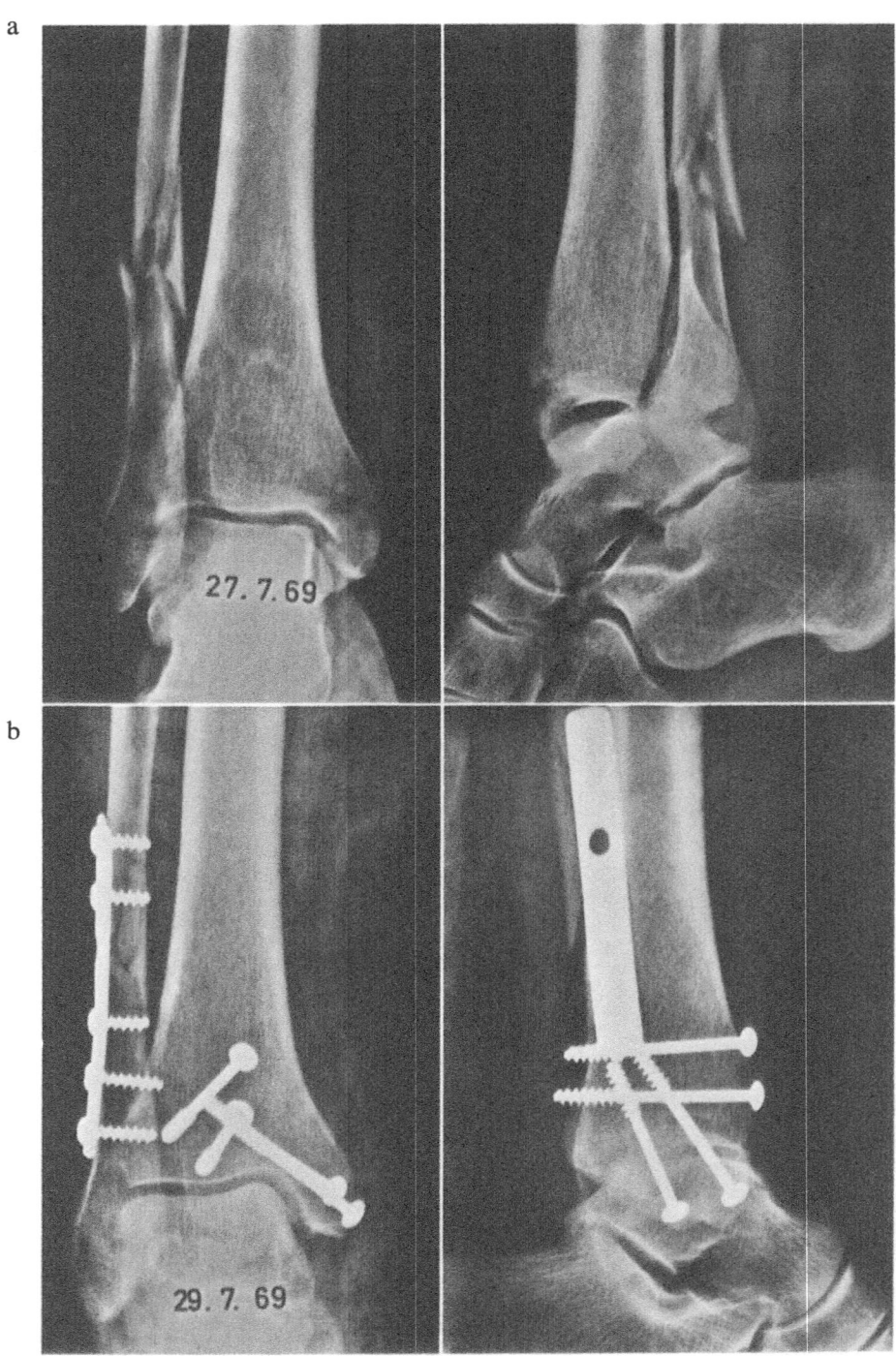

Fig. 122 Clinical example: The high malleolar fracture of type C with postero-lateral fragment detached from the tibia (Volkmann)

Patient was a housewife, aged 68 who had fallen on the stairs

a A high fracture of the fibula of type C. Large postero-lateral triangular fragment of Volkmann. Rupture of the anterior tibio-fibular ligament. Oblique fracture of the medial malleolus

b Emergency internal fixation: Reduction of the fibula with a small semi-tubular plate (6 holes), and repair of the ligament. Screw fixation of the fracture of the medial malleolus and posterior triangle with two small cancellous screws in each. Post-operative plaster splint replaced later with a complete plaster cast. Anticoagulation

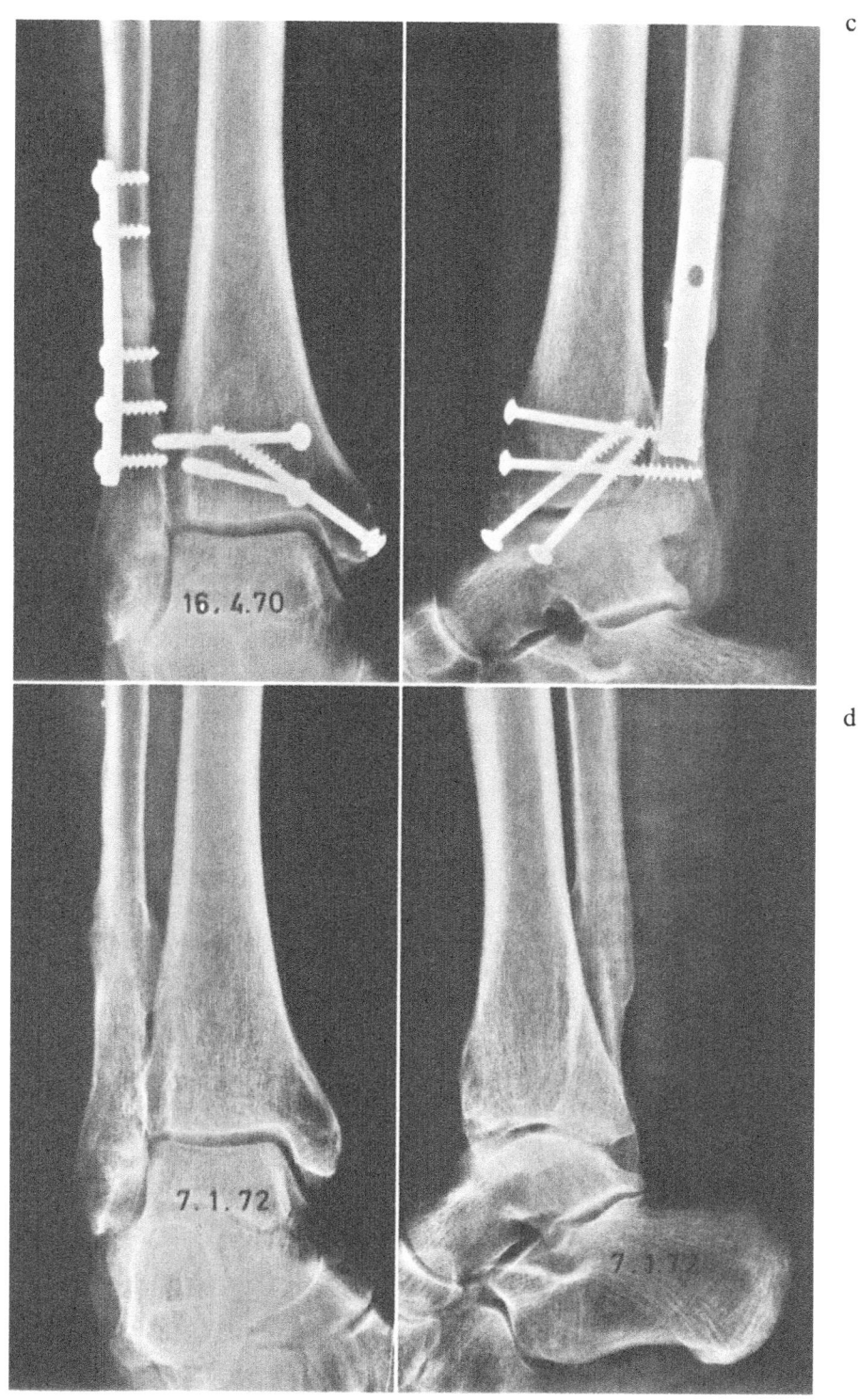

c

d

Fig. 122   **c**   No complications. Weight bearing from the 12th week. Removal of metal at the end of 9 months. A small loss of stability at the level of the fibular fracture was disregarded

    d   Final review at $1^1/_2$ years: No symptoms, mobility in the ankle joint identical with that on the normal side, slightly limited in the mid-tarsal joint. After removal of the metal, callus with slight shortening had developed level with the fibula fracture, producing mild signs of arthrosis in the region of the tibio-fibular joint

Fig. 123   Technical example: Transfixion in malleolar fracture, type C
The patient was a female injured in a skiing accident

  a Oblique fracture of the fibula type C with small posterior Volkmann triangle

  Emergency internal fixation:

  b Laterally: Screw fixation of the main fragment, with an additional neutralization plate in the form of a small semi-tubular plate with 5 holes. Repair of the anterior ligament. Since instability was still present after the repair of the ligament, the second screw was replaced by a transfixing screw getting a purchase on three cortices
  On the medial side: Intraosseous suture of the deltoid ligament which had been avulsed from the tibia

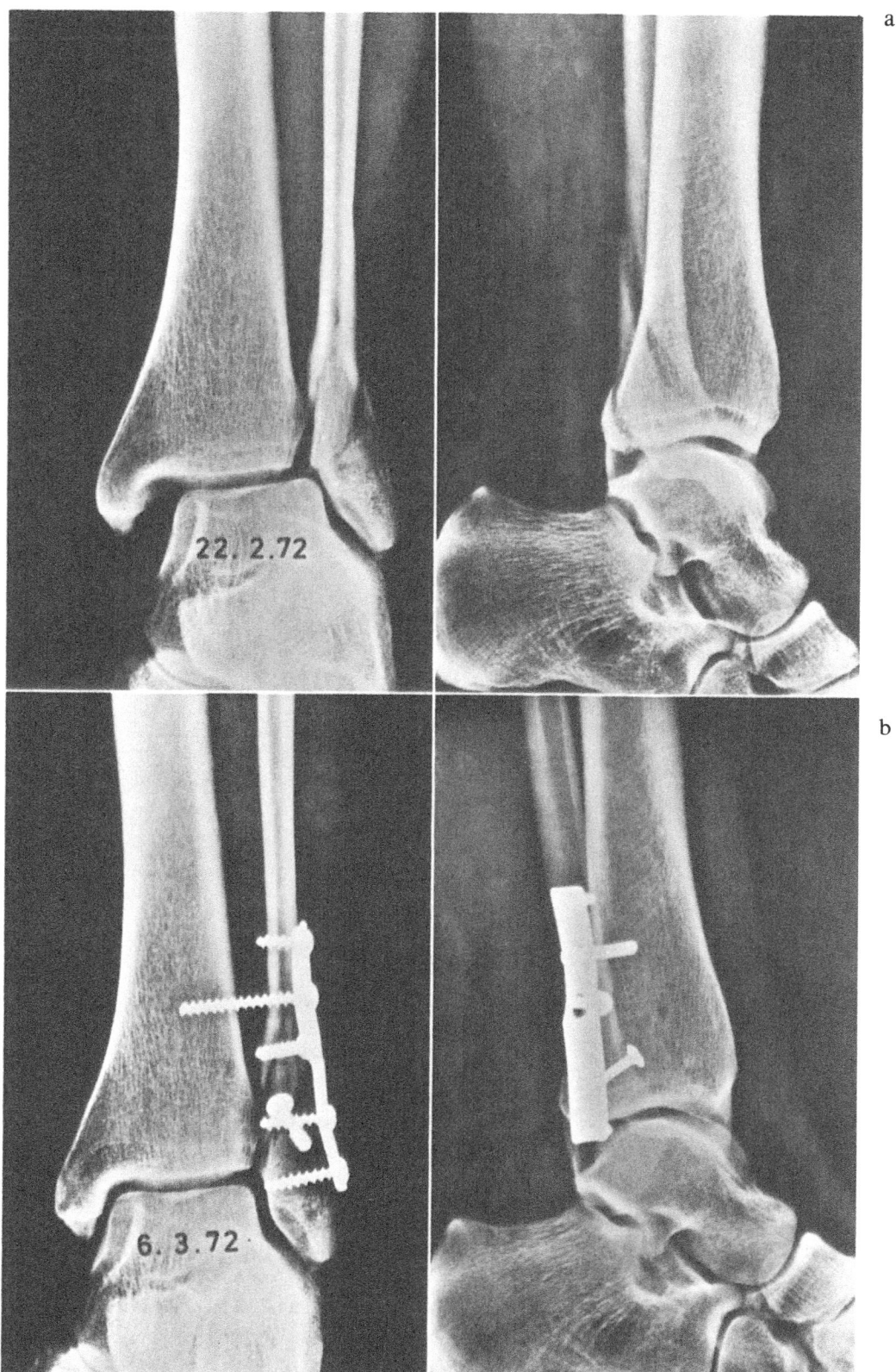

Fig. 124 Technical example: Malleolar fracture of type C with small avulsion from the medial side
The patient was a male injured in a skiing accident

a Comminuted fracture of the fibula type C. Fragment avulsed from the medial malleolus

Emergency internal fixation:

Laterally: Screw fixation of the large wedge shaped fragment and the main fragments. Long neutralization plate in the form of a small semi-tubular plate of 6 holes. Repair of the anterior syndesmotic ligament

b Medially: Kirschner wires with tension wiring and suture of the joint capsule

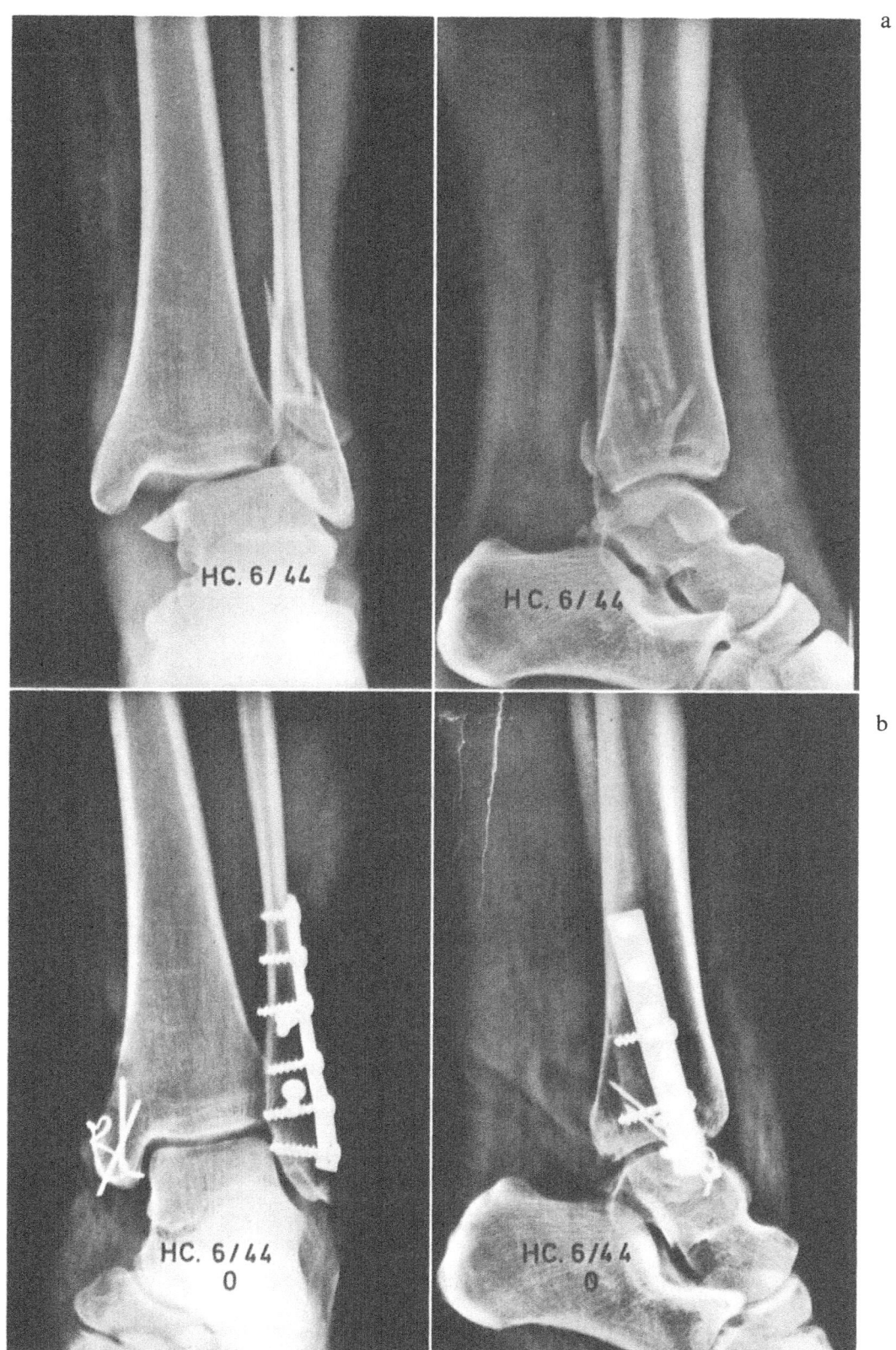

Fig. 125 Technical example: Malleolar fracture type B associated with a medial comminuted fracture
The patient was a female injured in a skiing accident

a Oblique fracture of the fibula of type B together with rupture of the anterior ligament. Comminuted fracture of the medial malleolus with extra-articular defects

Emergency internal fixation:

Laterally: Screw fixation of the fibular fracture and a neutralization plate in the form of a small semi-tubular one with 5 holes. Intraosseous suture of the ligaments; the boat-shaped fragment of the fibula was fixed back with flexible wire

b Medially: Internal fixation of the comminuted fracture by a screw together with Kirschner wires and tension-band wiring

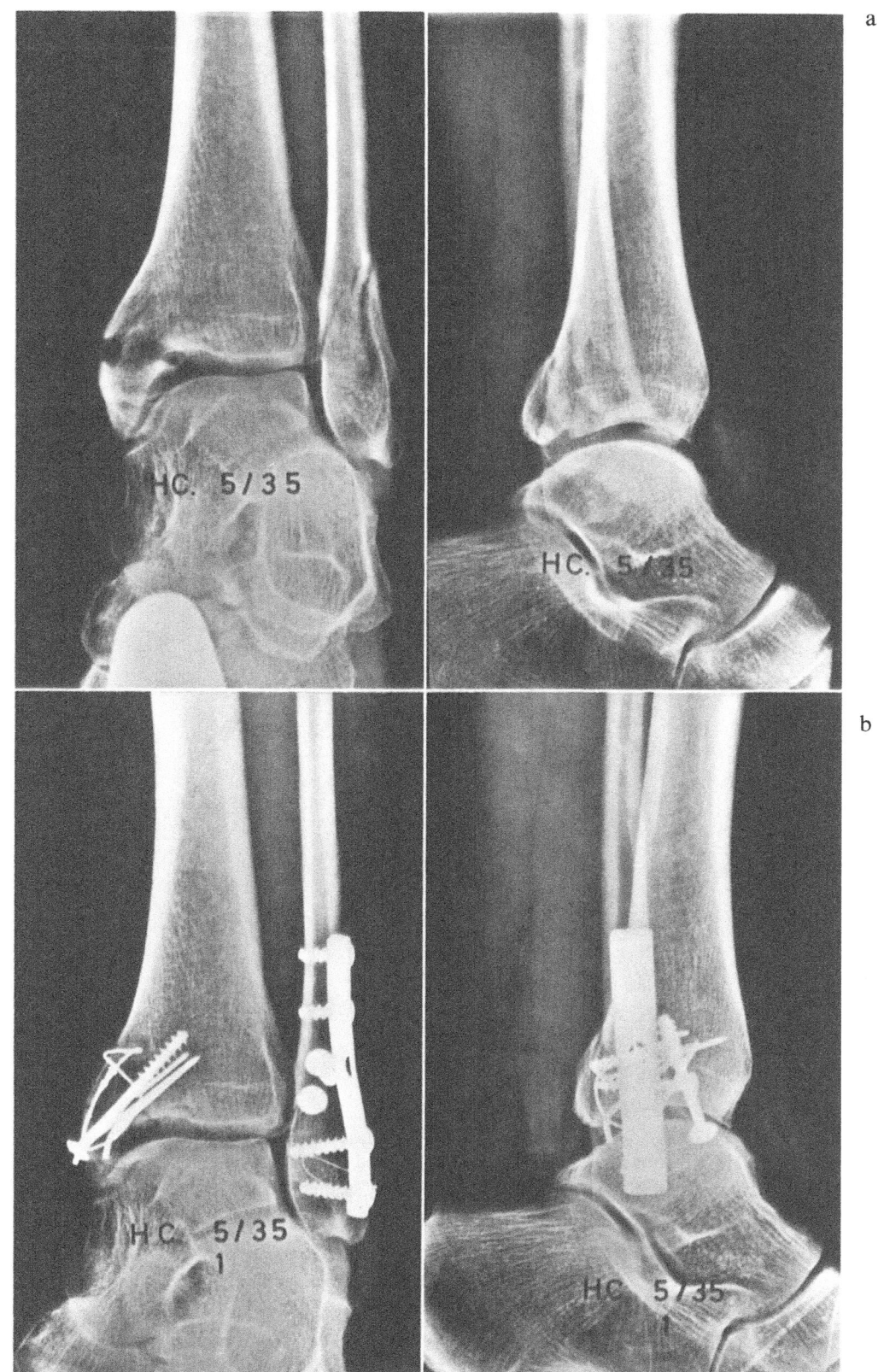

Fig. 126 Clinical example: Adduction fracture with impaction of the joint surface
The patient was a housewife, aged 28, injured in a skiing accident

a Adduction fracture of the medial malleolus with an articular fragment impacted upwards, an undisplaced avulsion fracture of the lateral malleolus of type A

Emergency internal fixation:

Medially: Accurate reconstruction of the articular surface by removing the impacted fragment. Fixation with two screws and a Kirschner wire

b Laterally: Simple Kirschner wire as the stability was restored by the medial internal fixation. A dorsal plaster slab replaced later by a complete cast. No complications. Full weight bearing at the 11th week

c Final review and removal of metal after 8 months: No symptoms, full mobility, and normal articular surface

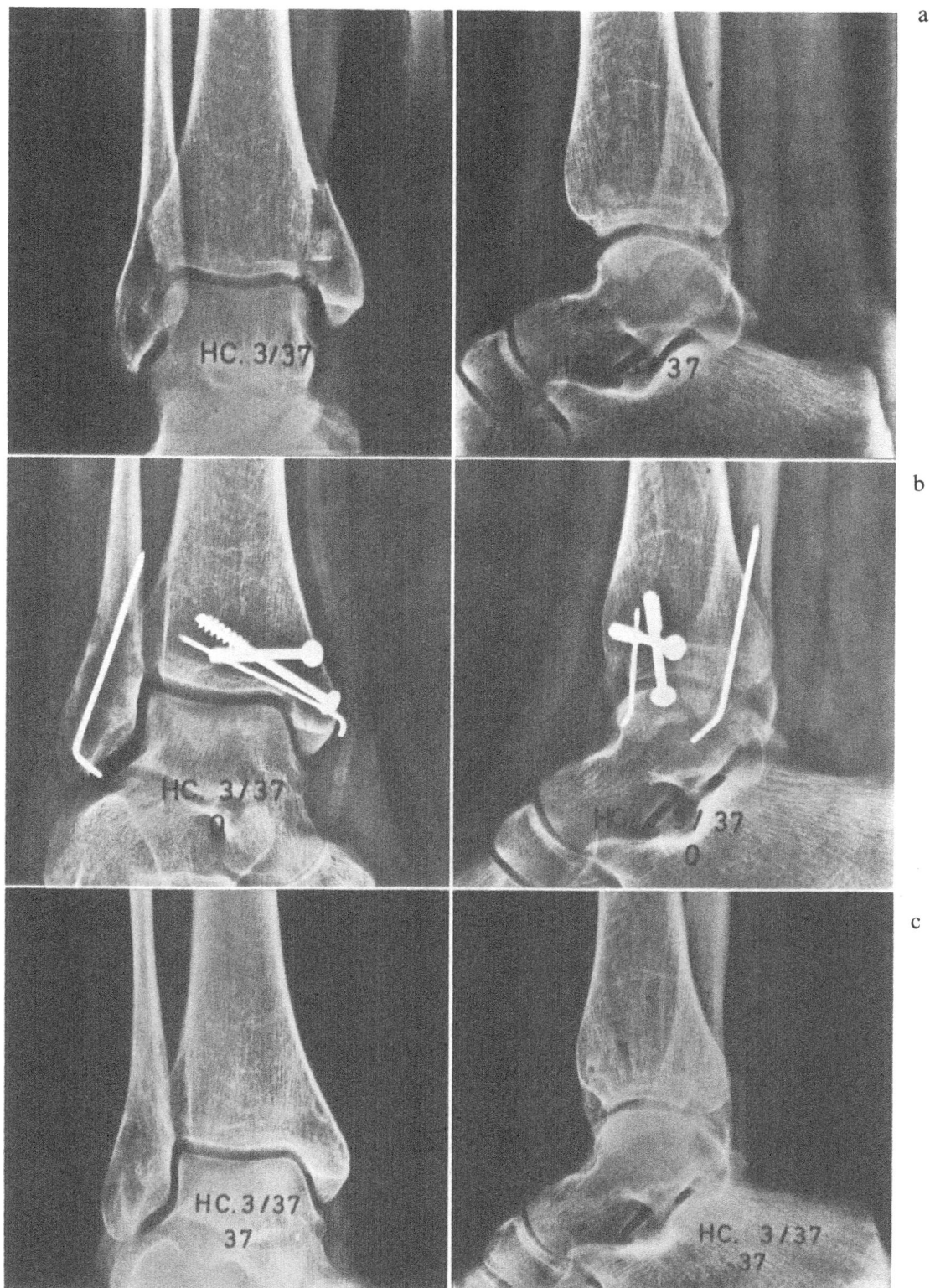

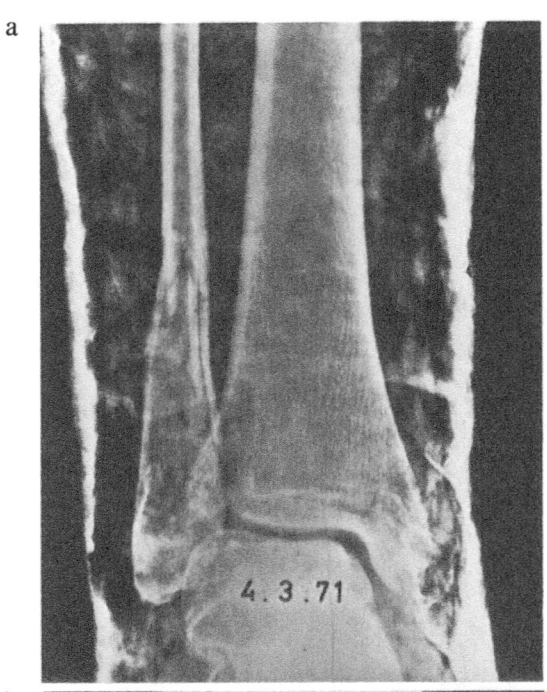

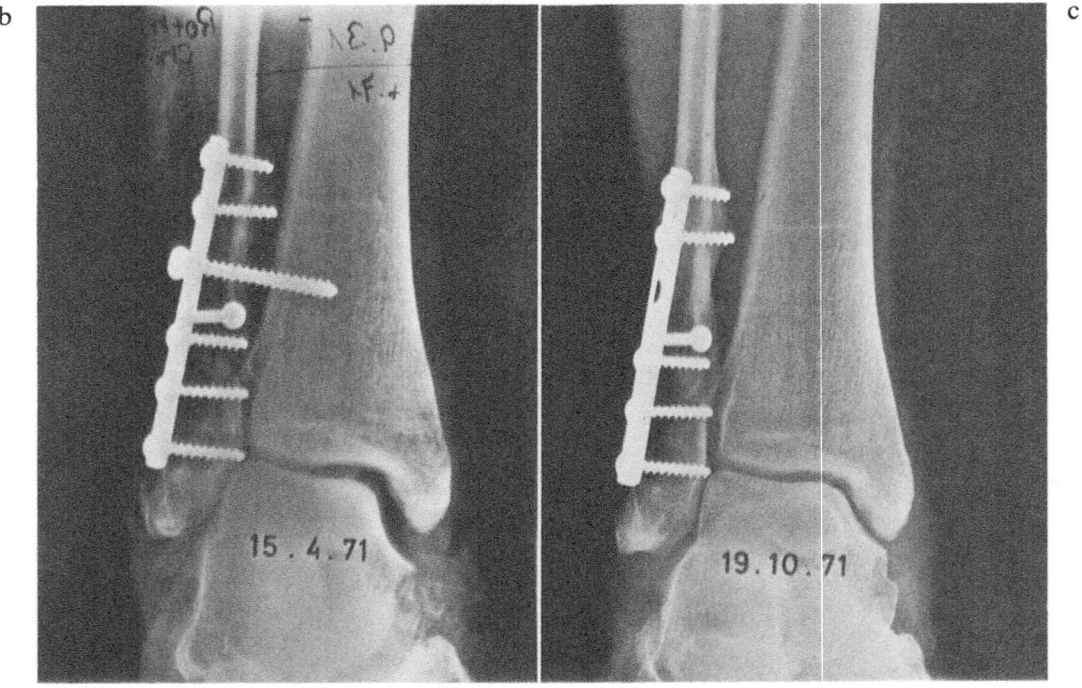

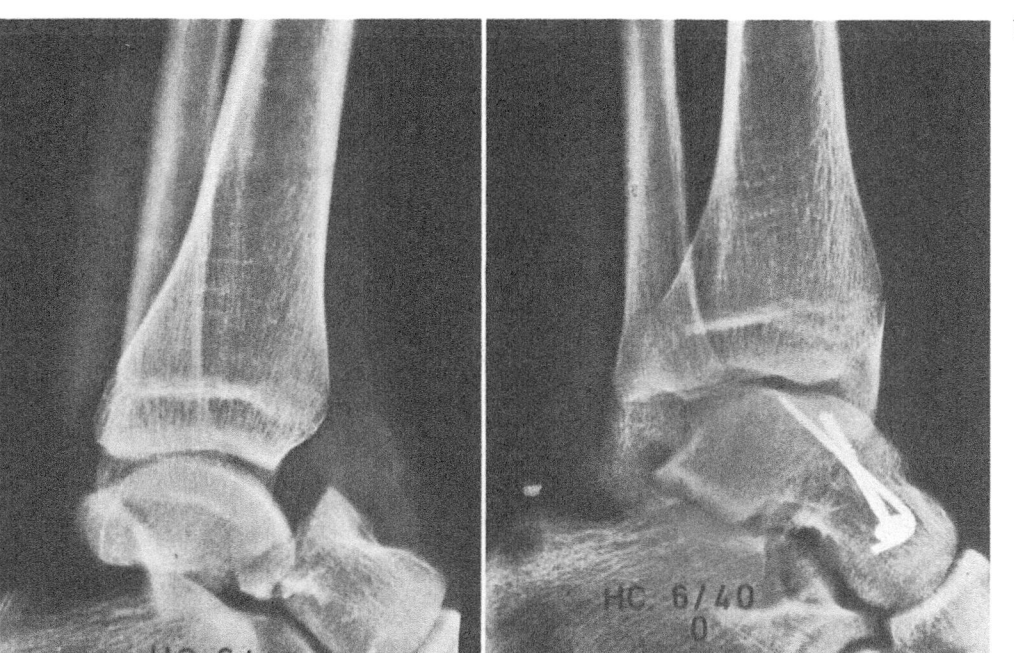

Fig. 128   Technical example: Fracture dislocation of the talus
The patient was a male injured at skiing

a   Fracture dislocation of the neck of the talus. Closed reduction was unsuccessful

b   Emergency internal fixation: Open reduction with exact adaptation of the fracture surfaces. Temporary fixation with 2 Kirschner wires, one of which was allowed to remain in place. Interfragmentary compression by a small cancellous screw

◁

Fig. 127   Clinical example: Secondary internal fixation in a malleolar fracture
The patient was a housewife, aged 40 injured while skiing. High spiral fracture of the lateral malleolus of type C

a   Conservative treatment with a plaster cast in another hospital. X-ray taken after 4 weeks showed considerable shortening of the fibula

Secondary internal fixation was undertaken 7 weeks after the accident:

b   Laterally: Removal of callus from the fibula and exact reduction. Stabilization with a small semi-tubular plate. Repair of the rupture of the anterior tibio-fibular ligament of the syndesmosis. Temporary transfixion with a large cortex screw
Medially: Repair of the torn deltoid ligament which had become interposed
Post-operative treatment: Early mobilization until the wound was healed and then a walking plaster cast for 6 weeks

c   Review at 8 months: No symptoms, movement identical with the other side. Booked for removal of metal

XII. The Forefoot

1. Tarsal Bones

Internal fixation in the tarsus is seldom indicated. Partial stabilization of larger fractures in the navicular and of some fracture dislocations in the mid-tarsal joint can sometimes be secured by screw fixation.

2. Metatarsus and Toes

a) Indications

The opinion that rigid internal fixation of marginal fractures in the forefoot is more effective than traditional treatment is beginning to gain ground. Its aim is the exact anatomical reconstruction of the plantar arch and particularly the functional post-operative treatment without any external support. These are the only methods that can reduce trophic changes and circulatory disturbances to a minimum. Compared with the hand, internal fixation in the metatarsus presents more difficulties since, for anatomical reasons, implants have to be sited on the dorsum of the foot. Here they cannot have the tension-band effect. Sometimes plates can be placed on the lateral side of tubular bones which improves their stabilizing effect, though a real tension-band effect cannot be achieved in this way. Early active movement which is quite possible in the hand, must in the foot entail partial weight-bearing and this cannot be allowed. In the presence of multiple injuries, we often find " vassal " fractures which only require a minimum of internal fixation.

b) Approaches

Postero-lateral incisions are made for the first and fifth metatarsals and for the big toe, similar to those in the hand. They must never extend downwards enough to reach the margin of the plantar surface of the foot, lest walking would be interfered with. Scars here would also be the subject of irritation because of wearing shoes. A transverse or Z-shaped incision on the dorsum of the foot has proved to give the best approach for fractures of the necks of the metatarsals (Fig. 129).

c) Shaft Fractures

Shaft fractures of the first metatarsals which are flexion fractures commonly occur in the middle third. Stabilization is obtained by small semi-tubular plates of 4 or 5 holes. Because of the considerable width of this strong tubular bone, proximal screws should be long enough (Fig. 130a).
Attention must be paid to small plantar wedge-shaped fragments or comminuted areas since they can delay healing. It is recommended that each fragment be removed and the defect filled with cancellous bone (Fig. 130b).

Fractures of the proximal phalanx of the big toe are usually somewhat displaced because of the strong tensile force of the tendons. Here is a good indication for internal fixation, but to get sufficient rigidity, plates must be used rather than screws alone. Small T-shaped or oblique L-shaped plates with cortex screws of 3.5 mm should be used.
It may sometimes be possible to reduce a *fracture-dislocation of the interphalangeal joint of the big toe* by screw fixation.

d) Articular Fractures

These fractures have to be reconstructed as exactly as possible. Simple fractures and isolated fragments can be reduced with a single screw, whereas this method of reduction is not feasible in comminuted fractures. Where these occur in the tarso-metatarsal and the interphalangeal joint of the big toe, the best solution may be a primary arthrodesis using plates or screws and cancellous bone grafting.

e) Middle Three Metatarsals

Fractures of the second to fourth metatarsals rarely need internal fixation with plates or screws. Here axial medullary wiring carried out at the same time as open reduction has proved to be the best method. Since the transverse arch must be maintained, exact reduction of such fractures is imperative (Fig. 131).

f) Fifth Metatarsal

Spiral and oblique fractures of the neck commonly occur with a vassal fracture of the fourth ray. If there is displacement, internal fixation with a finger L-plate is recommended. It may be necessary to open the proximal joint. Healing here may be interfered with not only by circulatory, but also by mechanical disturbances, especially the lack of stability provided by the plaster cast. Primary internal fixation is thus often indicated even when there is only mild displacement.

The *apophyseal fracture of the fifth metatarsal* is one of the most frequent fractures in the foot. This bone is particularly exposed to injury which may occur in two different ways: 1. Either an avulsion fracture (Jones) is produced by the sudden pull of the peroneus brevis muscle which has its insertion at this point. In this case there is a small displaced fragment. 2. or the fracture may be caused by excessive weight bearing on the outer side of the foot or by direct trauma. Here the fracture is of larger size and may include several fragments. Conservative treatment often results in a pseudarthrosis. In our opinion, such fractures should be reduced by primary operation and fixation.

It depends on the size of the fracture whether a small tension-band wire should be used or screw fixation. It may be necessary to repair the fibular ligaments in the ankle joint which may be involved in the injury (Fig. 132).

3. Secondary Operation on the Forefoot

a) Pseudarthroses

In the forefoot are rather common. They are usually situated in weight bearing areas such as the proximal phalanx of the big toe and the fifth metatarsal. Because of the poor circulation in this area, metal fixation alone is insufficient as a rule. It is recommended that bone grafting also be undertaken either by a bone peg or by a compressed bridging graft. The choice of implant depends upon the location of the non-union. As these tubular bones are so short, operation may need to involve a neighbouring joint and arthrodesis may be required, especially in the big toe.

b) Arthrodeses

In comminuted articular fractures, either a primary or secondary arthrodesis is required. Whenever possible, resection of the tarso-metatarsal joint and the proximal phalanx of the big toe should be avoided. The best method is internal fixation with plates combined with cancellous bone graft. Screw fixation is suitable for the interphalangeal joint of the big toe.
In some cases of hallux valgus and hallux rigidus, screw fixation is also useful for arthrodesis of the metatarso-phalangeal joint (Geiser).

4. Clinical X-Ray Examples

Figs. 133–138, pages 248–255

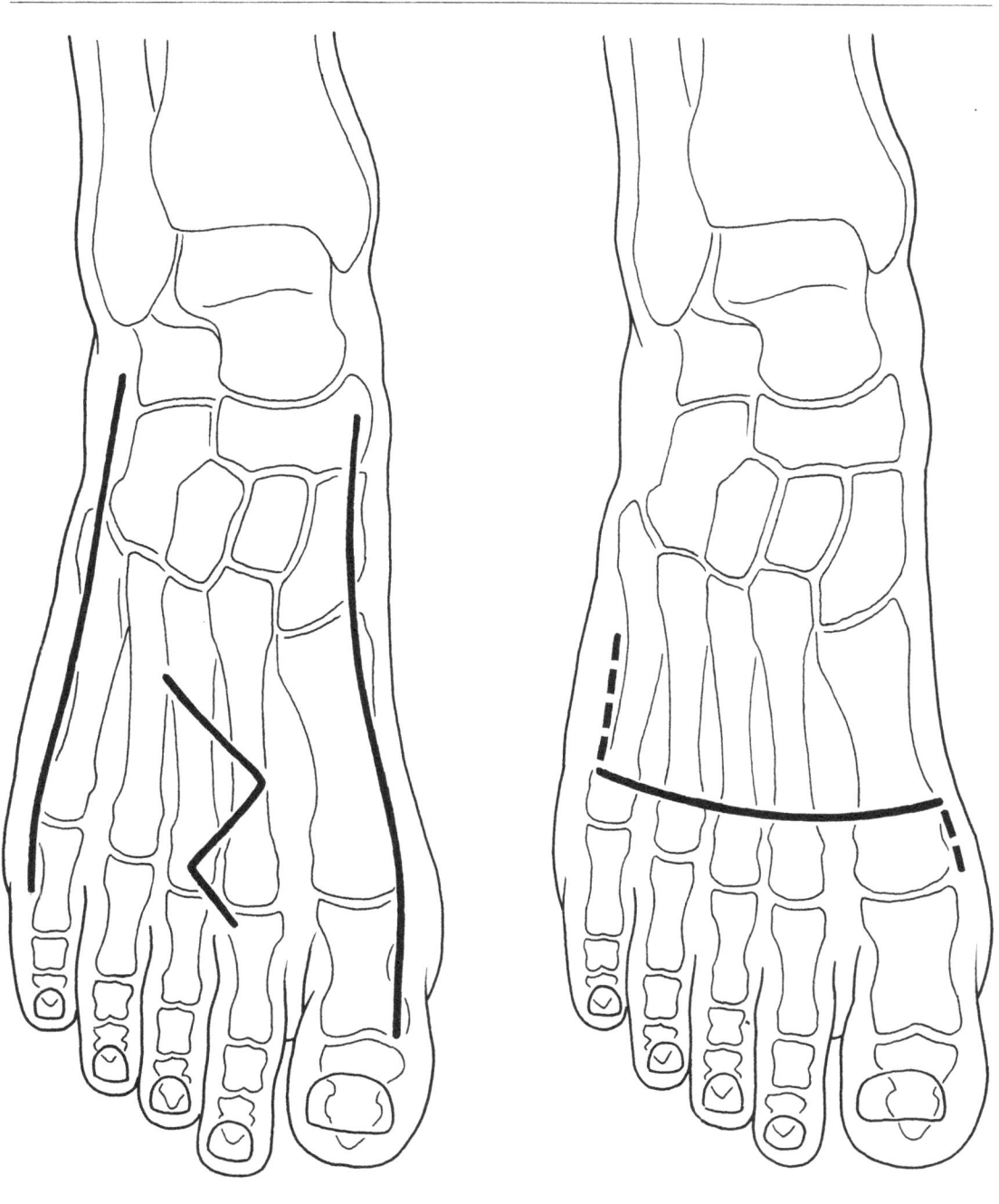

Fig. 129 Incisions for internal fixation of the forefoot

Fig. 130 **Typical internal fixation in the forefoot**

a Internal fixation of the first metatarsal with a small semi-tubular plate, of the fifth metatarsal and proximal phalanx of the big toe with small finger plates

b Small cancellous grafts in a comminuted fracture of the first metatarsal

c Lateral position of the plate which is mechanically better in the first metatarsal

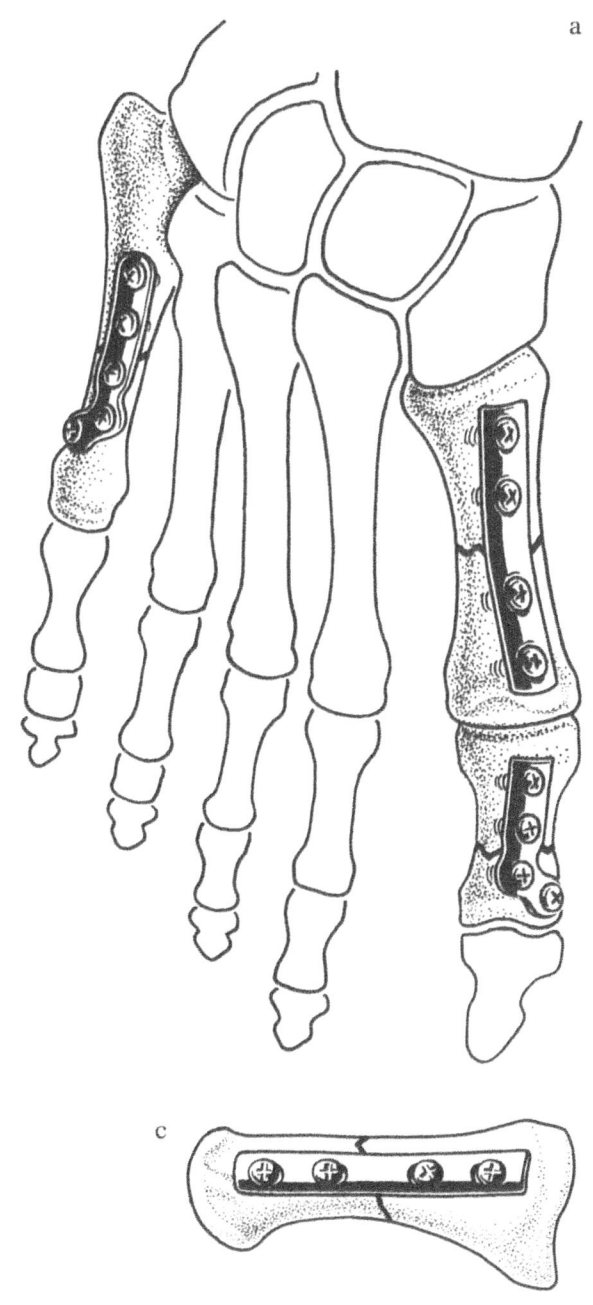

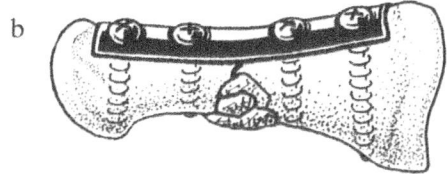

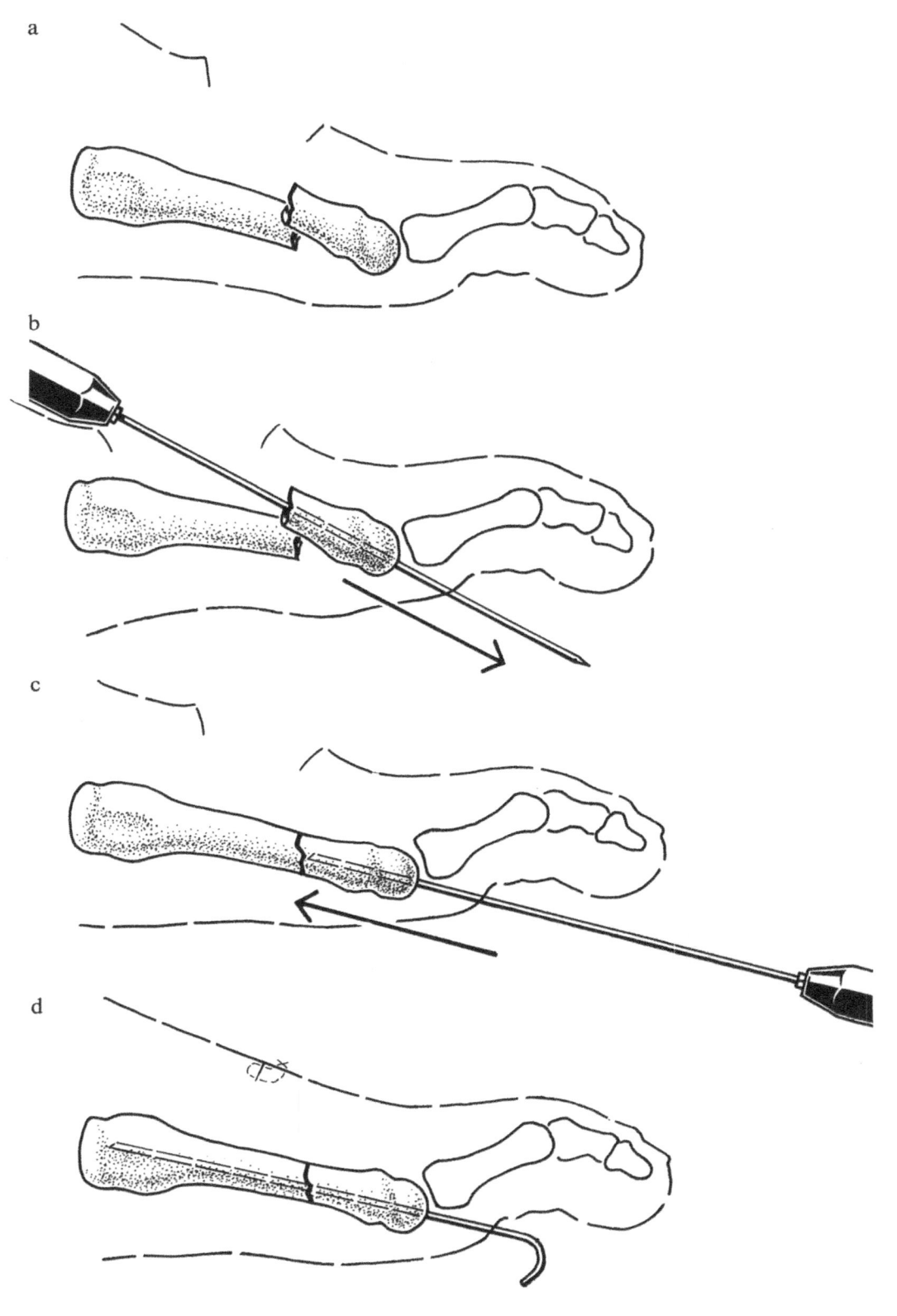

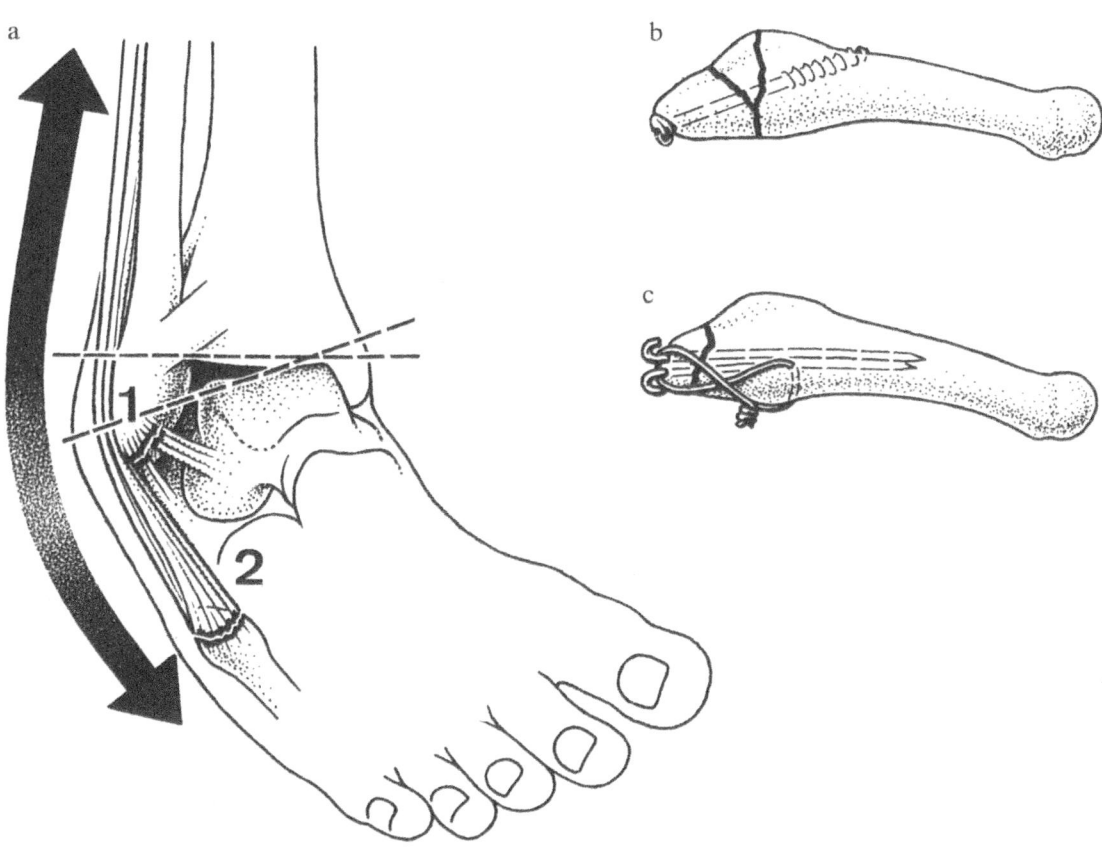

Fig. 132 Fracture of the base of the V metatarsal

  a Rupture of the fibulo-talar and fibulo-calcaneal ligaments often associated with avulsion fracture of the apophysis in inversion injuries

  b Screw fixation of larger fragments

  c Tension-wiring of small avulsion fracture

◁

Fig. 131 Open medullary wiring in fractures of the 2nd to 4th metatarsals

  a Initial position and approach

  b Insertion of a Kirschner wire dorsally from proximal to distal through the distal fragment and out through the plantar surface

  c Reduction of the fracture and drilling of the wire backwards into the proximal fragment

  d The end of the wire is not buried under the skin

a

9 . 6. 68

9 . 6. 68

b

29 . 11. 68

29 . 11. 68

248

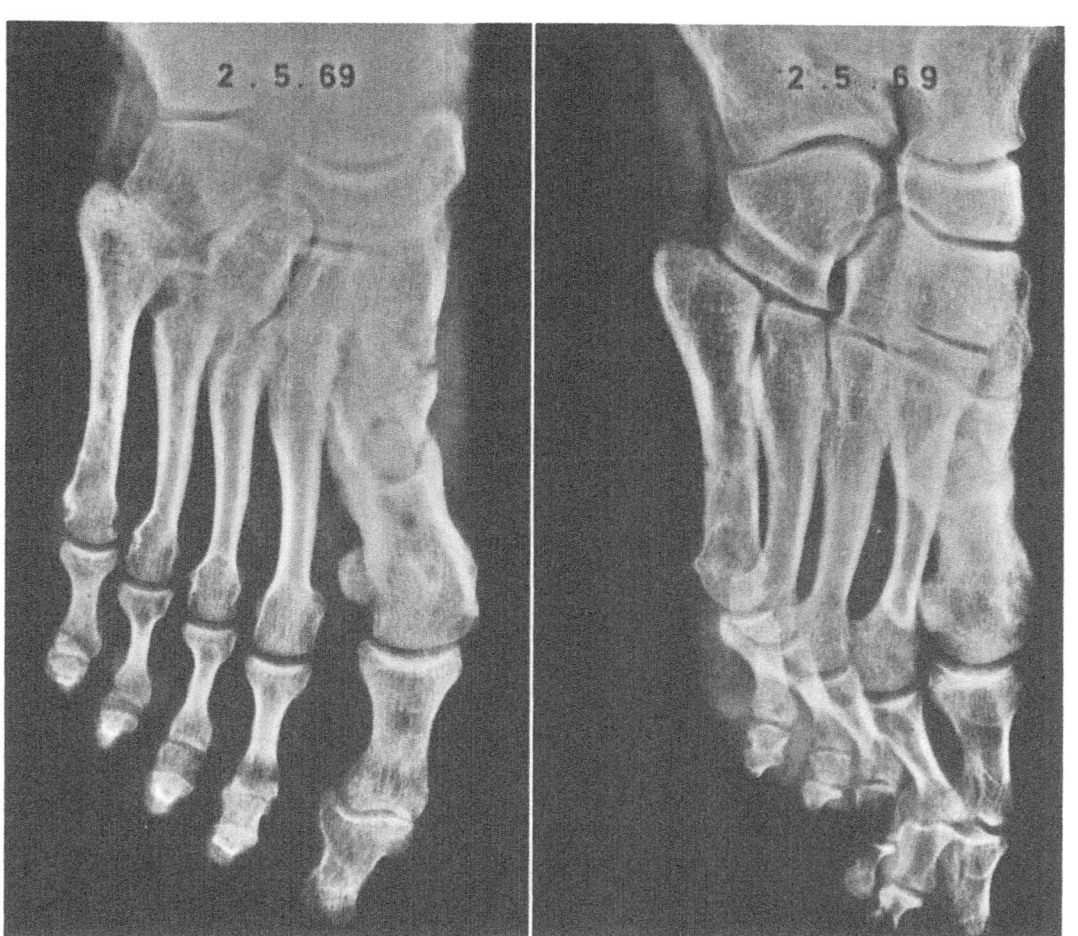

Fig. 133   Clinical example: Transverse fractures of metatarsals I and V

   The patient was a building labourer, aged 32. His foot had been squeezed in the shovel of an excavator

a   Transverse fractures of the 1st and 5th metatarsal. Severe local swelling. The limb was elevated

b   Internal fixation after 10 days: A finger L-plate on the 5th metatarsal. A small semi-tubular plate on the 1st metatarsal. The comminuted area at the base of the first metatarsal is disregarded. After operation treatment was without plaster cast
   Healing process: Primary fracture healing of the 5th metatarsal, the healing of the first metatarsal was accompanied by considerable callus formation

c   Removal of metal and final review at 8 months: Symptom-free, full working capacity. The movement on this side was identical with that on the other and the fractures had healed

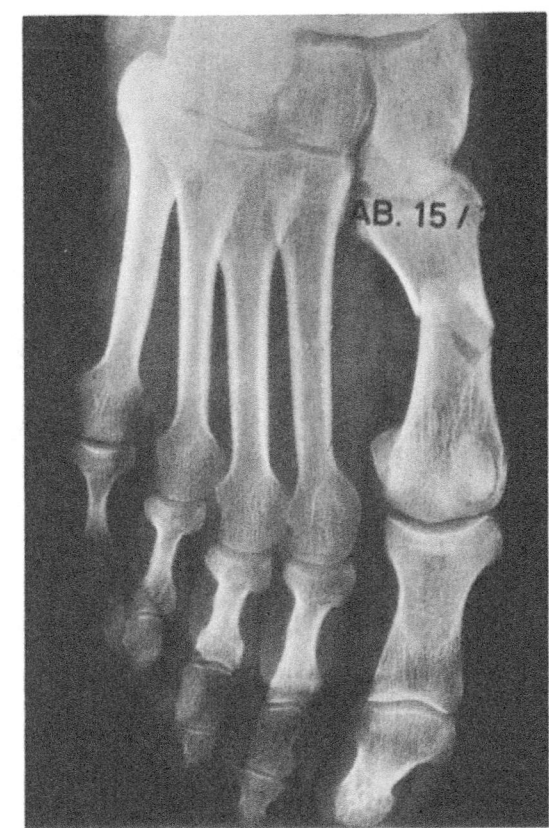

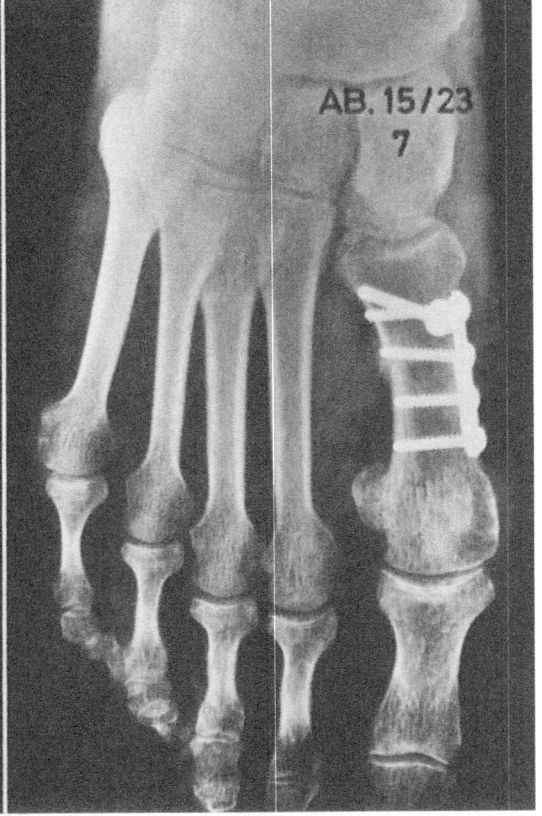

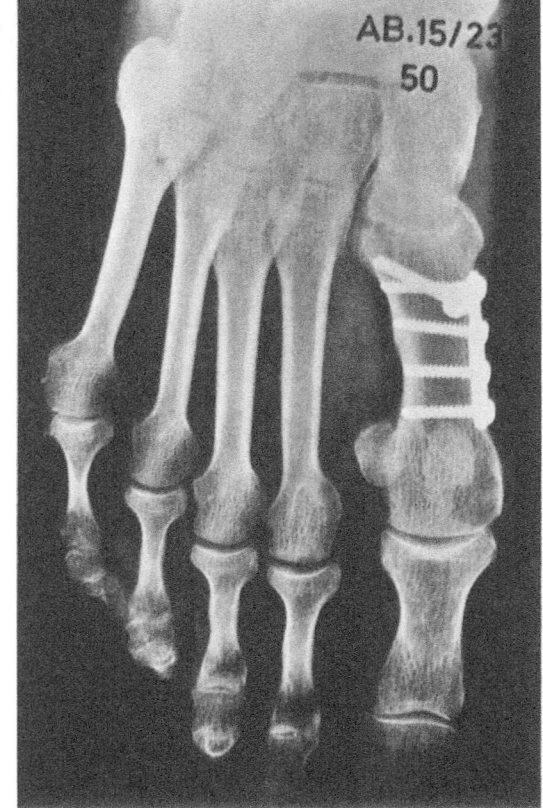

Fig. 134 Clinical example: Transverse fracture of first metatarsal
The patient was an unskilled worker, aged 38. A load had dropped on his foot

a Transverse fracture of first metatasal without any comminution

b Internal fixation with a finger plate applied laterally
No complications. Plaster free treatment after operation. Weight bearing began at four weeks. Full weight bearing at eight weeks

c Final review at one year: Symptom-free, full working ability, and identical function on both sides. The patient declined to have the metal removed

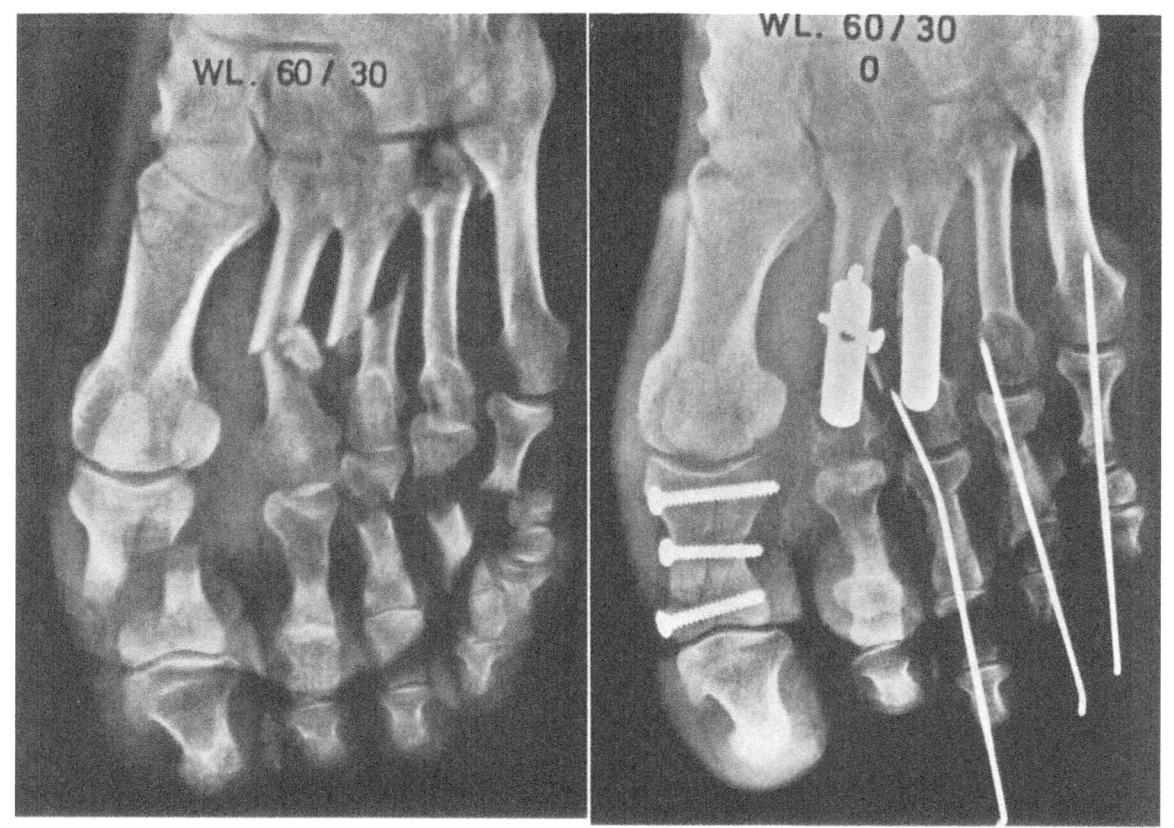

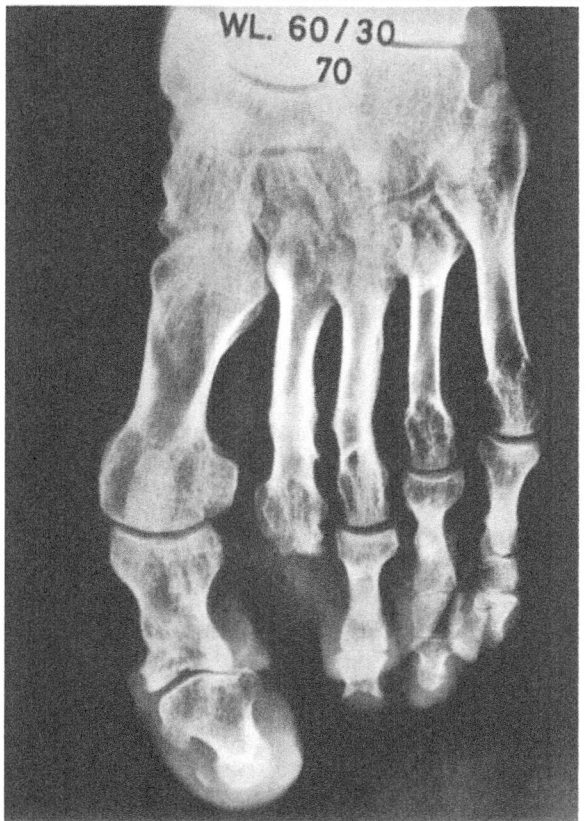

Fig. 135
Clinical example: Multiple open injuries of the forefoot

The patient was a driver of 33. A very heavy load had dropped on his foot

a Multiple open fractures of the metatarsals and phalanges. Severe lacerations of the foot and impairment of the blood supply

b after two weeks: Screw fixation of the proximal phalanx of the big toe, small straight plates applied to the shafts of the 2nd and 3rd metatarsal, axial medullary wiring of the proximal phalanges of the 3rd to 5th toes. Impacted fractures of the base of the 1st metatarsal are not amenable to operative treatment. The treatment after operation was without plaster cast

Healing process: Amputation of the terminal phalanx of the 3rd toe after 6 weeks, amputation of the 2nd toe after three months because of infected necrosis. The other fractures healed. Full weight-bearing at the end of three months. The metal was removed after 5 months. He was able to return to partial work after 5 months and was fully working at the end of 7 months

c Final review after 16 months: Symptom-free and full working capacity. Full function and he can join in sports. The fractures had healed

251

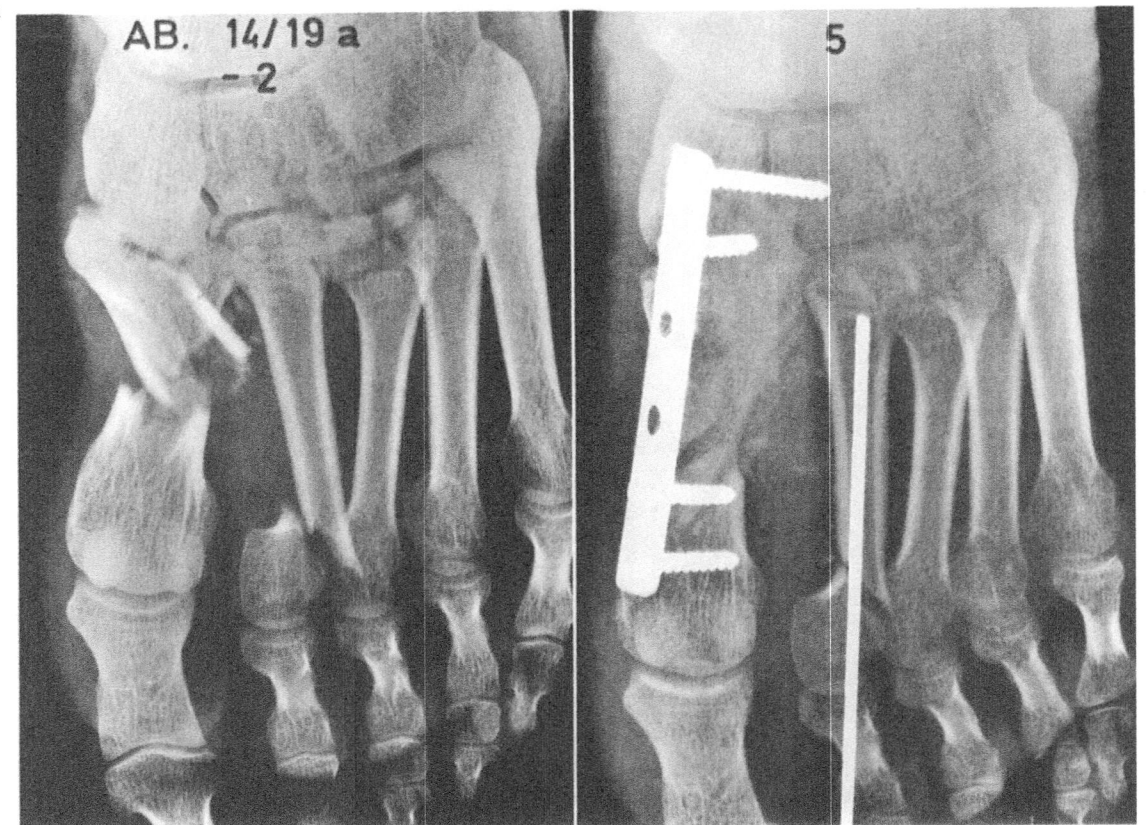

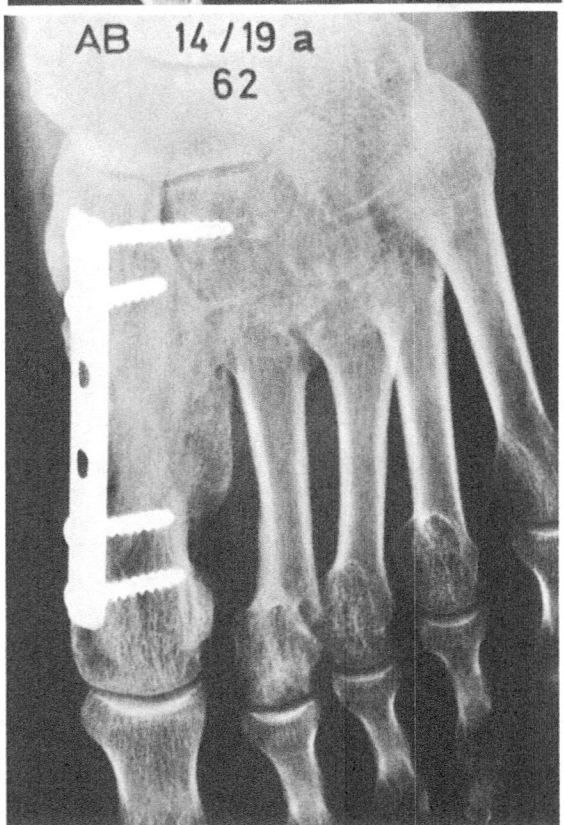

Fig. 136 Clinical example: Fracture of the base of the first metatarsal

The patient was an electrician, aged 28, who had fallen from scaffolding

a Comminuted articular fracture of the 1st metatarsal together with a fracture of the neck of the 2nd metatarsal (vassal fracture)

b Operation after 2 weeks: Arthrodesis of the 1st tarso-metatarsal joint with a small semi-tubular plate and cancellous bone graft. Medullary wiring of the second metatarsal

No complications. Removal of the medullary wire at the end of 4 weeks. Walking caliper used for 3 months. Temporary walking plaster cast

c Removal of the metal at 13 months, when the fracture had healed

Final review: No symptoms, full working ability, full movement of the ankle joint and the mid-tarsal joint

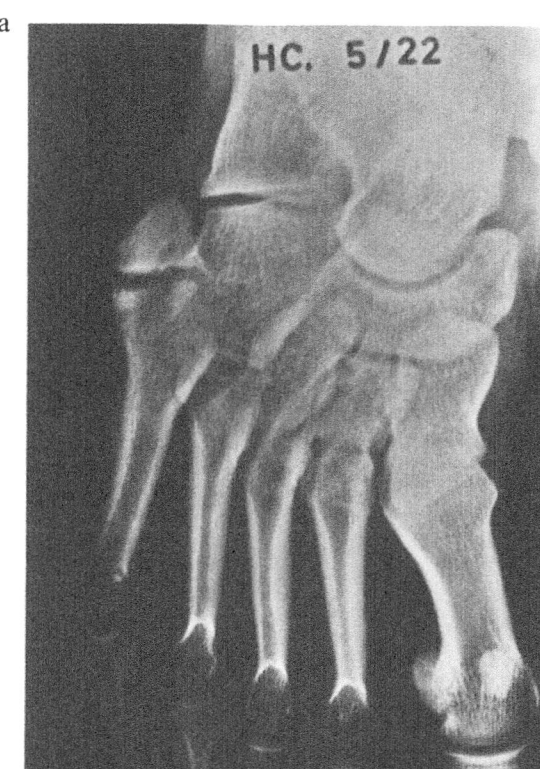

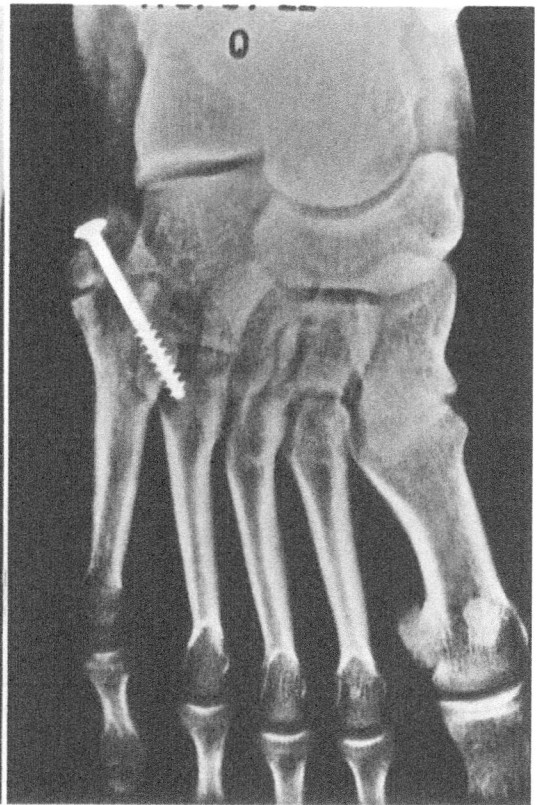

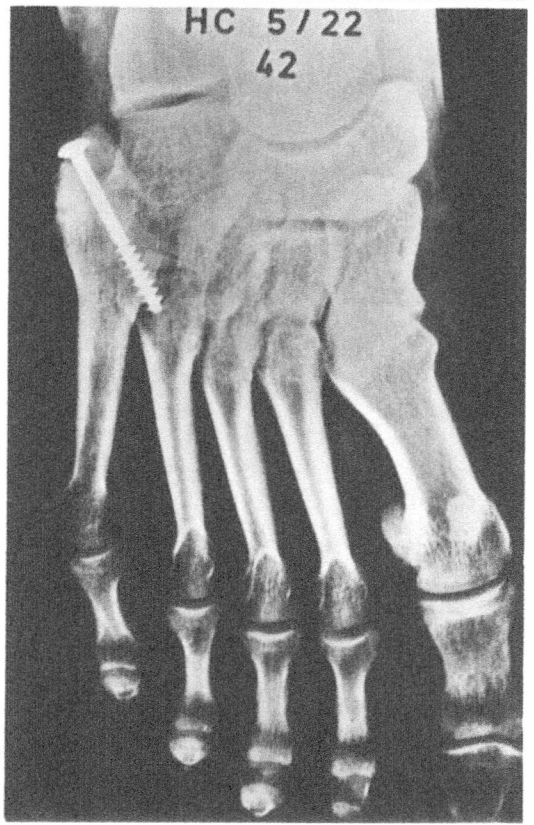

Fig. 137 Clinical example: Pseudarthrosis at the base of the 5th metatarsal

The patient was a building labourer, aged 36. Lateral margin of the foot had been injured on a stone. He had continued moderate symptoms and had received no treatment

a Pseudarthrosis was diagnosed at 8 months

b Rigid internal fixation with a small cancellous screw and without bone graft

Post-operative complete plaster cast applied and was worn for 3 months. The pseudarthrosis consolidated progressively

c Review at the end of 10 months: Full function, mild symptoms depending on the change in the weather. Full working ability and the pseudarthrosis had consolidated. He was booked for metal removal

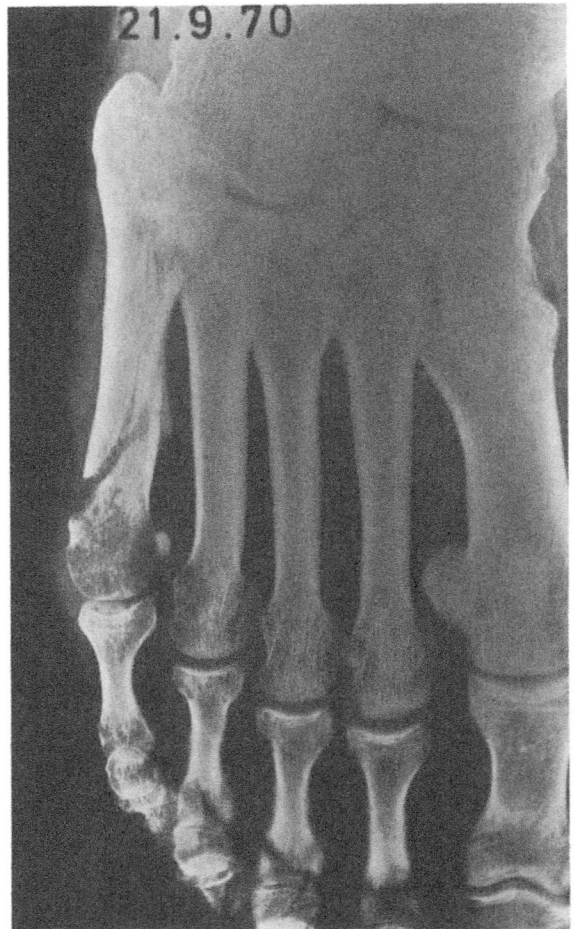

a

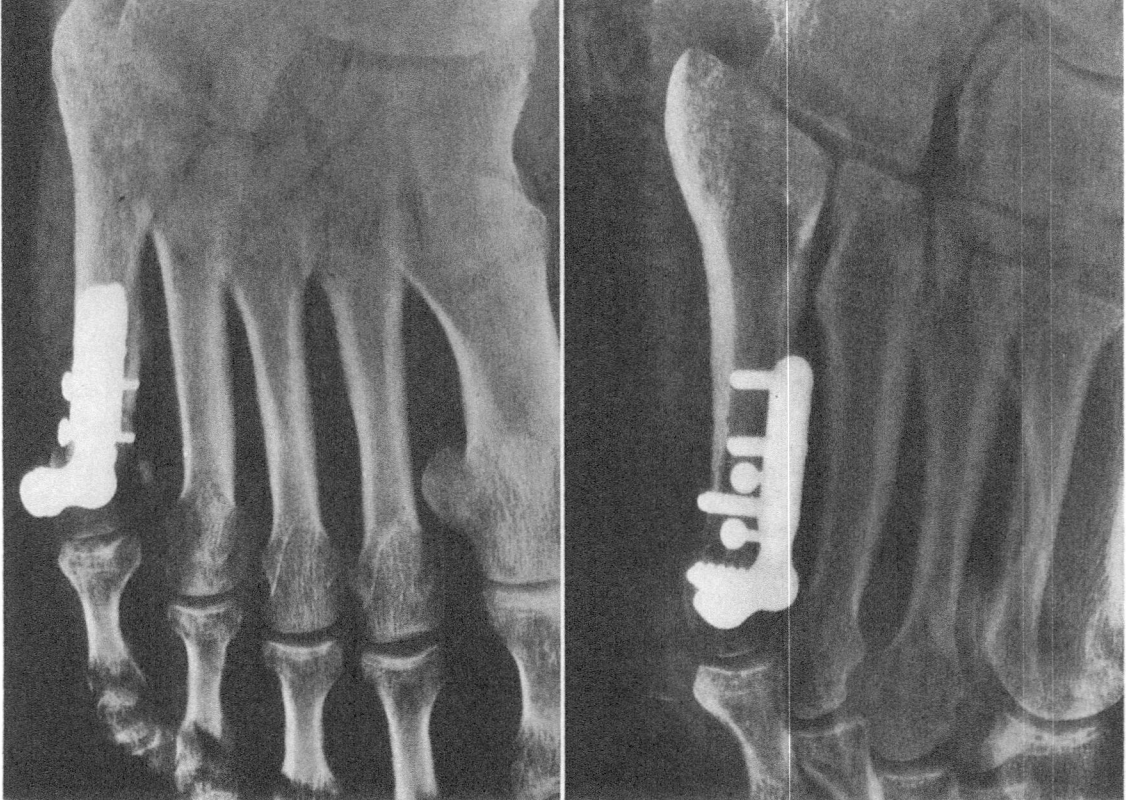

b

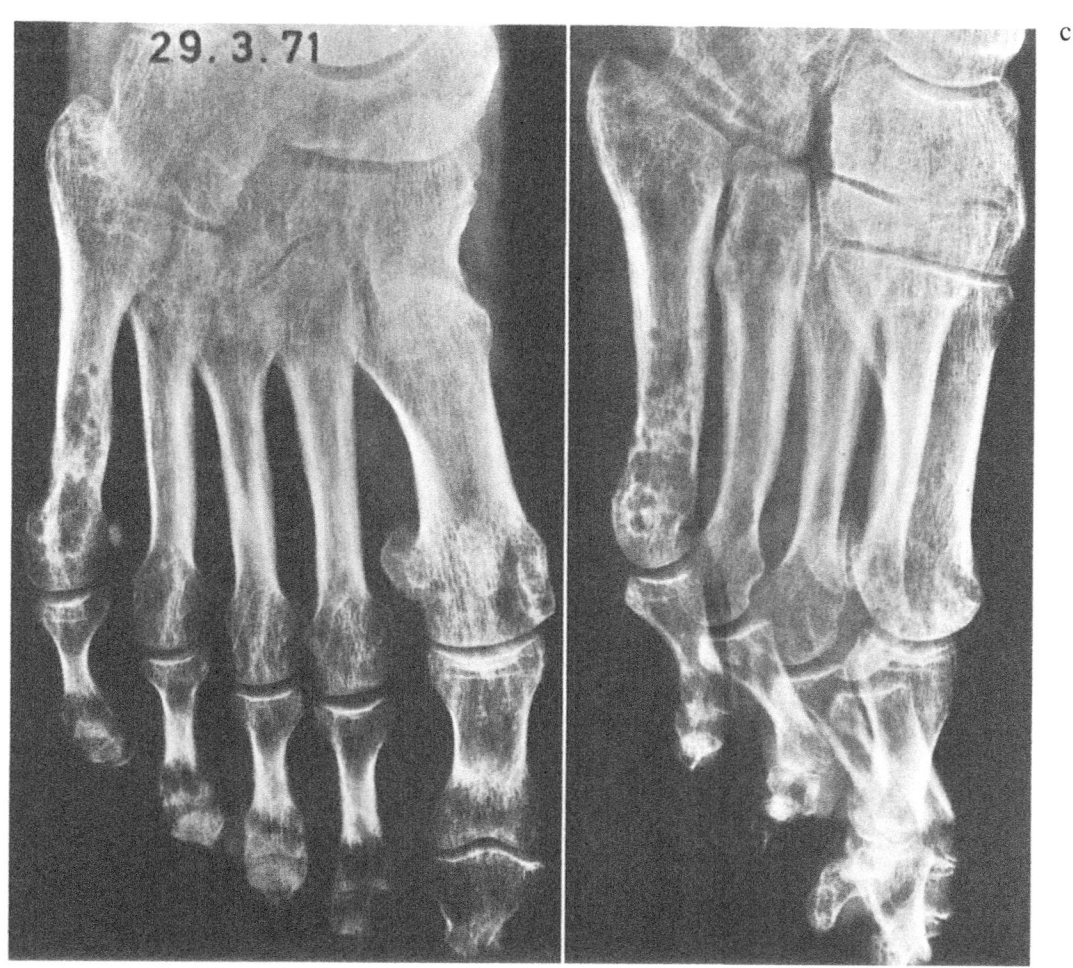

Fig. 138   Clinical example: Pseudarthrosis of the distal end of the 5th metatarsal
The patient was an interior decorator, aged 47 who had fallen off a ladder. He had a fracture of the neck of the 5th metatarsal in satisfactory position

a   A walking plaster produced no union and he had increasing osteoporosis peripherally

b   Two months after the accident: Internal fixation with a bone peg, finger L-plate and screws
No complications. Post-operative treatment without plaster. The fracture had consolidated at 10 weeks

c   Removal of the metal at 6 months
Final review at 9 months: symptom-free, full function

XIII. Special Locations

The use of small implants in more proximal areas of the skeleton is indicated for various reasons. Isolated fractures in minor tuberosities of long bones can usually be fixed with small implants and these give sufficient stability. Sometimes individual elements of comminuted fractures need to be fixed and this can be done with both large and small implants. Here we shall only mention a few typical examples, but will not embark upon a comprehensive description.

A. Upper Limb

1. Clavicle

Operation on the middle third of the clavicle is only indicated for non-union of badly displaced fractures, for injuries to vessels or nerves and for pseudarthrosis. In the oblique fractures, screw fixation together with a neutralization plate has proved to be effective. To give good stability, semi-tubular plates are usually applied to pseudarthroses whereas small semitubular plates are only used exceptionally. Here the small cortex screws are of particular value since the flat screw-head does not stand proud under the skin.

2. Scapula

Fractures of the scapula, especially those of the lower and anterior border of the glenoid, can easily be fixed with small semi-tubular plates and screws (see AO Manual, Figs. 97 and 105).

3. Humerus

a) Avulsion of the Tuberosity

An isolated avulsion of the tuberosity displaced under the acromion is successfully fixed with small cancellous screws. Sutures must be placed into the bone for the repair of the capsule (Fig. 139a).

b) Comminuted Fracture of the Surgical Neck of the Humerus

The clover leaf plate has proved to be appropriate for fixing this type of fracture, as we can thus obtain a congruous fixation as here there is loose cancellous bone as in the pilon tibial fracture (Fig. 139b).

B. Lower Limb

1. Knee

a) Fractures of the Tibial Spine

These isolated fractures are sometimes caused by frontal injury to the knee joint. Since the size of the fracture area and the instability are always considerable, operation should be carried out, even if only small displacements are visible on the X-ray. The insertion of the cruciates to the tibia must be exactly reduced and individually fixed. Stability is usually obtained by the use of a cerclage wire which is passed through anterior drill holes and round the tibial spine. The fixation achieved by open reduction, however, is limited. In compact fragments, fixation with small cancellous screws is best (Fig. 140). Because of the strong tensile properties of the ligaments, post-operative immobilization in a plaster with slight flexion is indispensable.

Screw fixation of the tibial spine can also be part of the internal fixation in complicated fractures of the tibial plateau.

b) Patella

The transverse fracture of the patella is reduced by tension-band wiring. Internal fixation with small implants is indicated in the following cases:

Vertical Fractures of the Patella

This uncommon type of fracture can be fixed simply by screws which allows active post-operative treatment (Fig. 141 a).

Associated Vertical Fissures

A transverse fracture of the patella is sometimes accompanied by additional vertical fissures, usually in the proximal fragment. Here the proximal complex should first be reduced with small cancellous screws. The transverse element may then be fixed with a tension-band wire (Fig. 141 b).

Avulsion of the Lower Pole

A small fragment avulsed from the patella, which is functionally the same as a rupture of the patella ligament, is fairly common in comminuted fractures. As there is usually a large fragment carrying most of the intact articular cartilage, there is no indication for primary patellectomy. A simple tension-band wiring rotates the distal fragment inwards as shown in Fig. 141 c. A screw can keep its surface in contact with the larger upper fragment. The anatomical connection between ligament and patella is thus restored. A temporary wire to relieve tension, anchored in the tibial tuberosity, is imperative if active post-operative treatment is to be allowed (Fig. 141 d).

This procedure is also recommended in cases of partial patellectomy, provided that the fragment attached to the patella tendon is of sufficient size (Fig. 141 c).

2. Tibial Shaft

In internal fixation of the tibia, the use of standard implants may sometimes be combined with individual small screws. This chiefly applies in three different situations:

a) Narrow Tips of Fragments

The small 3.5 mm cortex screw is especially appropriate for the fixation of such tips. It is available in lengths up to 40 mm. The procedure is the same as that with large cortex screws. Make a gliding hole with drill bit of 3.6 mm and the drill sleeve of 3.5 mm into the anterior cortex; then make a thread hole with the drill bit of 2 mm, tapping the thread with a 3.5 mm tap; in an oblique insertion the countersink tool should be used (Fig. 142 a).

b) Separated Oval Fragments

In the presence of comminuted fractures, small detached fragments should be accurately reduced. This helps in the reduction of the remaining fracture components and, in addition, can improve and guarantee the stability of the whole complex. These fragments can be re-vascularized from neighbouring bones (Schenk, Perren), and their fixation with small cortex screws avoids any damage to soft tissues. In the shaft, we use the small 3.5 mm cortex screw lag-wise, while the small cancellous screw of 4 mm is often used distally in cancellous bone (Fig. 142 b).

c) Small Butterfly Fragments

Similar experience has led to increasing use of small lag screws to fix small butterfly fragments. The flat screw heads never produce infractures and do not damage the periosteum (Fig. 142 c).

C. Mandible

A transverse fracture of the edentulous jaw is a good indication for the use of a tension-band plate for which Spiessl has produced a special design.

D. Clinical X-Ray Examples
Figs. 143–147, pages 265–273

258

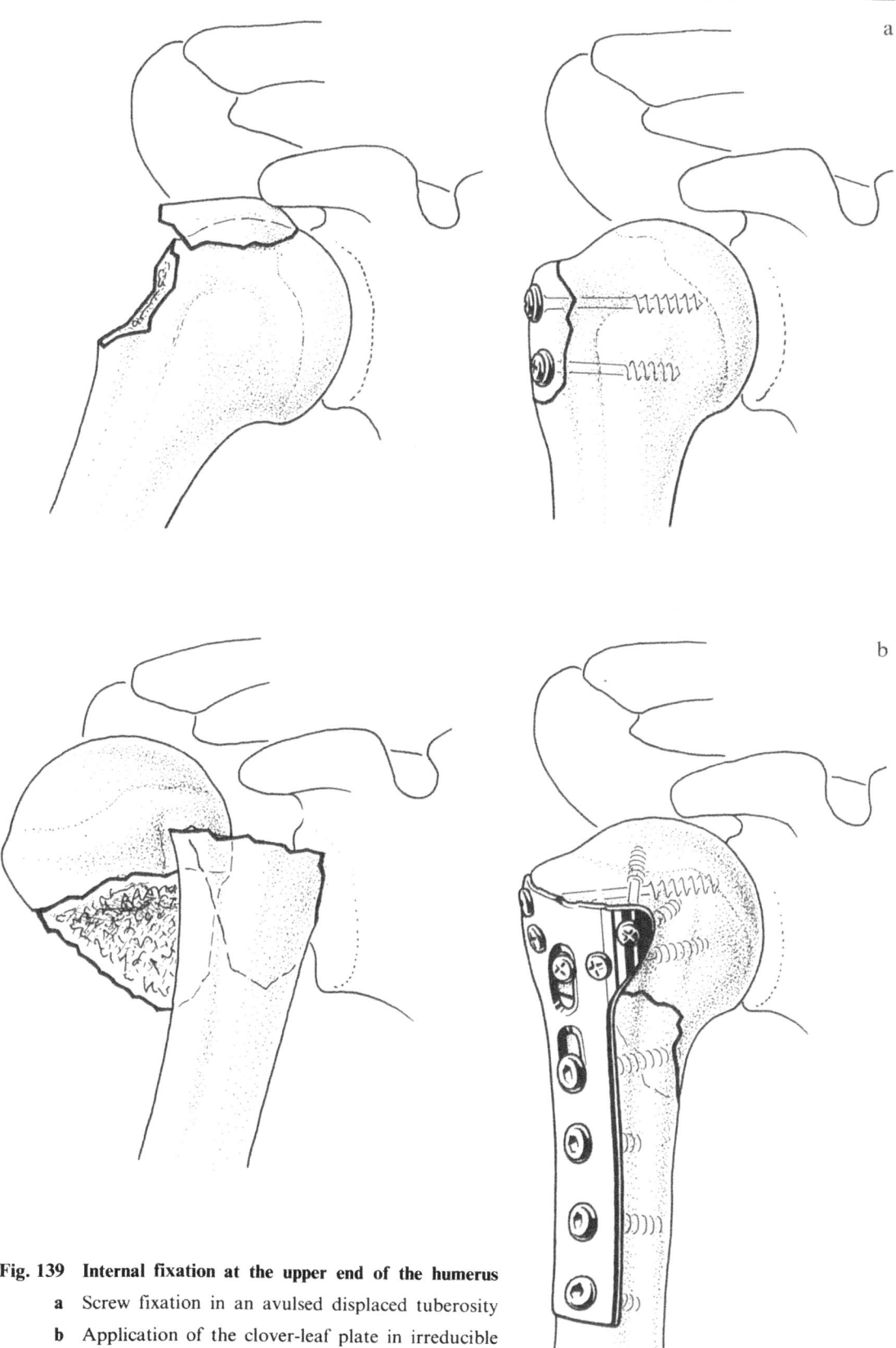

Fig. 139   Internal fixation at the upper end of the humerus

  a Screw fixation in an avulsed displaced tuberosity

  b Application of the clover-leaf plate in irreducible and unstable fractures of the surgical neck of the humerus

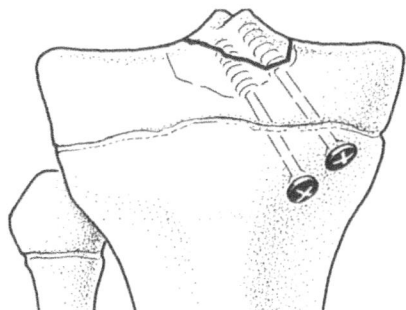

Fig. 140 Fracture of the tibial spine

Screw fixation

Fig. 141 **Internal fixation in fractures of the patella** ▷

   a Screw fixation in a vertical fracture of the patella

   b Screw fixation combined with tension-band wiring in a transverse patellar fracture with a vertical component

   c With a small distal fragment, tension-band wiring tips backwards the lower fragment

   d Axial screw fixation combined with the tension-band wiring is effective, but the wires must be anchored in the tibial tubercle

   e Comminuted fracture of the lower pole of the patella: Partial patellectomy. The small remaining fragment attached to the patellar ligament is fixed to the proximal main fragment with a screw and tension-band wiring, which must be anchored in the tibial tubercle

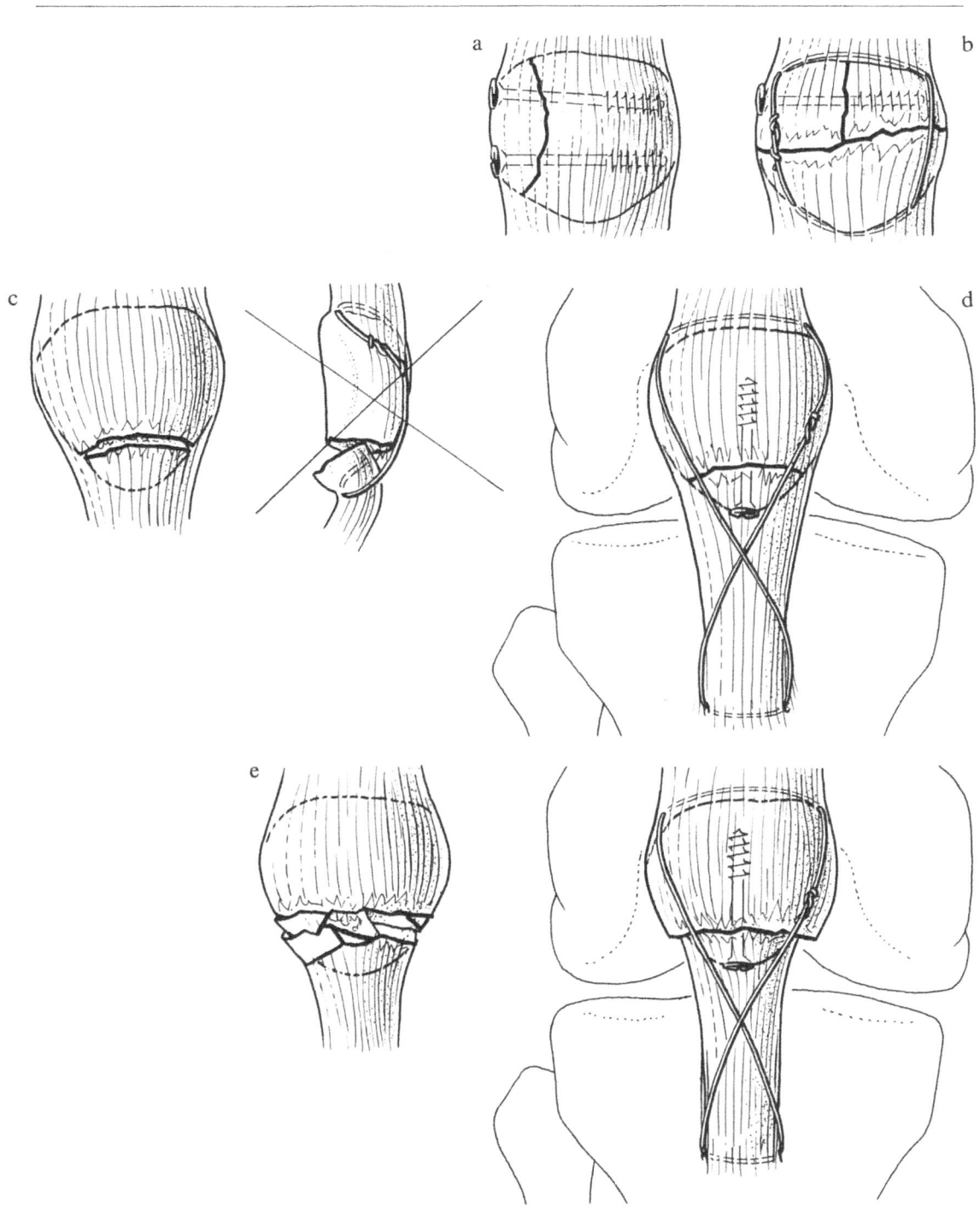

Fig. 142 Use of the small cortex lag screw for internal fixation of the tibia

   a For fixation of the tips of narrow fragments

   b For the fixation of detached cortex fragments

   c For the fixation of thin butterfly fragments

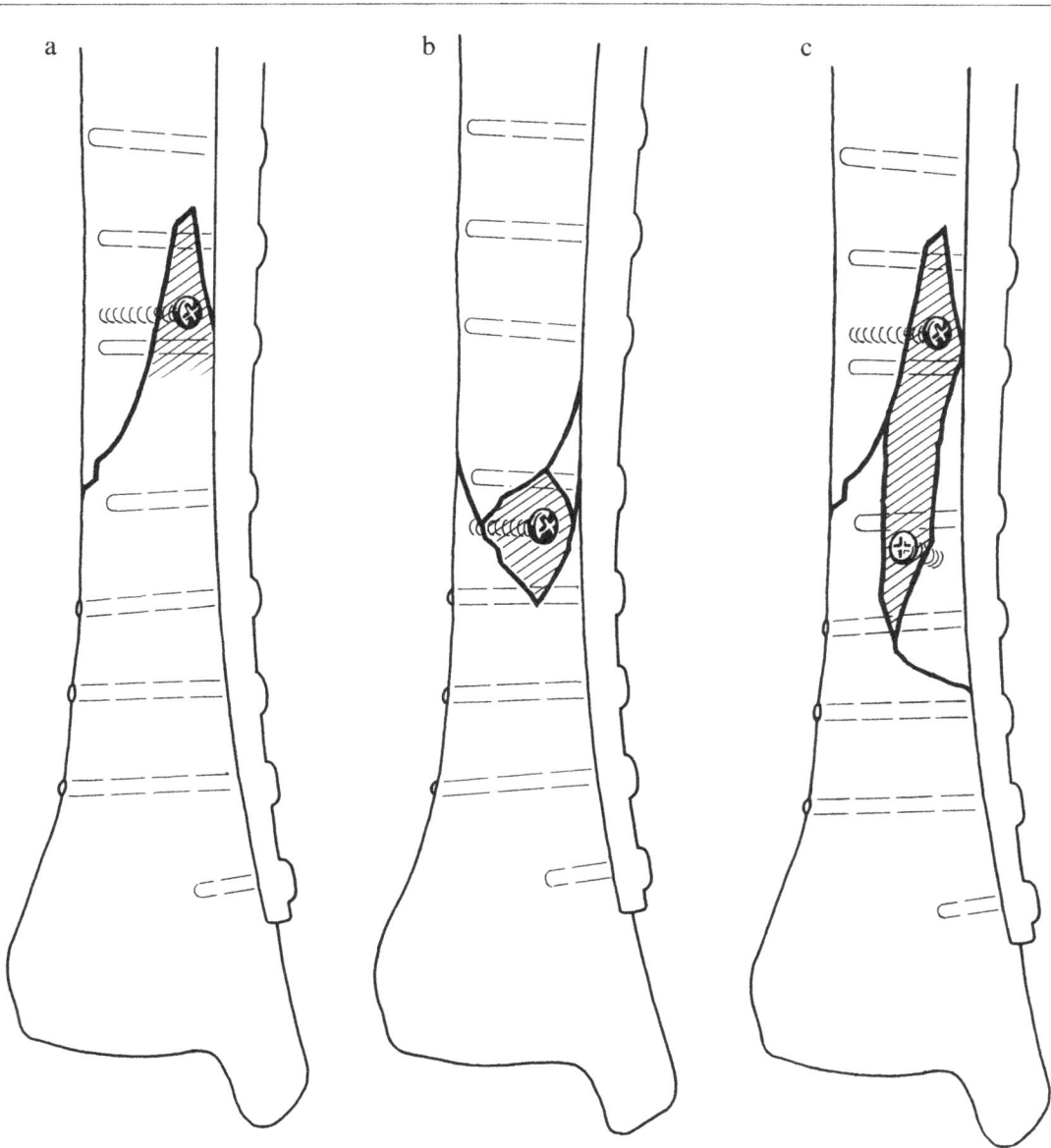

Fig. 143 Clinical example: Secondary internal fixation of the clavicle
A mechanic, aged 19, who had fallen on his left shoulder

a Reduction and the application of a figure-of-eight bandage did not secure union. There was no visible callus

b Internal fixation four weeks after the accident. Small semi-tubular plate with 7 holes was screwed on and a separate lag screw applied to get interfragmentary compression
No complications. Active movement after operation. Consolidation confirmed by X-ray at ten weeks

c Final review and removal of metal at five months. Symptom-free, function identical to the normal side, fracture consolidated

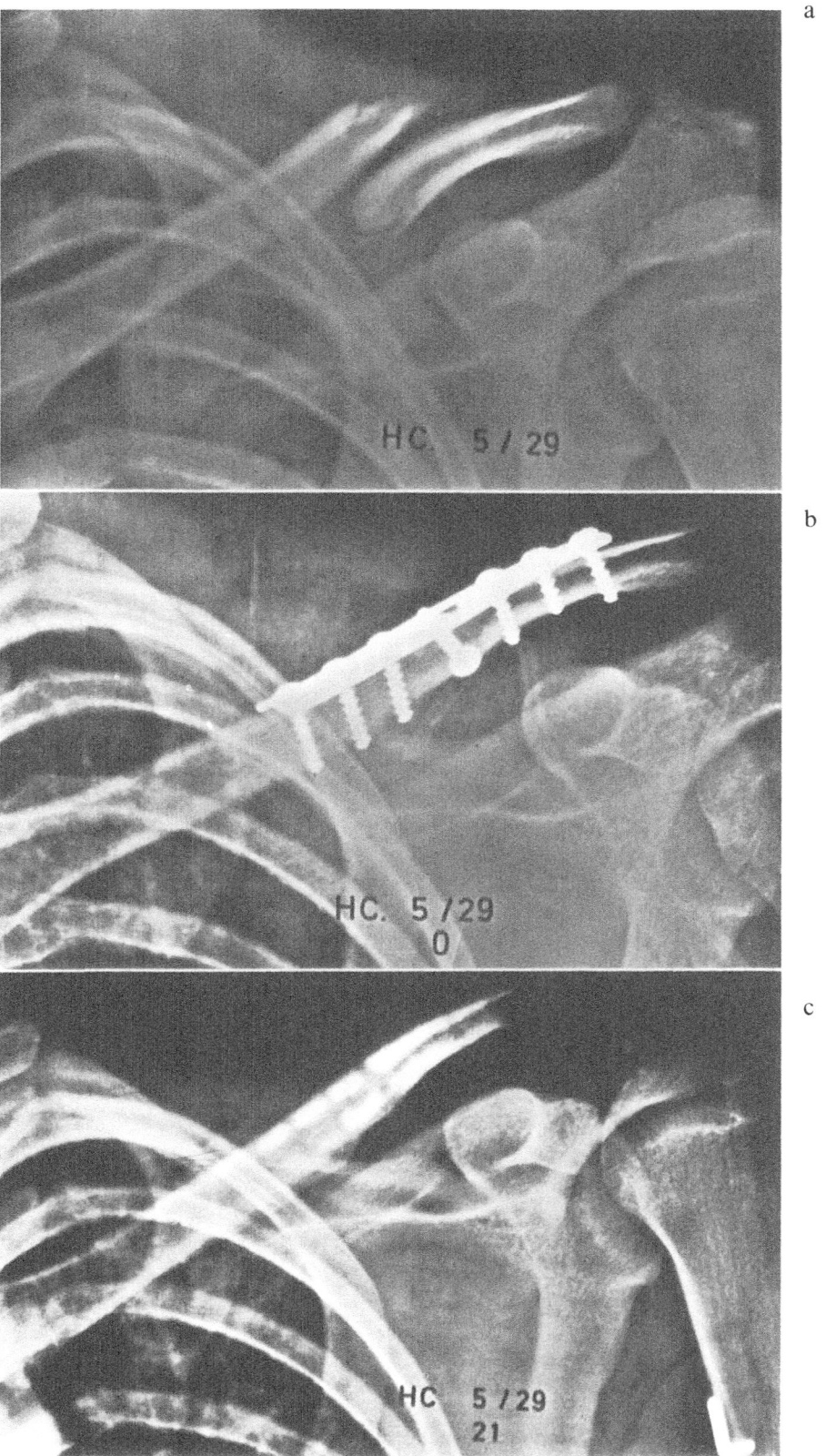

a

b

c

265

Fig. 144 Technical example: Internal fixation in a fracture of the surgical neck of the humerus

   a A severely displaced and fully mobile fracture of the surgical neck of the humerus. An unhealed fracture of the radius in the same arm with limited movement and circulatory disturbance

   b Internal fixation with the clover-leaf plate. Post-operative treatment included early movement

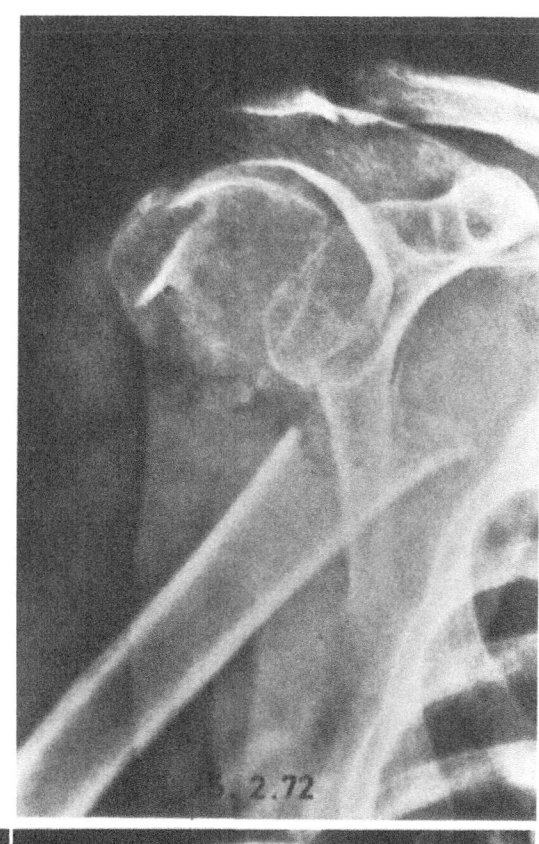

a

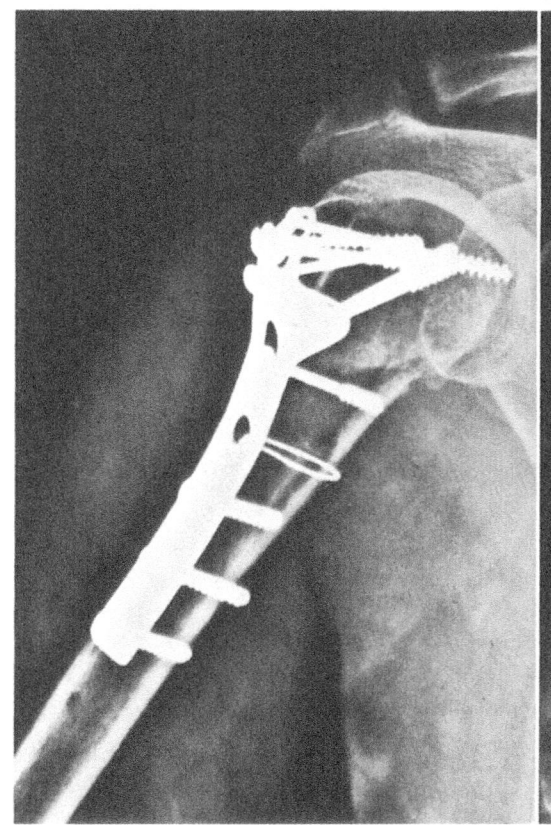

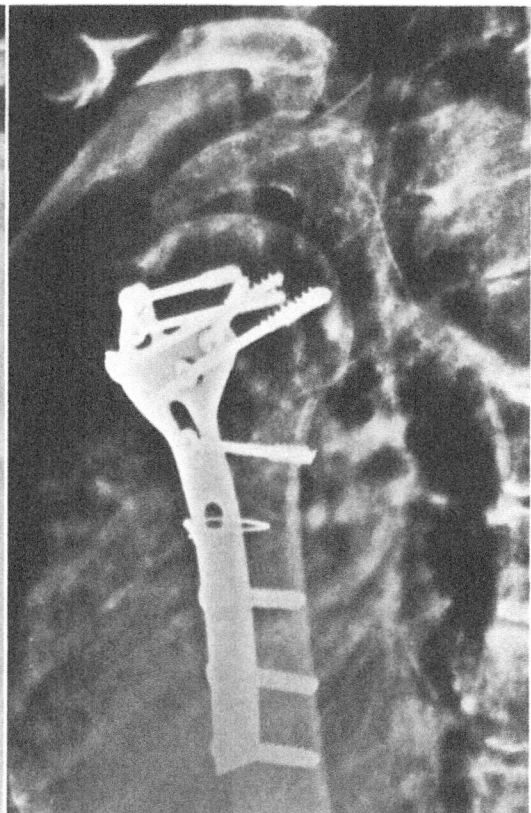

b

267

Fig. 145 Clinical example: Vertical fracture of the patella
The patient was a merchant, aged 38, who had fallen on a stone

a Vertical fracture of the patella; correct diagnosis can only be made with the help of an axial X-ray

b Internal fixation with two small cancellous screws
No complications

c Final review and removal of the metal at one year: Full function. No physical signs

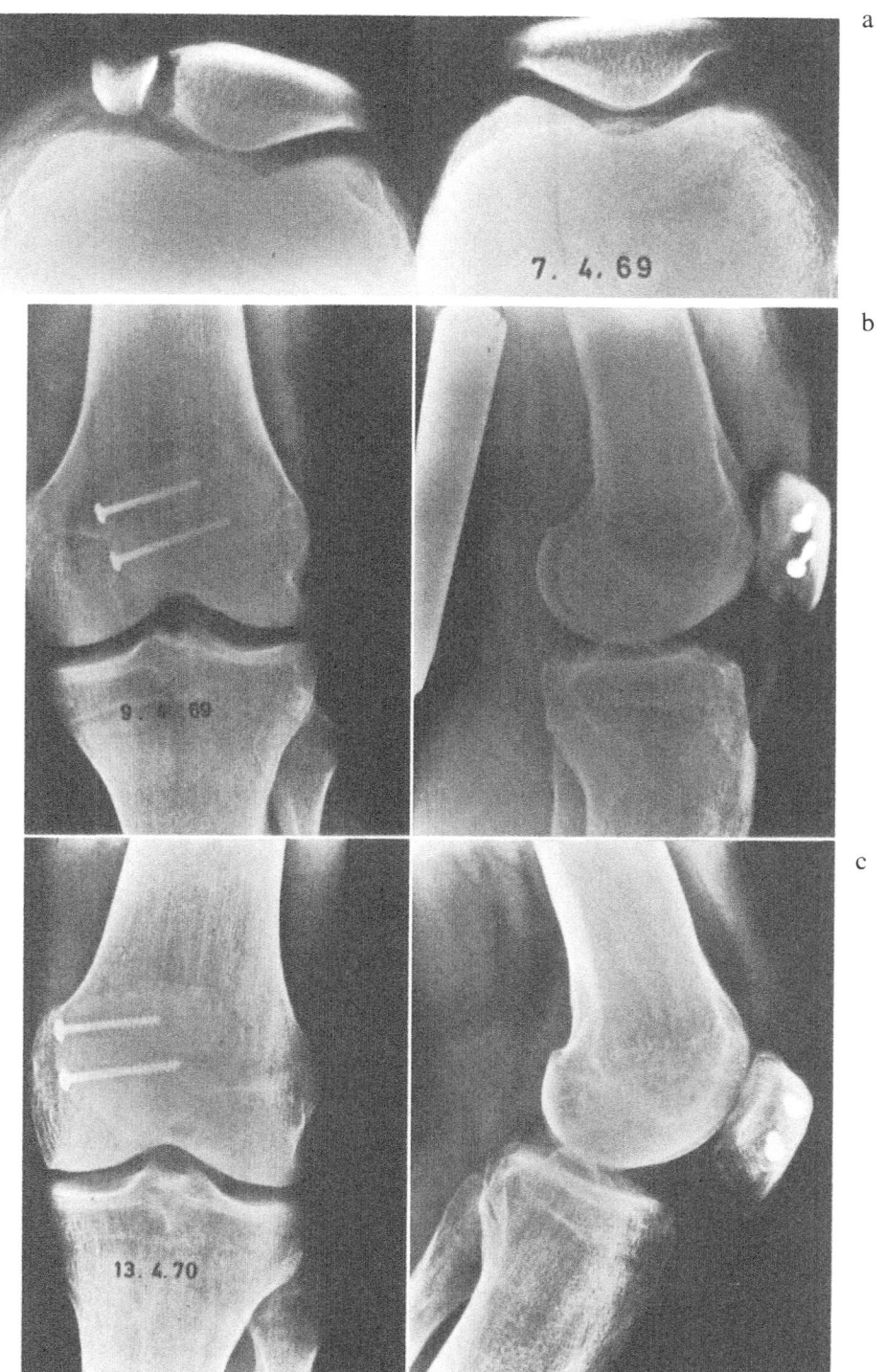

Fig. 146 Clinical example: Transverse fracture of the patella with a vertical component
The patient was a housewife, aged 57, injured in a traffic accident

a The patient had concussion. There was a comminuted fracture of the lower third of the patella. The large proximal fragment had a vertical fissure

b Emergency internal fixation: Partial patellectomy, preserving the large proximal fragment and with screw fixation of the vertical fissure. Figure-of-eight tension-band wiring anchored in the tibial tubercle
No complications. Plaster cast worn for two months. Removal of the metal at eight months

c Final review at sixteen months: Symptom-free, full movement, no arthrosis

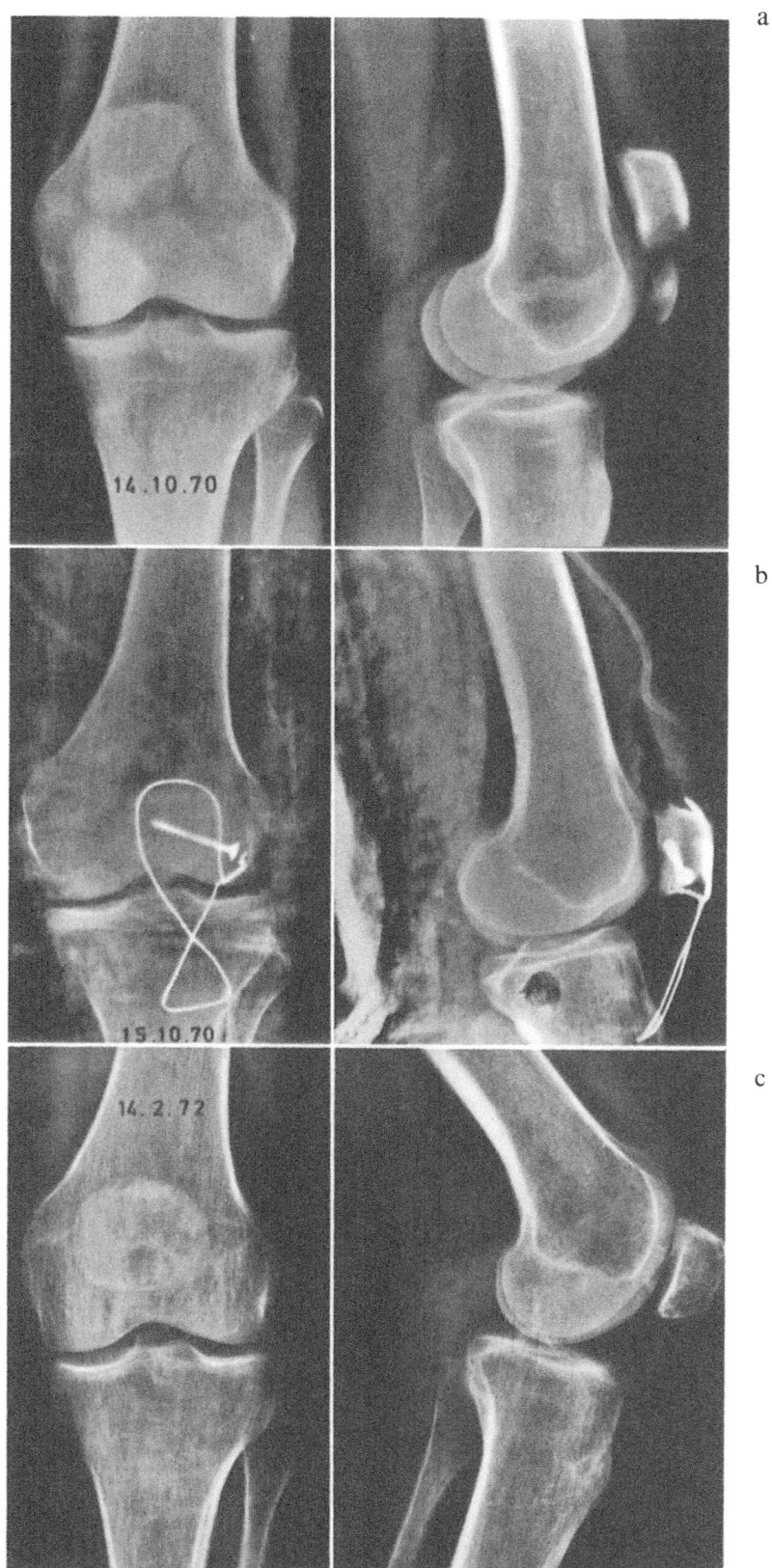

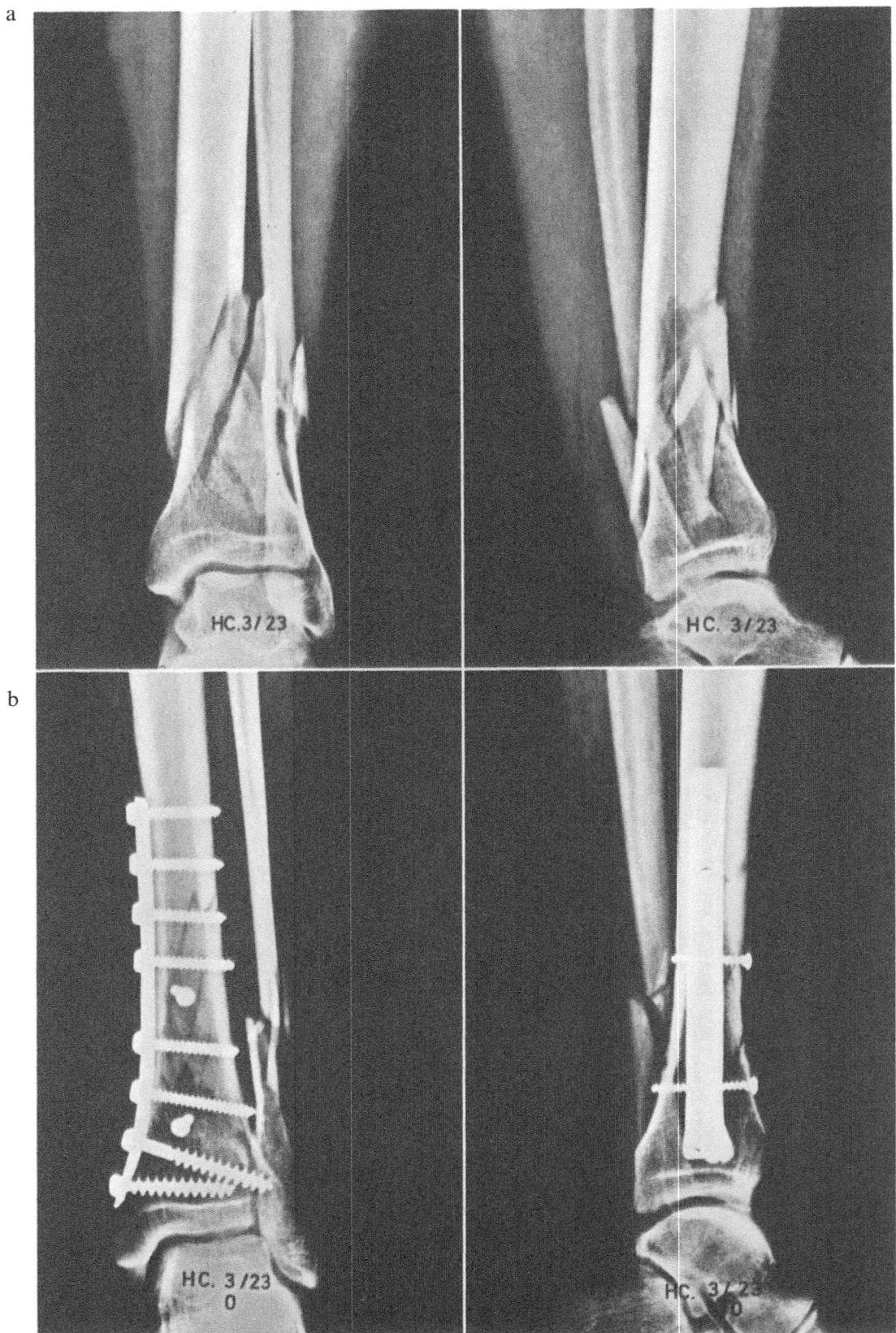

a

b

272

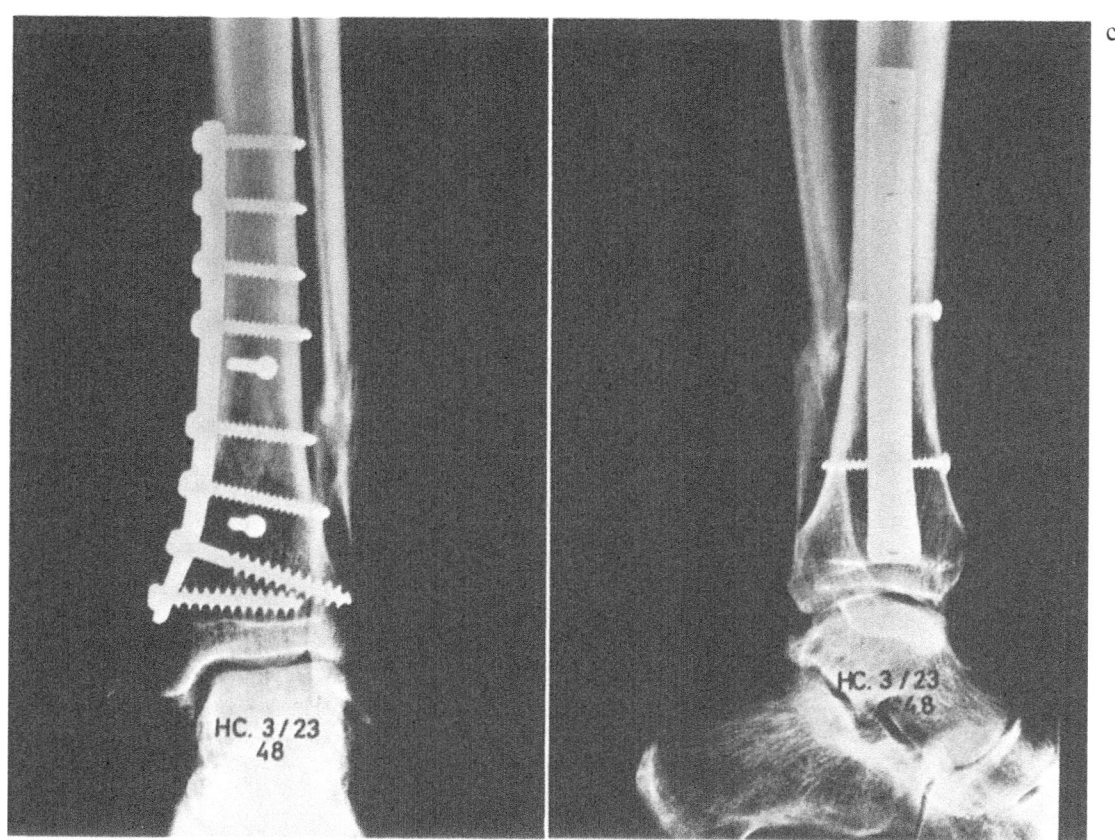

Fig. 147 Clinical example: Use of small ASIF Screw in internal fixation of the tibia

The patient was a pharmacist, aged 42, injured in skiing

a Comminuted fracture of the lower part of the tibia and fibula

b Emergency internal fixation: Semi-tubular plate with additional small lag screws used to fix the small fragment tips
Active post-operative movement. Superficial infection, arising after four months, healed early. Consolidation of the fracture was somewhat delayed. Weight bearing began at the twelfth week

c Final review after one year: Symptom-free, full function, fully consolidated. Booked for removal of metal

XIV. Special Indications

Besides the standard location and others where the use of small implants are sometimes appropriate, there is a series of special indications which include internal fixation in children, open fractures, and some orthopaedic operations especially involving rheumatoid surgery which have become more important recently.

1. Internal Fixation in Children

This is only indicated where there are irreducible or otherwise mobile fractures through the shaft of a long bone, especially in slipped epiphyses following trauma as well as fractures of the epiphyses themselves (Süssenbach).

As there is scarcely any danger of post-traumatic ankylosis in children, which allows the use of external splints with impunity, these operations are more in the nature of accurate open reductions. Nevertheless, biomechanichal relationship between implant and bone must be carefully considered.

In such cases the delicate implants of the SFS are especially appropriate and small semi-tubular plates are used most often. Washers should be used when using screws independently, as the screw heads may otherwise sink into the rather soft childhood bone (Fig. 148).

Implants must be removed early, which means immediately after consolidation has been confirmed by X-ray.

2. The Use of the SFS in Open Fractures

Primary internal fixation of fragments in open fractures should be untertaken with the smallest amount of metal (AO Manual), so that it may sometimes be looked upon as provisional internal fixation. Even in large fractures, small plates can be useful, though they must be replaced by standard implants of greater load-bearing capacity after the damaged soft parts have healed.

3. Special Orthopaedic Indications

a) Osteochondritis Dissecans

Replacing and fixing large loose bodies is now generally approved (Smillie). Larger defects can also be filled with an osteo-chondral graft (Wagner). Previously, fixation was undertaken with thin autogenous cortical nail-shaped grafts which were introduced through drill holes and pressed into the cancellous bone of the condyles (Bandi and Allgöwer). Recent experience has shown that such fixation can be more easily obtained with small screws which provide reliable compression and the early incorporation of the sequestra. As these methods are little known, details will now be given:

Technique of Simple Fixation

— Remove the loose bodies.
— Freshen the bed with a sharp spoon.
— Where a step develops, the defect must be lined with cancellous bone.
— Fix the fragment back with 1–3 screws. Screw heads should not prodrude beyond the surface of the cartilage (Fig. 149a and b).

Technique of Osteo-Chondral Grafting

— Freshen the bed.
— Take an osteo-chondral graft of sufficient size from the posterior surface of the

femoral condyle which is subjected to little if any load-bearing.

— Fix the graft into its bed with 1 or 2 screws (Fig. 149 c).

Post-Operative Treatment

Active movement must be begun when the wound has healed. Weight-bearing should be avoided for the first three months. In most cases, screws can be removed six months after the operation. The screw heads may then be covered with cartilage and, therefore, difficult to find.

b) Tibial Tuberosity

Displacement of the tibial tuberosity is often required in secondary operations on the knee joint.

When the tuberosity needs to be *replaced in a medial and distal direction* (Roux, Hauser) most authors recommend a bone-plasty, but the tuberosity can be just as well fixed with a screw. The large cancellous or malleolar screws used up till now have been replaced by the small cancellous screw of which the traumatizing effect is much less (Fig. 151 a). A small tension-band plate which counteracts the pull of the patella ligament (Fig. 151 b) allows early flexion.

When *anterior displacement of the tuberosity* is required for relaxation of the patellar ligament (Bandi), an interposed cancellous bone graft can easily be fixed with a small cancellous screw, the flat head of which causes no disturbance under the skin. Where the periosteum and cortical connections between the reflected tuberosity and the tibia is preserved, the screw is not subjected to any bending stress. Active movement is then possible (Fig. 151 c).

c) Kelly's Operation

Damage to the ankle joint associated with rupture of the synovial sheaths may lead to chronic displacement of the peroneal tendons at the lateral malleolus. Correction of such displacement is achieved by Kelly's operation. By means of a sagittal osteotomy, a flat cortical disc of bone is raised from the fibula and displaced posteriorly. The wide posterior pulley of the malleolus that results keeps the tendons in their right position and prevents displacement. Two short small cancellous screws are adequate to fix the disc in its new position (Fig. 150 b).

d) Reconstruction of the Limbus in the Recurrent Dislocation of the Shoulder

The use of small screws has proved to be adequate for the reconstruction of the limbus here (Fig. 150 a).

4. The Use of the SFS in the Surgery of Rheumatoid Deformities

Here the metal implants are especially used for arthrodesis, the techniques of which are described in the general section. The brittle and delicate bones of the rheumatoid patient often require especially thin implants.

The small semi-tubular plate must thus be used in most cases for arthrodesis of the wrist joint, although they give less rigidity than the standard ASIF plate. Additional external support is, therefore, sometimes unavoidable. On the other hand the small fragment set allows us to obtain a wide range of internal fixations.

5. Clinical X-Ray Examples
Figs. 152–157, pages 282–289.

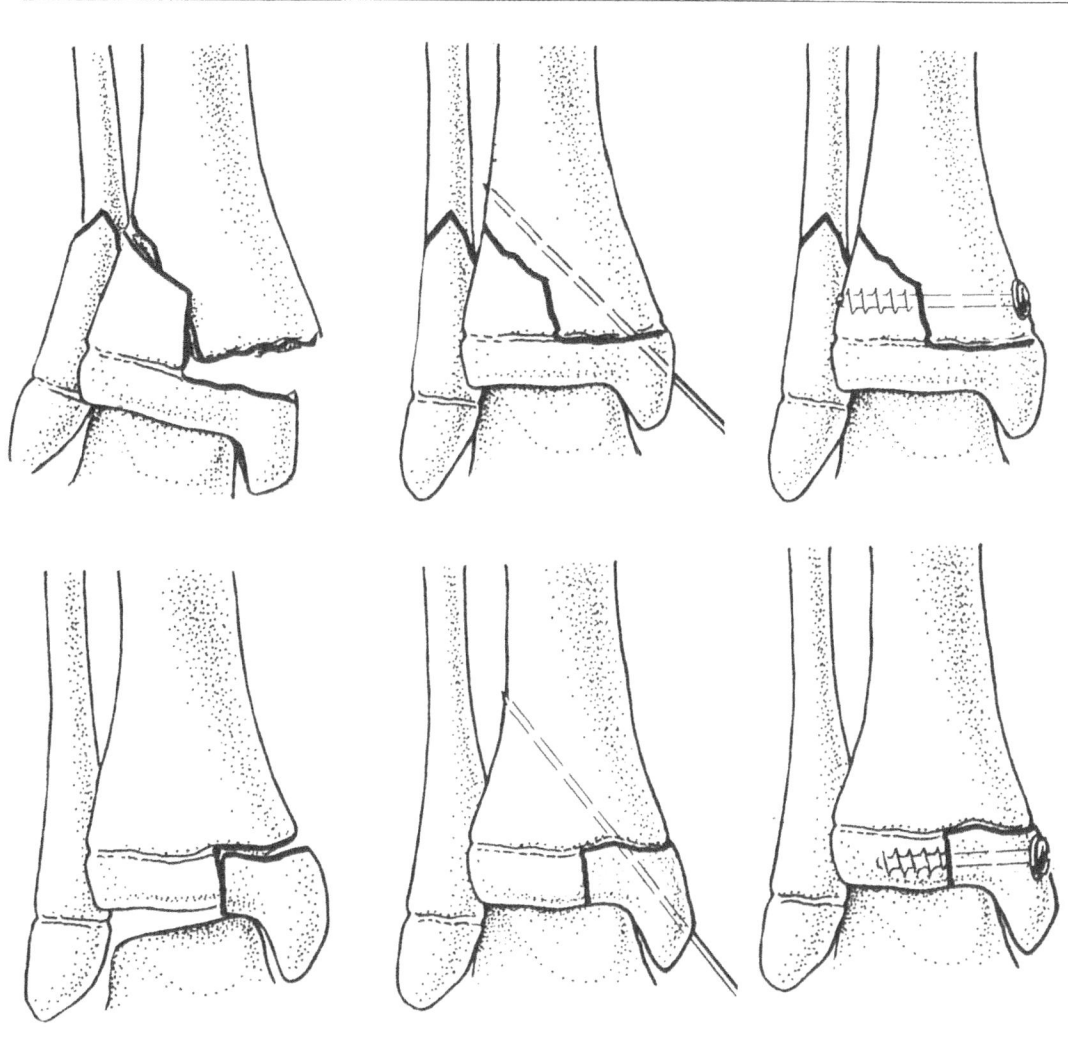

Fig. 148 Internal fixation in children

Two examples of screw fixation in fractures of the epiphysis as an alternative to open reduction and fixation with Kirschner wire

Fig. 149 Screw fixation in osteochondritis dissecans

   a Fixation in the bed of the loose body with small cortex screws

   b Reduction and fixation of the loose body fragment with small cancellous screws

   c Osteo-chondral graft taken from the posterior surface of the femoral condyle fills in the defect and can be fixed with small cancellous screws

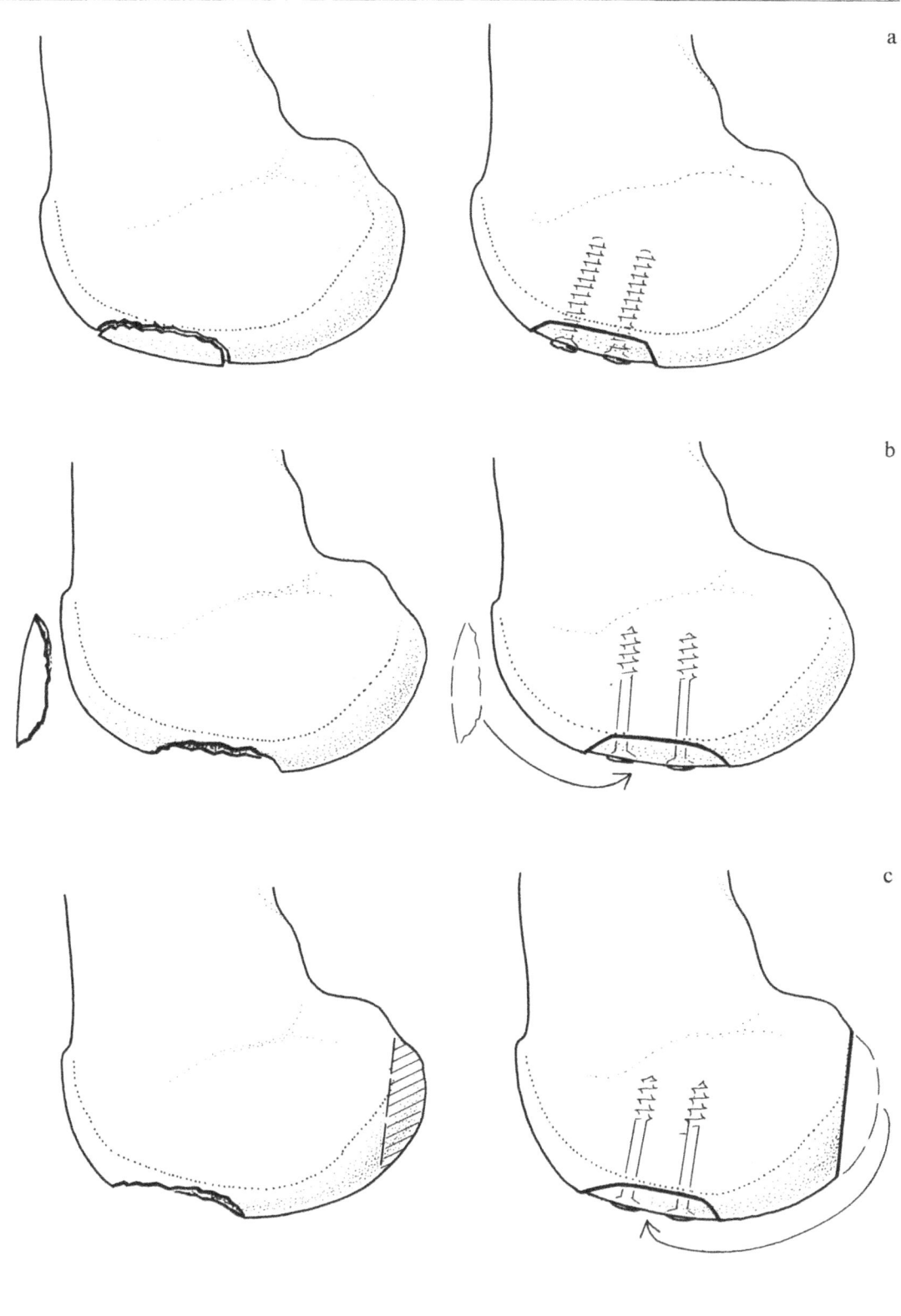

Fig. 150 **Various orthopaedic operations**

  a Screw fixation of the limbus in recurrent dislocation of the shoulder

  b Kelly's operation. Dorsal displacement of a cortical disc and its fixation with two small cancellous screws

Fig. 151 **Operations on the tibial tuberosity**

  a Roux's operation with medial and distal displacement of the tuberosity. Fixation with small cancellous screws

  b Small tension-band plate is used instead of the screw alone

  c Displacement of the tibial tubercle by an interposed graft fixed with small cancellous screw

280

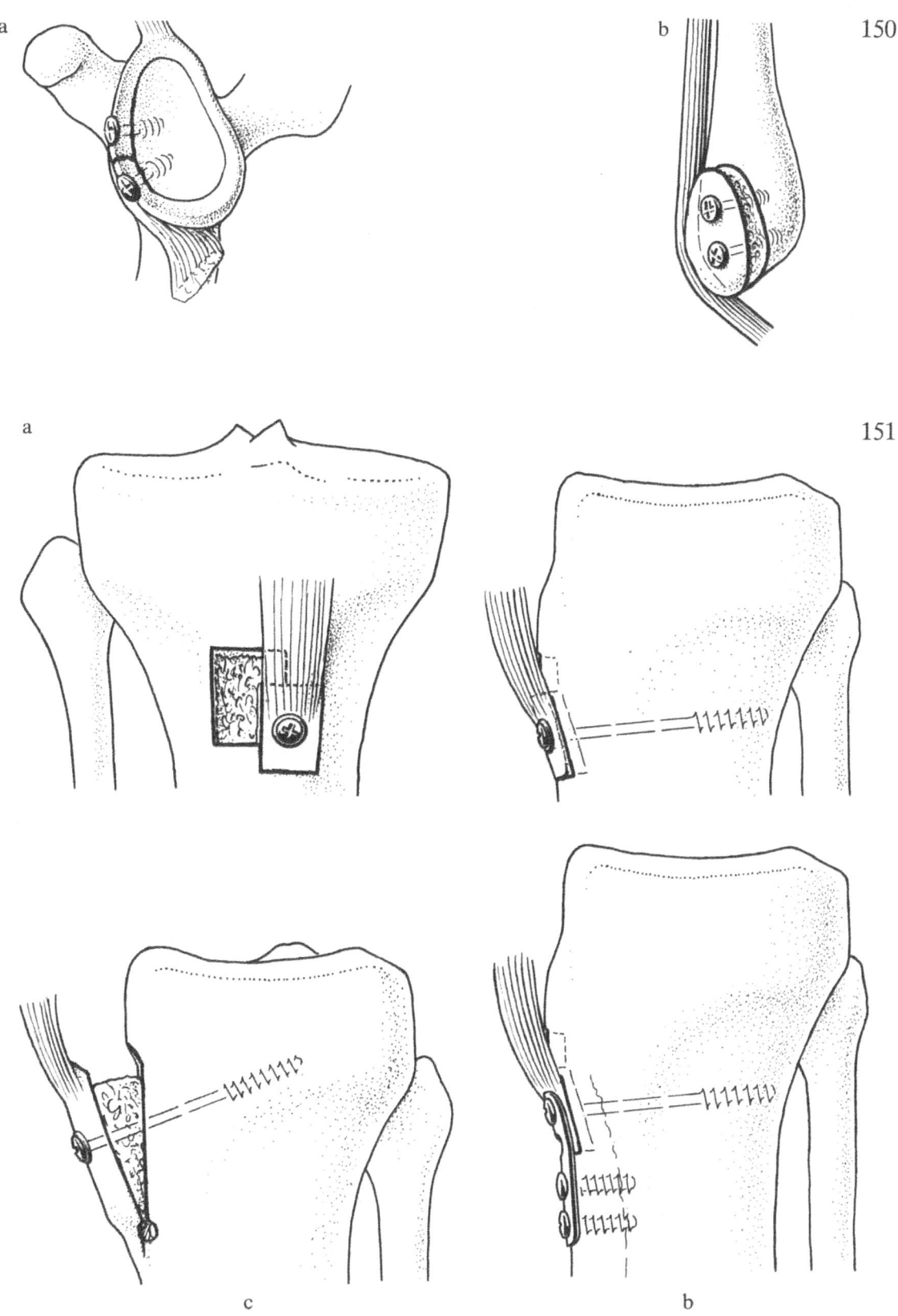

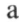

a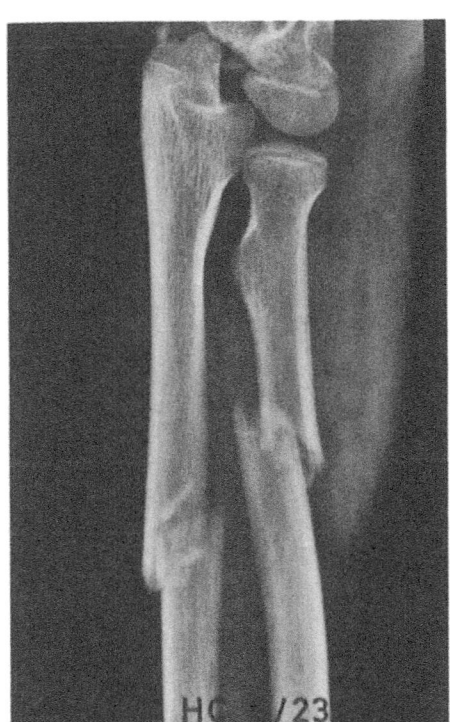

Fig. 152 Clinical example: Internal fixation of fracture of the forearm

The patient was a 12 year-old boy who had fallen from a height of 6 feet

a Open fracture of the shaft of both forearm bones

b Emergency internal fixation with two small semi-tubular plates
No complications. A posterior plaster splint was applied for three weeks

c Removal of the metal at three months. Mild limitation of pronation and supination

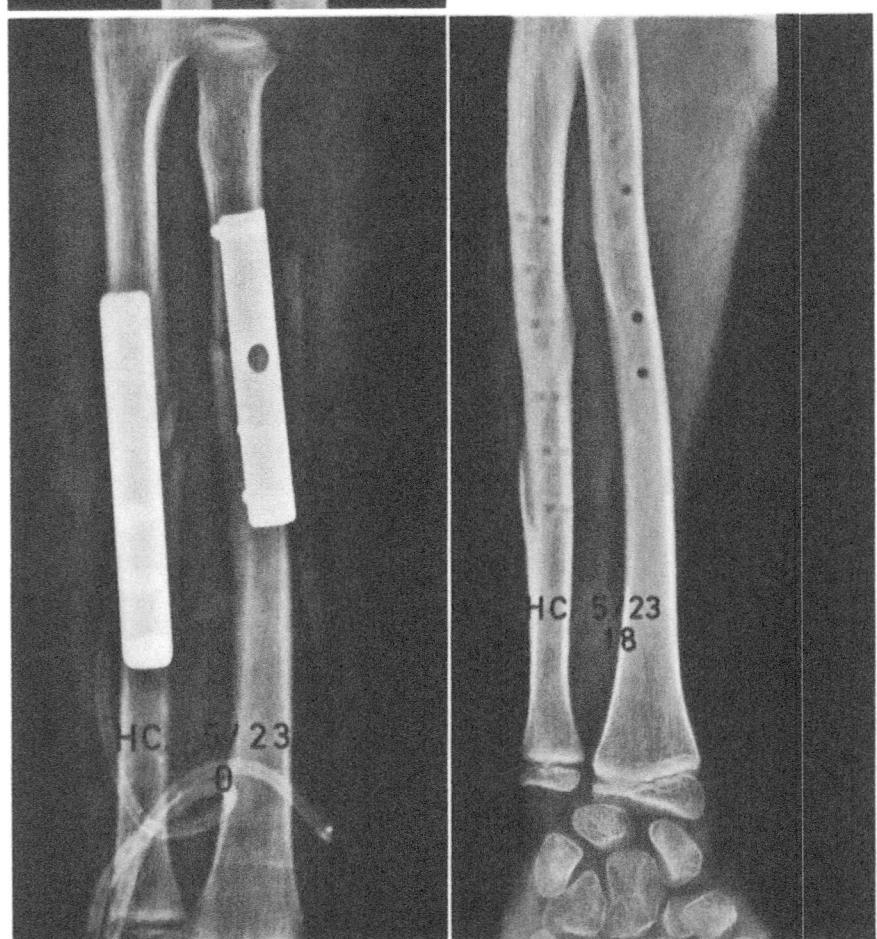

b

c

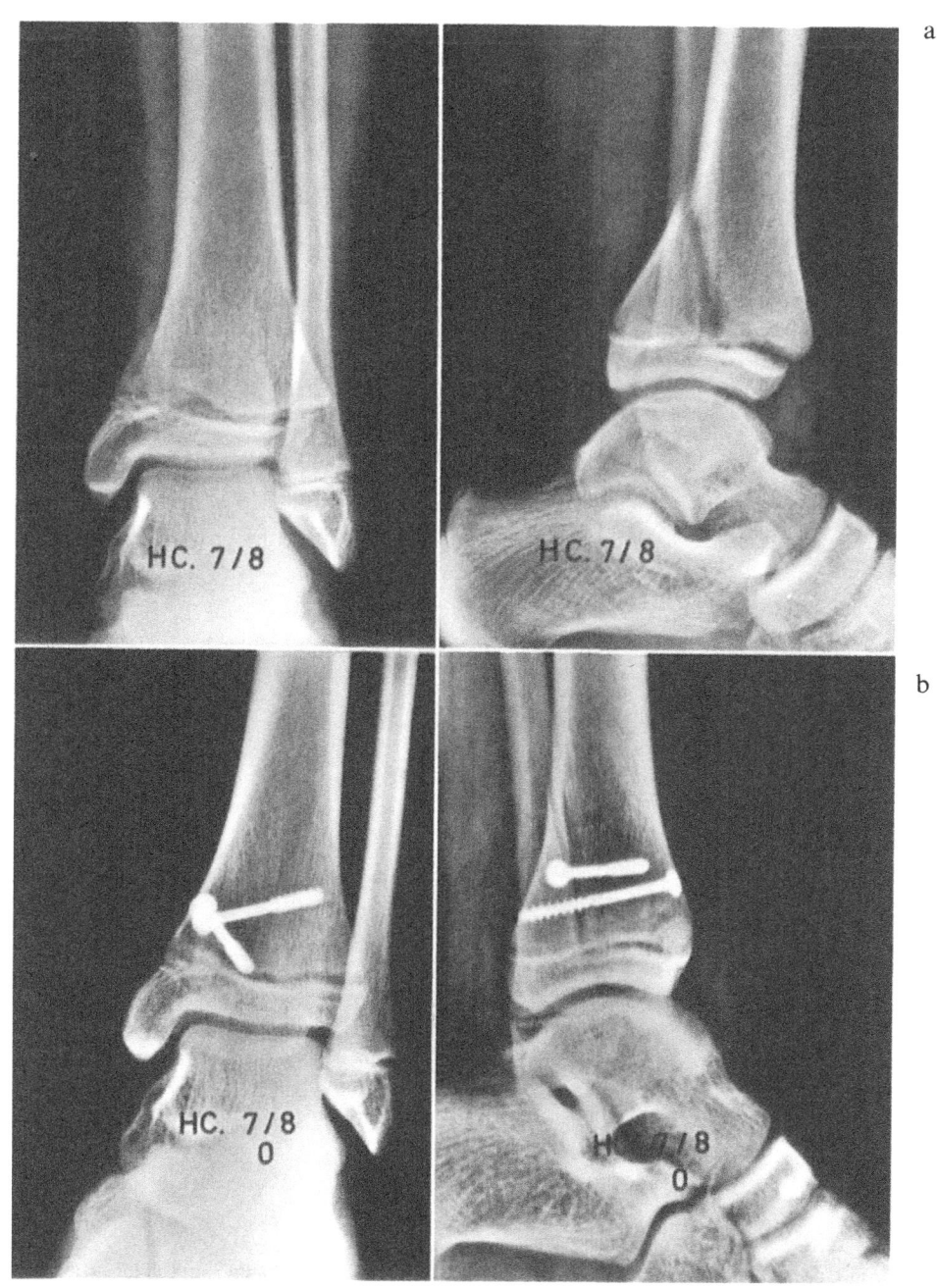

Fig. 153 Technical example: Traumatic separation of epiphyseal plate
The patient was injured in a skiing accident

a Traumatic epiphyseal plate displacement of the lower tibia

b Rigid internal fixation with two cancellous screws inserted in different directions from the medial side

Fig. 154 Clinical example: Screw fixation of a loose body in the knee joint, resulting from osteochondritis dissecans

The patient was an unskilled worker in the building trade, aged 25

a He had been shooting a football with a slightly twisted left knee which then became locked. Extension was limited to 30° and there was a slight effusion. A loose body was found to be avulsed from the medial femoral condyle and was lying in the intercondylar notch

Arthrotomy two days later. It was found that a loose body had been avulsed from an area of the medial condyle of the femur: it was fixed back in place with a small cancellous screw. He was immediately mobilized. A week later a plaster cast was applied and left in place for six weeks without any weight-bearing. He was then mobilized without weight-bearing and was able to return to full work $4^1/_2$ months later

b Review at eleven months: he was symptom-free and had function in this knee equal to that on the other side. X-ray shows that the loose body had been re-incorporated

c Removal of the metal at sixteen months. X-ray showed no sign of arthrosis

284

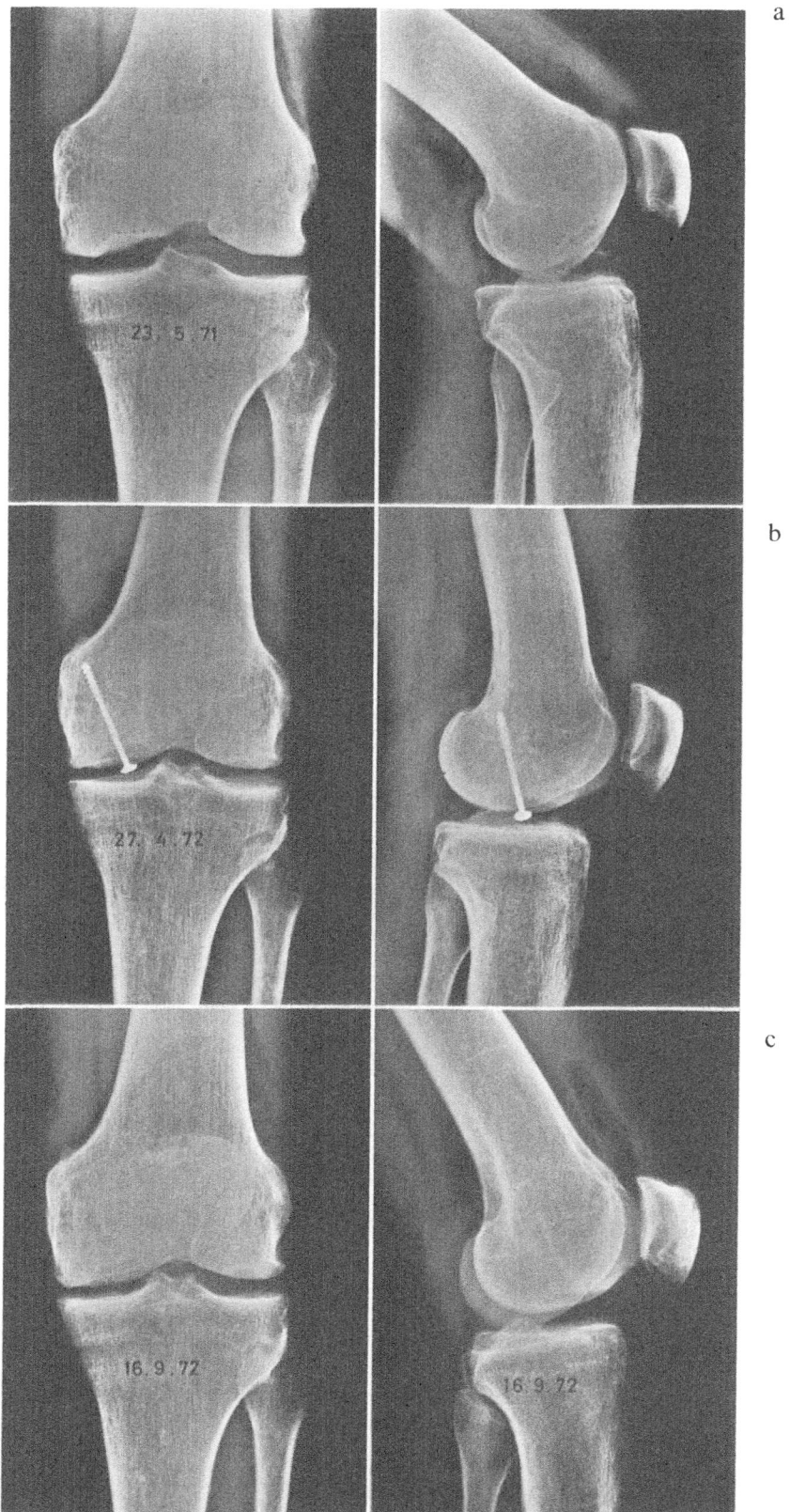

285

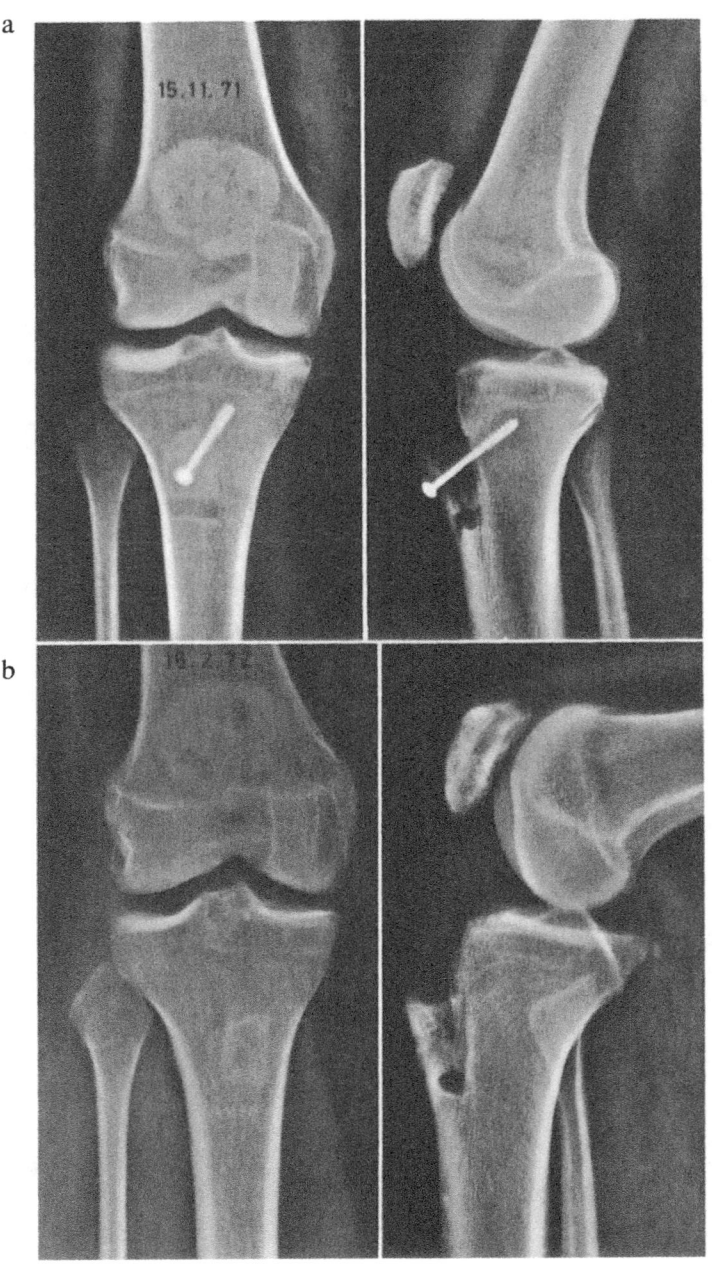

Fig. 155 Clinical example: Anterior displacement of the tibial tuberosity
The patient was a female office clerk, aged 24. She had chondromalacia of the patella

a The tibial tuberosity was displaced forwards with an interposed graft and fixed with a small cancellous screw. Beck's drilling was carried out
No complications after operation. Mobilization was begun at three weeks

b Final review at three months. Full movement, symptom-free, the graft was fully settled and the metal was removed

286

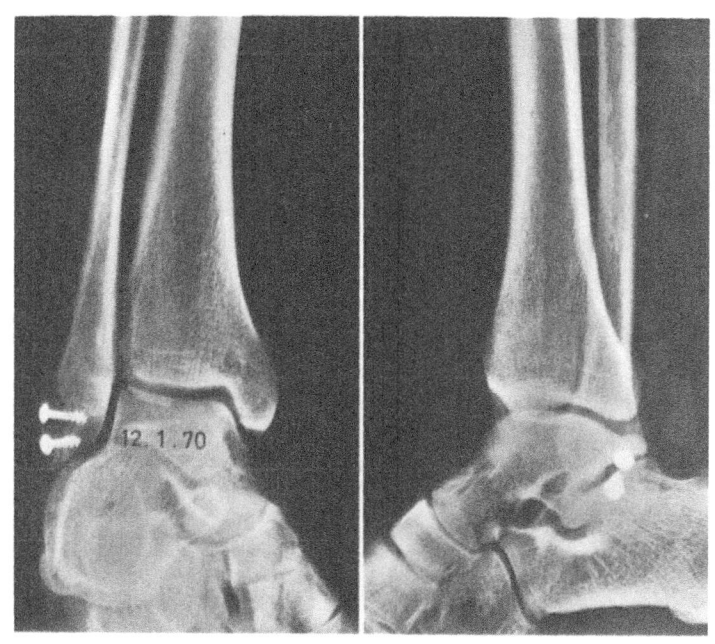

Fig. 156 Technical example: Kelly's operation

Kelly's operation: Fixation of the displaced disc of bone with two small cancellous screws. Removal of metal four months after the operation

a

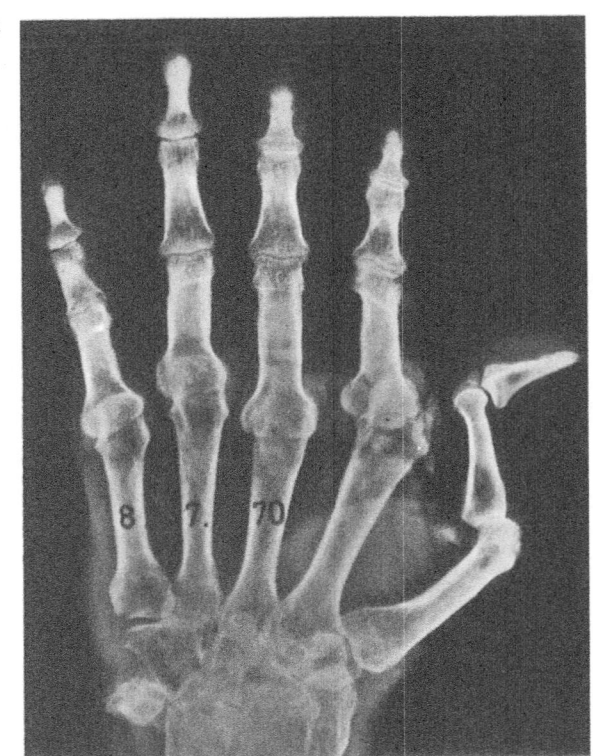

b

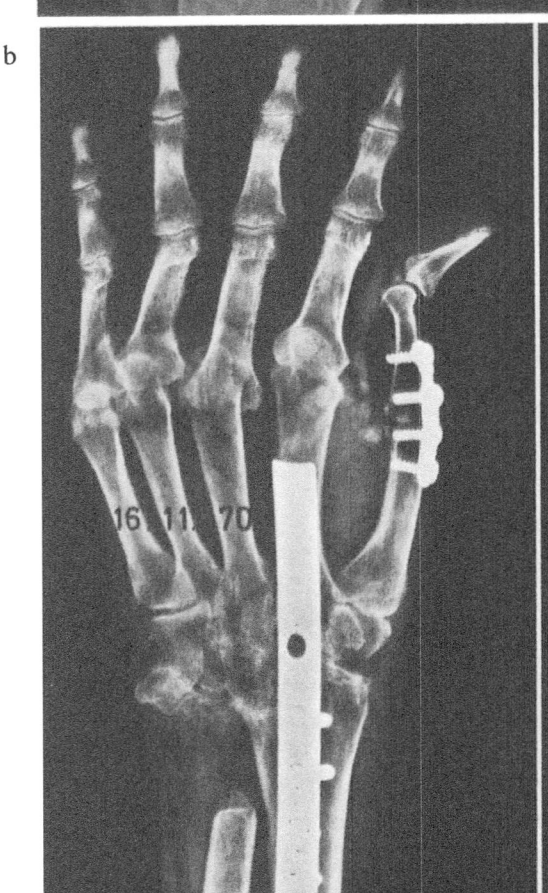 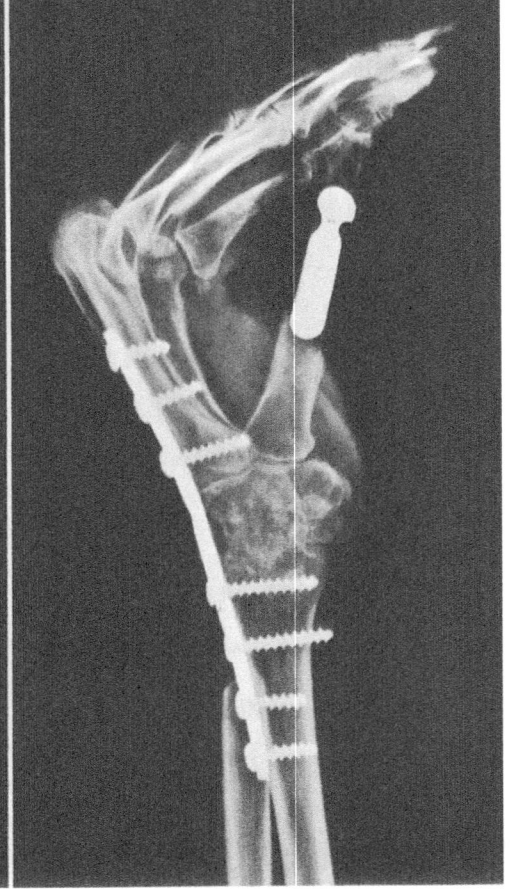

c   d

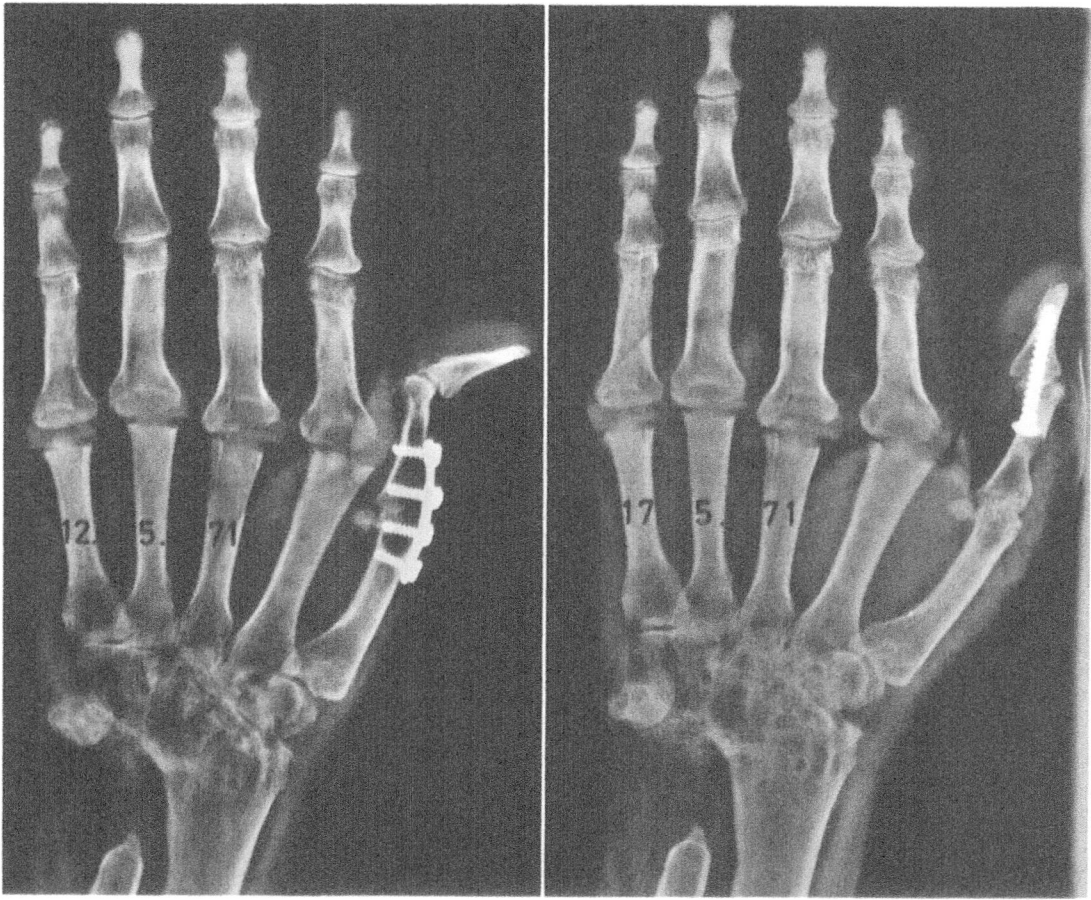

Fig. 157   Technical example: Use of small ASIF implants in rheumatoid surgery
The patient was a housewife, aged 48. Example of a severely altered hand due to rheumatoid arthritis and the various stages of functional reconstruction

  a   Initial position: Multiple subluxations and erosions in the wrist joint, metacarpo-phalangeal joints, and interphalangeal joint of the thumb

  b   Arthrodesis of the wrist with a small semi-tubular plate and resection of the lower end of the ulna. At the same time arthrodesis of the metacarpo-phalangeal joint of the thumb

  c   Arthroplasty of the metacarpo-phalangeal joints of the fingers with silastic prostheses of Swanson

  d   After removal of the implants from the wrist joint and metacarpo-phalangeal joint of the thumb, screw arthrodesis was carried out in the interphalangeal joint of the thumb

289

References

Allgöwer, M., Huggler, A., Segmüller, G.: Innere Fixation bei Achsenkorrektur am unteren Tibiaende, S. 137. In: Posttraumatische Achsenfehlstellungen an den unteren Extremitäten, Hrsg. M. E. Müller. Bern-Stuttgart: Huber 1967.

Bandi, W.: Zur Mechanik der supramalleolären, intraartikulären Schienbeinbrüche des Skifahrers. Kongreßbericht 9. Internat. Kongreß für Ski-Traumatologie u. Wintersportmedizin, S. 74, Hrsg. J. Heinkelein u. F. Lechner. Garmisch-Partenkirchen: Nebel-Verlag 1970.

Bandi, W.: Die posttraumatische Chondropathia patellae und Femoropatellararthrose. Hefte z. Unfallheilk. 1972.

Bandi, W.: Chondromalacia patellae und femoropatellare Arthrose. Helv. chir. Acta 1972.

Baumann, H.: Ellbogen. In: Spezielle Frakturen- und Luxationslehre, Bd. II/1, Hrsg. H. Nigst. Stuttgart: Thieme 1965.

Bernett, P., Krueger, P., Proschka, G., Wiendl, H. J.: Ergebnisse konservativer und operativer Behandlung distaler, intraartikulärer Tibiafrakturen. Kongreßbericht 9. Intern. Kongreß für Ski-Traumatologie und Wintersportmedizin, S. 108, Hrsg. J. Heinkelein und F. Lechner. Garmisch-Partenkirchen: Nebel-Verlag 1970.

Bonnin, J. G.: Injuries to the ankle. London: Heinemann 1950.

Buck-Gramcko, D.: Zur Technik der Trapeziumexstirpation. Handchirurgie 1972.

Burri, C., Rüedi, Th., Matter, P., Pfeiffer, K. M., Pusterla, C.: Stabile Osteosynthese: Frakturen im Handbereich. Akt. Chir. **4**, 305 (1969).

Danis, R.: Théorie et pratique de l'ostéosynthèse. Paris: Masson 1949.

Decoulx, P., Razemon, J.-P., Rouselle, Y.: Fractures du pilon tibial. Rev. Chir. orthop. **47**, 563 (1961).

Doliveux, P.: Table ronde sur les fractures des métacarpiens et des phalanges. Bull. Soc. orthop. Ouest 1972.

Durband, M. A.: Metacarpalefrakturen unter besonderer Berücksichtigung der therapeutischen Möglichkeiten aus neuester Sicht. Inauguraldissertation, Zürich 1969.

Flemming, F.: Versorgung komplizierter Mittelhandfrakturen mittels Pull-out-wire-Technik. Mschr. Unfallheilk. **65**, 112 (1962).

Gasser, H.: Delayed union and pseudarthrosis of the carpal navicular: treatment by compression-screw osteosynthesis. J. Bone Jt Surg. A **47**, 249 (1965).

Gay, R., Evrard, J.: Les fractures récentes du pilon tibial chez l'adulte. Rev. Chir. orthop. **49**, 397 (1963).

Gedda, K. O., Moberg, E.: Open reduction and osteosynthesis of so-called Bennett's fracture in the carpo-metacarpal joint of the thumb. Acta orthop. scand. **22**, 249 (1953).

Geiser, M.: Erfahrungen mit der Arthrodese des Großzehengrundgelenkes, S. 110. In: Der Vorfuß, Hrsg. P. Scholder. Bern-Stuttgart-Wien: Huber 1970.

Heim, U.: Die Technik der operativen Behandlung der Metacarpalefrakturen. Helv. chir. Acta **36**, 619 (1969).

Heim, U.: Zur operativen Technik der distalen, intraartikulären Tibiaimpressionsfrakturen. Kongreßbericht 9. Internat. Kongreß für Ski-Traumatologie u. Wintersportmedizin, S. 91, Hrsg. J. Heinkelein und F. Lechner. Garmisch-Partenkirchen: Nebel-Verlag 1970.

Heim, U.: Die Behandlung von Frakturen der Metatarsalia und Zehen unter besonderer Berücksichtigung der Osteosynthese. Z. Unfallmed. Berufskr. **63**, 305 (1970).

Heim, U.: Le matériel AO dans le traitement chirurgical des fractures des phalanges et métacarpiens. Chirurgie de la main, Paris **32**, 3 (1971).

Heim, U., Pfeiffer, K. M., Meuli, H. Ch.: Resultate von 332 AO-Osteosynthesen des Handskelettes. Handchirurgie **5**, 71 (1973).

Herold, H., Heim, U.: Desinfektion der Haut mit der Spritzpistole. Helv. chir. Acta **35**, 188 (1967).

Hunter, J. M., Cowen, N. J.: Fifth metacarpal fractures in a compensation clinic population. J. Bone Jt Surg. A **52**, 1159 (1970).

Iselin, M., Blanguernon, S., Benoist, D.: Fractures de la base du 1er métacarpien. Mém. Acad. Chir. **82**, 771 (1965).

Iselin, M., Iselin, F.: Traité de chirurgie de la main. Paris: Flammarion 1967.

Jahna, H.: Behandlung und Behandlungsergebnisse von 734 frischen einfachen Brüchen des Kahnbeinkörpers der Hand. Wien. med. Wschr. **104**, 1023 (1954).

Jahna, H.: Erfahrungen und Nachuntersuchungsergebnisse von 47 De Quervain'schen Verrenkungsbrüchen. Arch. orthop. Unfall-Chir. **57**, 51 (1965).

Kilbourne, B., Paul, E.G.: The use of small bone screws in the treatment of metacarpal, metatarsal and phalangeal fractures. J. Bone Jt Surg. A **40**, 375 (1958).

Koob, E.: Die Verschraubung der Kahnbeinpseudarthrose der Hand. Hefte z. Unfallheilk. **91**, 190 (1967).

Koob, E., Goymann, V., Haas, H.G.: Ergebnissen nach Verschraubung der Kahnbeinpseudarthrose der Hand. Handchirurgie **2**, 205 (1971).

Leach, R.E., Bolton, P.E.: Arthritis of the carpometacarpal joint of the thumb; results of arthrodesis. J. Bone Jt Surg. A **50**, 1171 (1968).

Matti, H.: Technik und Resultate meiner Pseudarthrosenoperation. Zbl. Chir. **63**, 1442 (1936).

Matti, H.: Über die Behandlung der Navicularefraktur und der Refractura patellae durch Plombierung mit Spongiosa. Zbl. Chir. **64**, 2353 (1937).

Maurer, G., Lechner, F.: Konservative und operative Behandlungsmöglichkeiten bei Stauchungsbrüchen des distalen Unterschenkels. Mschr. Unfallheilk. **68**, 207 (1965).

McLaughlin, H.L.: Fracture of the carpal navicular (scaphoid) bone. Some observations based on treatment by open reduction and internal fixation. J. Bone Jt Surg. A **36**, 765 (1954).

McLaughlin, H.L., Perkes, J.C.: Fracture of the carpal navicular (scaphoid) bone: gradations in therapy based upon pathology. J. Trauma **9**, 311 (1969).

Moberg, E.: Aseptische Knochennekrosen. Langebeck's Arch. klin. Chir. **319**, 429 (1967).

Moberg, E., Henricksson, B.: Technique for digital arthrodesis. A study of 150 cases. Acta chir. scand. **118**, 331 (1960).

Müller, M.E.: Les fractures du pilon tibial. Rev. Chir. orthop. **50**, 557 (1964).

Müller, M.E.: Posttraumatische Fehlstellungen an der unteren Extremität. Bern-Stuttgart: Huber 1967.

Müller, M.E., Allgöwer, M., Willenegger, H.: Technik der operativen Frakturbehandlung. Berlin-Heidelberg-New York: Springer 1963.

Müller, M.E., Allgöwer, M., Willenegger, H.: Manual der Osteosynthese. Berlin-Heidelberg-New York: Springer 1969.

Mumenthaler, M.: Die Ulnarisparesen. Stuttgart: Thieme 1961.

Pannike, A.: Handchirurgische Osteosynthesen. Habilitationsschrift, Tübingen 1971.

Pannike, A., Meyer, J.: A new method of bone stabilisation in reconstructive surgery of the hand. Excerpta Med. Intern. Congr. Series **174**, 946 (1969).

Pauwels, F.: Gesammelte Abhandlungen zur funktionellen Anatomie des Bewegungsapparates. Berlin-Heidelberg-New York: Springer 1965.

Pearson, J.R.: Combined fracture of the base of the fifth metatarsal and the lateral malleolus. J. Bone Jt Surg. A **43**, 513 (1961).

Perren, S.M., Allgöwer, M., Mathys, R., Schenk, R., Willenegger, H., Müller, M.E.: The reaction of cortical bone to compression. Acta orthop. scand., Suppl. **125**, 19 (1969).

Perren, S.M., Russenberger, M., Steinemann, S., Müller, M.E., Allgöwer, M.: A dynamic compression plate. Acta orthop. scand., Suppl. **125**, 31 (1969).

Pfeiffer, K.M.: Zur Frage der primären Schraubenosteosynthese von Navicularefrakturen. Helv. chir. Acta **39**, 471 (1972).

Pfeiffer, K.M., Nigst, H.: Schraubenarthrodese von Fingergelenken. Handchirurgie **2**, 149 (1970).

Ricklin, P.: Entbehrliche Knochen. Helv. chir. Acta **27**, 397 (1960).

Rüedi, Th., Burri, C., Matter, P., Allgöwer, M.: Operationstaktik bei Frakturen des Pilon tibial. Kongreßbericht 9. Internat. Kongreß für Skitraumatologie u. Wintersportmedizin, S. 87, Hrsg. J. Heinkelein u. F. Lechner. Garmisch-Partenkirchen: Nebel-Verlag 1970.

Rüedi, Th., Burri, C., Matter, P., Allgöwer, M.: Spätresultate nach Pilon-Tibial-Frakturen. Kongreßbericht 9. Internat. Kongreß für Ski-Traumatologie u. Wintersportmedizin, S. 114, Hrsg. J. Heinkelein u. F. Lechner. Garmisch-Partenkirchen: Nebel-Verlag 1970.

Rüedi, Th., Burri, C., Pfeiffer, K.M.: Stable internal fixation of fractures of the hand. J. Trauma **11**, 381 (1971).

Rüedi, Th., Matter, P., Allgöwer, M.: Die intraarticulären Frakturen des distalen Unterschenkelendes. Helv. chir. Acta **35**, 556 (1968).

Russe, O.: Erfahrungen und Ergebnisse bei der Spongiosafüllung der veralteten Brüche und Pseudarthrosen des Kahnbeins der Hand. Wiederherstellungschir. u. Traum. **2**, 175 (1954).

Russe, O.: Nachuntersuchungsergebnisse von 22 Fällen operierter, veralteter Brüche und Pseudarthrosen des Kahnbeins der Hand. Z. Orthop. **93**, 5 (1960).

Russe, O.: Fracture of the carpal navicular. Diagnosis, non-operative treatment and operative treatment. J. Bone Jt Surg. A **42**, 759 (1960).

Schenk, R., Willenegger, H.: Morphologic findings in primary fracture healing. Symp. biol. Hung. **7**, 75 (1967).

Segmüller, G.: Operative Stabilisierung am Handskelett. Bern-Stuttgart-Wien: Huber 1973.

Segmüller, G., Schönenberger, F.: Technik der Kompressionsarthrodese am Finger mittels Zugschraube. Handchirurgie **2**, 218 (1971).

Simonetta, C.: The use of AO plates in the hand. Hand **2**, 43 (1970).

Smillie, I.S.: Osteochondritis dissecans. Edinburgh-London: Livingstone 1960.

Smillie, I.S.: Treatment of osteochondritis dissecans. J. Bone Jt Surg. B **39**, 248 (1967).

Spiessl, G., Schargus, G., Schroll, K.: Die stabile Osteosynthese bei Frakturen des unbezahnten Unterkiefers. Schweiz. Mschr. Zahnheilk. **81**, 39 (1971).

Spycher, E.: Untersuchungen mit Drehmomentschlüssel an verschiedenen Schraubentypen. Inauguraldissertation, Bern 1971.

Suessenbach, F., Weber, B.G.: Epiphysenfugenverletzungen am distalen Unterschenkel. Bern-Stuttgart-Wien: Huber 1970.

Swanson, A.B.: Silicone-rubber implants for replacement of arthritic or destroyed joints in hand. Surg. Clin. N. Amer. **48**, 1113 (1968).

Trojan, E.: Die operative Behandlung des veralteten Kahnbeinbruches der Hand. Verh. dtsch. orthop. Ges. **43**, 160 (1955).

Truchet, P.: Fractures du pilon tibial. Kongreßbericht 9. Internat. Kongreß für Ski-Traumatologie u. Wintersportmedizin, S. 69, Hrsg. J. Heinkelein u. F. Lechner. Garmisch-Partenkirchen: Nebel-Verlag 1970.

Wagner, H.: Operative Behandlung der Osteochondritis dissecans des Kniegelenkes. Z. Orthop. **98**, 333 (1964).

Weber, B.G.: Behandlung der Sprunggelenks-Stauchungsbrüche nach biomechanischen Gesichtspunkten. H. Unfallheilk. **81**, 176 (1965).

Weber, B.G.: Die Verletzungen des oberen Sprunggelenkes, 2. Aufl. Bern-Stuttgart-Wien: Huber 1972.

Weber, M.: Operative Behandlung von Navicularepseudarthrosen der Hand. Erfahrungen der Schweizerischen Unfallversicherungs-Anstalt aufgrund von 345 Fällen. Inauguraldissertation, Zürich 1970.

Wilhelm, K.: Die stabile Osteosynthese bei offenen Handskelettfrakturen. Arch. orthop. Unfall-Chir. **71**, 6 (1971).

Wilhelm, K.: Die stabile Osteosynthese bei Frakturen des Handskelettes. Arch. orthop. Unfall-Chir. **70**, 275 (1971).

Willenegger, H.: Die Behandlung der Luxationsfrakturen des oberen Sprunggelenkes nach biomechanischen Gesichtspunkten. Helv. chir. Acta **28**, 225 (1961).

Willenegger, H.: Spätergebnisse nach konservativ und operativ behandelten Malleolarfrakturen. Helv. chir. Acta **38**, 321 (1971).

Willenegger, H., Guggenbühl, A.: Zur operativen Behandlung bestimmter Fälle von distalen Radiusfrakturen. Helv. chir. Acta **26**, 81 (1959).

Willenegger, H., Weber, B.G.: Malleolarfrakturen. Langenbecks Arch. klin. Chir. **318**, 489 (1965).

Zimmermann, H.: Frakturen des Vorfußes, S. 204. In: Der Vorfuß, Hrsg. P. Scholder. Bern-Stuttgart-Wien: Huber 1970.

Subject Index

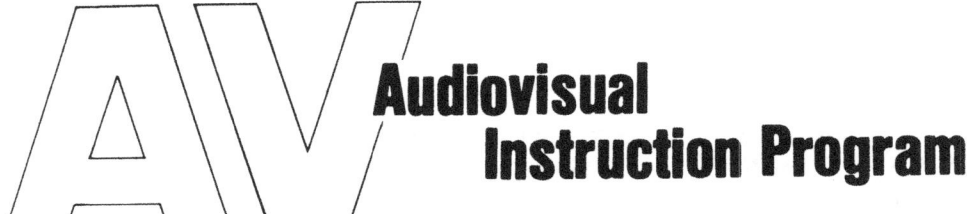

Audiovisual Instruction Program

Film Series "Internal Fixation of Fractures":

Internal Fixation. Basic Principles and Modern Means
M. Allgöwer, Basle; S. M. Perren, Davos

Internal Fixation of Forearm Fractures
Th. Rüedi, Basle; M. Allgöwer, Basle; A. v. Hochstetter, Basle

Internal Fixation of Noninfected Diaphyseal Pseudarthroses
M. E. Müller, Bern; R. Ganz, Bern

Internal Fixation of Malleolar Fractures
B. G. Weber, St. Gall

Internal Fixation of Patella Fractures
B. G. Weber, St. Gall

Medullary Nailing
S. Weller, Tübingen; F. Schauwecker, Tübingen

Internal Fixation of the Distal End of the Humerus
C. Burri, Ulm; A. Rüter, Ulm

Internal Fixation of Mandibular Fractures
B. Spiessl, Basle; J. Prein, Basle; B. A. Rahn, Davos

Corrective Osteotomy of the Distal Tibia
M. Allgöwer, Basle; Th. Rüedi, Basle

The Biomechanics of Internal Fixation
S. M. Perren, Davos; B. A. Rahn, Davos; J. Cordey, Davos

Films on "Allo-Arthroplasty":

Total Hip Prostheses (3 parts)
Part 1: Instruments. Operation on Model.
Part 2: Operative Technique
Part 3: Complications. Special Cases
M. E. Müller, Bern; R. Ganz, Bern

Elbow-Arthroplasty with the New GSB-Prosthesis
N. Gschwend, Zurich; H. Scheier, Zurich

Slide series:

Manual of Internal Fixation
Book and slides by M. E. Müller, Bern; M. Allgöwer, Basle; H. Willenegger, Liestal

Small Fragment Set Manual
Technique Recommended by the AO-Group
Book and slides by U. Heim, Chur; K. M. Pfeiffer, Basle

Total Hip Prostheses
Instruments
Operative Technique
Complications. Special Cases
M. E. Müller, Bern; R. Ganz, Bern

■ Further films and slide series in preparation

■ Technical data:
16 mm, Super-8 (Eastmancolor, magnetic sound / optical sound) EVR, VCR, TED-videodisc

■ All films available in English and German, several in French

■ Please ask for special brochure

Sales:
Springer-Verlag,
D-1 Berlin 33, Heidelberger Platz 3

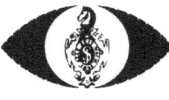 **Springer-Verlag Berlin Heidelberg New York**

Made in the USA
Las Vegas, NV
07 November 2024

11217314R10175